T0391188

Inflammatory Breast Cancer: An Update

Naoto T. Ueno • Massimo Cristofanilli
Editors

Inflammatory Breast Cancer: An Update

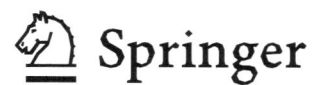 Springer

Editors

Naoto T. Ueno, M.D., Ph.D., F.A.C.P.
Morgan Welch Inflammatory Breast
Cancer Program and Clinic
Department of Breast Medical Oncology
The University of Texas
MD Anderson Cancer Center
Unit 1354, Holcombe Blvd. 1515
Houston, TX, USA

Massimo Cristofanilli
Department of Medical Oncology
Fox Chase Cancer Center
Cottman Avenue, Room C315 333
Philadelphia, PA, USA

ISBN 978-94-007-3906-2   ISBN 978-94-007-3907-9 (eBook)
DOI 10.1007/978-94-007-3907-9
Springer Dordrecht Heidelberg New York London

Library of Congress Control Number: 2012935582

Printed on acid-free paper

Springer is part of Springer Science+Business Media (www.springer.com)

Contents

Chapter 1
Introduction: Why IBC Now?

Naoto T. Ueno and Massimo Cristofanilli

We are truly honored to provide the first textbook related to inflammatory breast cancer. This inflammatory breast cancer is rare but the most aggressive form of breast cancer. Despite it has a distinct clinical presentation, we have yet to establish the pathogenesis of this disease. The disease does not have molecularly defined diagnostic criteria and we are not able to establish the definitive inflammatory breast cancer specific treatment. Therefore, there is a strong need for a clinical and a scientific advancement of this disease.

The aggressiveness of this disease stems from its rapid locoregional recurrence and distant metastasis. Therefore, this disease is an excellent disease model to understand the biology of metastasis, epithelial-mesenchymal transition, stem cell, microenvironment, etc. Further, the diffuse redness resembling inflammation allows speculating immunological and inflammatory processes are involved in the pathogenesis of this disease. If we could understand this biology of the disease, it not only helps inflammatory breast cancer but other noninflammatory breast cancer disease.

Each chapter of this textbook will offer a detailed, comprehensive most up to date description of inflammatory breast cancer. We will provide not only the existing information about this disease but also how this can be incorporated into your routine clinical practice. This textbook covers imaging, pathology, basic research, clinical trials, clinical practice, genetic predisposition, and epidemiology. Further, we have had a special chapter from the patient advocacy perspective of this deadly

N.T. Ueno, M.D., Ph.D., F.A.C.P. (✉)
Morgan Welch Inflammatory Breast Cancer Program and Clinic, Department of Breast
Medical Oncology, The University of Texas, MD Anderson Cancer Center,
Unit 1354, Holcombe Blvd. 1515, Houston, TX, USA
e-mail: nueno@mdanderson.org

M. Cristofanilli
Department of Medical Oncology, Fox Chase Cancer Center,
Cottman Avenue, Room C315 333, Philadelphia, PA, USA
e-mail: Massimo.Cristofanilli@fccc.edu

N.T. Ueno and M. Cristofanilli (eds.), *Inflammatory Breast Cancer: An Update*,
DOI 10.1007/978-94-007-3907-9_1, © Springer Science+Business Media B.V. 2012

disease. It is always an enthusiastic welcome for cancer survivor, which includes cancer patients, family and their friend, to participate in the fight of this disease. It is important for the healthcare providers to learn the perspective of cancer survivors. We hope that this textbook will provide the opportunities to our readers to see who are in the forefront of this disease research. We highly encourage your participation and contacting these authors to form collaboration so that we can eliminate the suffering from this disease.

At the end, we believe that this will be a valuable resource for those who are taking care of breast cancer. This work is supported in part by The State of Texas Grant for Rare and Aggressive Cancers through the Morgan Welch Inflammatory Breast Cancer Research Program. We would also like to thank Jenna Boatright and, Danielle Walsh for organizing this book as well as MD Anderson Cancer Center Scientific Publications for its editing assistance.

Chapter 2
Epidemiology of Inflammatory Breast Cancer

Shannon Wiggins, Sarah Taylor, and Melissa Bondy

Abstract Inflammatory breast cancer (IBC) is the most aggressive and fatal form of invasive breast cancer. The disease affects approximately 2.5% of breast cancer patients in the United States typically with younger age of onset and higher incidence in African-Americans. Incidence rates vary due to the clinical nature, rather than pathological, of the diagnosis. Changes to the SEER coding rules will also likely have an impact on IBC reporting rates. Epidemiological observations have also suggested geographic differences in the incidence of IBC but without resulting in the identification of risk factors. Few risk factors have been established but associations have been noted with African American race and younger age of onset, as well as high BMI. Decreased survival rates in patients with ER-negative tumors have also been noted. An ongoing registry is being conducted at The University of Texas MD Anderson Cancer Center to address this issue. It is a prospective registry, and although relatively small, some observations of note can be made. The patients enrolled on the registry have a mean age at diagnosis of 55 years and over half of the patients present with ER-negative tumors. Also 18% of the patients reported a first-degree relative with breast cancer. The majority was overweight or obese and were former or still currently smokers. The registry includes sites in both the United States and internationally and information collected in the registry will be used in order to further elucidate the etiology and risk factors for IBC.

S. Wiggins, M.P.H. • M. Bondy, Ph.D.
Dan L. Duncan Cancer Center, Baylor College of Medicine,
Houston, TX, USA
e-mail: swiggins@bcm.edu; mbondy@bcm.edu

S. Taylor, M.P.H. (✉)
Department of Tumor Registry, The University of Texas MD Anderson Cancer Center,
Houston, TX, USA
e-mail: shtaylor@mdanderson.org

N.T. Ueno and M. Cristofanilli (eds.), *Inflammatory Breast Cancer: An Update*,
DOI 10.1007/978-94-007-3907-9_2, © Springer Science+Business Media B.V. 2012

Keywords Inflammatory breast cancer • Risk factors • Incidence rates • Epidemiology • Survival • Tumor registry • MP/H coding rules • Cancer • Multiple primary rules • Abstracting rules

2.1 Introduction and Definition of Inflammatory Breast Cancer

Inflammatory breast cancer (IBC) is the most aggressive and fatal form of invasive breast cancer. The median overall survival among women with IBC is less than 4 years, even with multimodality treatment options [1]. According to the Surveillance, Epidemiology, and End Results (SEER) registries of the National Cancer Institute (NCI), the incidence of breast cancer decreased significantly in 2003 and has leveled off since then [2, 3]. The NCI estimates that approximately 200,000 new cases of breast cancer will be diagnosed this year and more than 40,000 people will die from the disease. Given the estimation that IBC comprises 2.5% of all incident breast cancer cases in the United States, we can approximate that 5,000 new cases are diagnosed each year. However, it is difficult to determine the incidence rate trends specifically for IBC because of the debatable case definitions that are used to diagnose this disease. The clinical signs used to diagnose IBC vary from the beginnings of edema (peau d'orange) and redness, up to that which covers the entire breast. Depending on the comprehensiveness of the case definition used (e.g., including pathological findings), the sample sizes for IBC cases can vary substantially, thereby significantly affecting the calculation of a true incidence rate. The American Joint Committee on Cancer defines IBC as diffuse erythema and peau d'orange over most of the breast, commonly without an underlying mass [4]; this definition is widely used in the United States. In a previous report, in which a comprehensive case definition comprising both clinical and pathological features was used, IBC incidence rates in the United States were significantly higher in African American women than in white women. In addition, African American women were diagnosed with IBC at a much earlier age, a finding that further emphasizes the considerable racial disparities that exist among patients with IBC compared to those that exist among patients with non-T4 breast cancer [5].

In January 2003, the SEER program formed the Multiple Primary and Histology (MP/H) Task Force to develop standardized methods for tumor registries to collect information for primary malignancies and coding histological types and subtypes. The result of the efforts of the task force was the creation of the 2007 MP/H Coding Rules, which apply to cases diagnosed on or after January 1, 2007. The rules have been adopted by all state cancer registries, the National Cancer Data Base of the American College of Surgeons, and the SEER registries. Included in the MP/H Coding Rules is a rule that specifically addresses the coding of IBC. The rule states that the International Classification for Oncology histology code 8530 for IBC should be used only "when the final diagnosis of the pathology report specifically states inflammatory carcinoma." Because IBC is typically diagnosed clinically rather than pathologically, most cases diagnosed on or after January 1, 2007, would not be identifiable using the International Classification for Oncology histology code for IBC [6].

2.2   IBC Coding at MD Anderson Cancer Center

To verify the notion that most IBC cases diagnosed on or after January 1, 2007, would not be identifiable using the International Classification for Oncology histology code, researchers used The University of Texas MD Anderson Cancer Center Tumor Registry database to identify 240 patients with IBC who had initially presented to the institution between 2005 and 2007. IBC was diagnosed pathologically in 73 patients and clinically in 167. Of the 167 patients with a clinical diagnosis of IBC, 164 patients also had a pathologic diagnosis of a non-IBC histology. Following the new rule, the non-IBC histology would have been recorded for these 164 patients.

These findings suggest that if the new SEER multiple primary guidelines were applied, the International Classification for Oncology-IBC histology code would be recorded for approximately 30% of patients with IBC. In the remaining 70%, the pathology report would have revealed only non-IBC malignancies, mainly invasive ductal carcinoma. If these guidelines were applied to the data from the SEER database from 2001 to 2005, as few as 144 cases may have been reported in 2007 [6, 7] (Fig. 2.1).

Searching by histology code has traditionally been the most straightforward and intuitive way to identify cases from tumor registries. With the implementation of the MP/H Coding Rules, this will no longer be true for the majority of IBC cases. Although IBC cases that have been pathologically diagnosed will still be identifiable using histology codes, clinically diagnosed cases are to be identified using the Collaborative Staging System extension codes [8] or the American Joint Committee on Cancer tumor-node-metastasis classification T4d [4]. The Collaborative Staging System is a method in which specific data items are coded and then an algorithm is

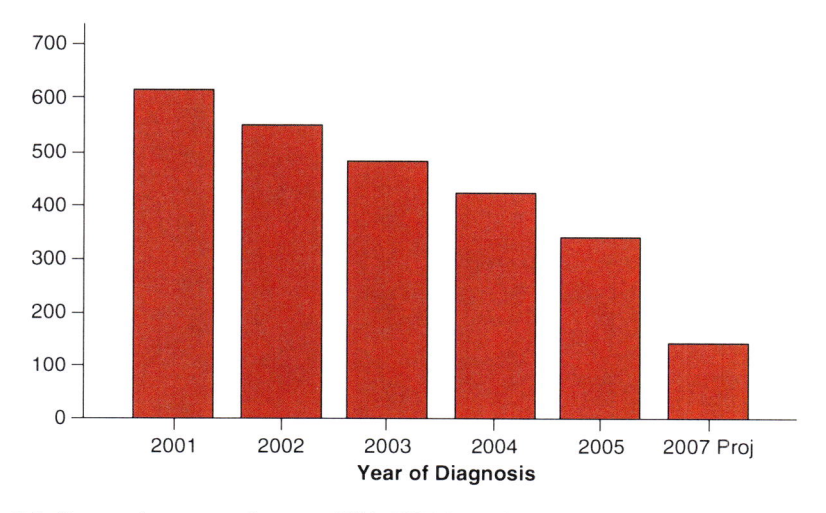

Fig. 2.1 Presented are counts for years 2001–2005 determined by using the SEER database. 2007 projected patients were based on The University of Texas M. D. Anderson Cancer Center data

used to combine the codes into various staging systems. The Collaborative Staging System is to be used for cases diagnosed on or after January 1, 2004. Researchers who work in the tumor registry field are aware of both the MP/H rules and the Collaborative Staging System values. However, researchers who are not directly involved in tumor registry procedures are not likely to be aware of either the MP/H rules or the Collaborative Staging System values. With datasets like SEER available to non-registry researchers, the researchers who are unaware of this caveat for IBC cases may likely search tumor registries according to histology only. The ultimate result may be the erroneous assumption that the number of IBC cases has decreased when in reality it may be that the change in abstracting rules is the only change that has occurred [6].

2.3 Epidemiologic Risk Factors

At present, few risk factors have been established for IBC. However, many distinguishable epidemiologic characteristics of IBC have been studied (Table 2.1). The risk factors with the strongest associations include African American race, high body mass index (BMI), and younger age at disease onset. African American women have been found to have at least a 50% increased incidence, to be diagnosed at earlier ages, and to have lower survival times compared to white women [9]. Additionally, patients with IBC who had estrogen receptor (ER)-negative tumors have been shown to have significantly lower survival rates than those with ER-positive tumors. Hance et al. reported a median survival time of 2 years for

Table 2.1 Selected risk factors for inflammatory breast cancer

Probable risk factors	Association[a]
Younger age at diagnosis	+++
Younger age at menarche	+
Younger age at live first birth	+
High BMI (≥ 30)	+++
Oral contraceptive use	+
Ever pregnant	+
Longer duration of breast feeding	+
White vs. African American ethnicity	+++
Hormone receptor status (negative)	+
Residence in Northern African countries	+
Too few studies to assess consistency	
Family history of breast cancer	
Carrier of HHV/HPV viruses	
Smoking status	
Alcohol use	
NSAID use	

[a]+++ Indicates relative risk >3; +, relative risk >1 and <3; −, relative risk >0.3 and <1

patients with ER-negative tumors and 4 years for patients with ER-positive tumors [5]. Moreover, IBC appears to have a prominent geographic pattern. North African countries have reported a high number of IBC cases, and the most studied and documented were reported in Tunisia [10]. Despite these epidemiologic considerations, limited research exists on the risk factors associated with this disease, particularly because of the ambiguous case definitions used for IBC [9] and the lack of an agreed-upon single definition.

2.4 MD Anderson Cancer Center IBC Registry

Although no risk factors for IBC have been clearly defined, some of the important findings related to IBC are in contrast to the risk factors for breast cancer in general. The MD Anderson Cancer Center established an IBC registry in April 2007 to address this issue [11]. The registry includes patients from institutions in the United States and internationally. The primary objective of the registry is to prospectively collect epidemiological, clinical, and imaging data from all patients diagnosed with IBC with the intent of establishing defined risk factors (Table 2.2). We have not observed a higher incidence rate in African American women at this time because of the small sample size of African American women enrolled in the registry and a

Table 2.2 Selected demographic factors from the M.D. Anderson Inflammatory Breast Cancer Registry[a]

Mean age at Dx	Mean age (years)		% of study population		
Overall	55		100		
Caucasian	55		77.1		
Hispanic	56		17.8		
African American	48		5.7		
Hormonal factors	**n**	**%**		**n**	**s.d.**
ER+/PR+	19	27.2	Mean age, menarche	12.6	1.6
ER−/PR+	1	1.4	Mean age, 1st pregnancy[b]	22.8	5.1
ER+/PR−	11	15.7	Mean no. live births	2.98	1.31
ER−/PR−	39	55.7	Mean age OCP started	21.4	4.9
HER2neu +	31	44.3			
Triple Negative	23	32.9			
Body mass index	**n**	**%**			
Normal (<25)	16	22.9			
Overweight (24–29)	19	27.1			
Obese (>30)	35	50.0			
Lifestyle factors	**n**	**%**			
Ever smoked	37	52.9			
Mean no. pack-years	22.7				

[a]n = 70 at time of data analysis
[b]Parous women only

possible referral bias at MD Anderson Cancer Center. The mean age of the patients is 55 years, which corroborates the previously assumed risk of younger age at diagnosis. More than half of the patients in the registry have presented with ER-negative tumors, and approximately 33% of those have presented as triple-negative (i.e., ER-negative-PR-negative-HER2-negative) tumors. Growing evidence in the literature also shows that high BMI may be positively associated with a diagnosis of IBC. An overwhelming 50% of registry patients at MD Anderson Cancer Center have a BMI of 30 or higher, marking them as obese. Over two-thirds of the women in the registry are also postmenopausal. The association does not vary by menopausal status, which differs from breast cancer in general [12].

A familial predisposition for IBC has not been reported in large epidemiological studies, but a matched case–control study in Pakistani women revealed that family history of breast cancer was significantly more prominent in IBC cases compared to non-IBC cases [13]. Approximately 40% of the MD Anderson Cancer Center registry patients reported having a family history of some form of breast cancer, and 18% reported having a first-degree relative with breast cancer. Although extremely rare, a small number of male IBC cases have been reported, dating back to 1953 [14]. Furthermore, a Tunisian study reported that rural residence was related to a rapid progression of breast cancer in both pre- and postmenopausal women, and early age at first live birth was associated with IBC [15]. However, Chang et al. reported contradictory findings in their research conducted in the United States. The current research at MD Anderson Cancer Center, however, reports a mean age of 22.8 years at first live birth, similar to the Tunisian findings. Rural residence and its relation to disease progression will be investigated in the future as the size of the registry and length of enrollment time increases.

Several other risk factors have shown some indication of being associated with a diagnosis of IBC, but future studies are warranted. Other reproductive factors including younger age at menarche and the use of oral contraceptives in comparison to non-IBC patients could prove to be of interest. Studies of the relationship between IBC and these factors, paired with other aspects such as menopausal status and hormone receptor status, in larger population groups would serve to further establish the associated risk. Likewise, continued research on the association between smoking and an IBC diagnosis may be informative. Over half of the MD Anderson Cancer Center registry patients reported being either a current or former smoker with a mean of 22.7 pack-years. Several of the aforementioned factors have been investigated in terms of their association with general breast cancer, but additional research within the specific subset of patients with IBC is necessary to help further elucidate the risk factors and etiology for this aggressive disease.

References

1. Anderson W et al (2005) Epidemiology of inflammatory breast cancer (IBC). Breast Dis 22:9–23
2. Kerlikowske K et al (2007) Declines in invasive breast cancer and use of postmenopausal hormone therapy in a screening mammography population. J Natl Cancer Inst 99(17):1335–1339

3. Ravdin P et al (2007) The decrease in breast-cancer incidence in 2003 in the United States. N Engl J Med 356(16):1670–1674
4. Greene FL et al (eds) (2002) AJCC, AJCC cancer staging handbook. Springer, New York
5. Hance K et al (2005) Trends in inflammatory breast carcinoma incidence and survival: the surveillance, epidemiology, and end results program at the National Cancer Institute. J Natl Cancer Inst 97(13):966–975
6. Taylor SH, Walters R (2010) Potential impact of tumor registry rule changes for recording inflammatory breast cancer. Cancer 116(suppl 11):2745–2747
7. Surveillance, Epidemiology, and End Results (SEER) Program (www.seer.cancer.gov) SEER*Stat Database: (1973–2005) National Cancer Institute, DCCPS, Surveillance Research Program, Cancer Statistics Branch, released April 2008, based on the November 2007 submission
8. Collaborative Staging Manual and Coding Instructions. Collaborative Staging Task Force of the American Joint Committee on Cancer. NIH Publication Number 04–5496. Bethesda, MD. Version 01.04.00. October 31, 2007 Revision, pt. II, 375
9. Levine P, Veneroso C (2008) The epidemiology of inflammatory breast cancer. Semin Oncol 35(1):11–16
10. Tabbane F et al (1977) Clinical and prognostic features of a rapidly progressing breast cancer in Tunisia. Cancer 40(1):376–382
11. Bondy M et al (2009) A progress review of the inflammatory breast cancer registry at The University of Texas MD Anderson Cancer Center [abstract]. Cancer Res 69(suppl 24): Abstract nr 2073
12. Chang S, Buzdar A, Hursting S (1998) Inflammatory breast cancer and body mass index. J Clin Oncol 16(12):3731–3735
13. Aziz S et al (2001) Case control study of prognostic markers and disease outcome in inflammatory carcinoma breast: a unique clinical experience. Breast J 7(6):398–404
14. Choueiri M et al (2005) Inflammatory breast cancer in a male. N Z Med J 118(1218):U1566
15. Mourali N et al (1980) Epidemiologic features of rapidly progressing breast cancer in Tunisia. Cancer 46(12):2741–2746

Chapter 3
Clinical Aspect of Inflammatory Breast Cancer: Diagnosis, Criteria, Controversy

Shaheenah Dawood and Vicente Valero

Abstract Inflammatory breast cancer (IBC) is a rare and aggressive subtype of breast cancer, and its diagnosis is primarily clinical. IBC follows an aggressive biological course that is typically associated with rapid onset of symptoms and signs, and it is associated with poor overall outcome. Diagnosis of IBC is based on a combination of information derived from medical history, physical examination, and biopsy-confirmed presence of invasive cancer. Patients with IBC typically present with a history of less than 6 months of rapid breast enlargement, erythema, skin ridging, and peau d'orange appearance of the overlying skin, with or without an underlying palpable mass. Because of a lack of consensus on IBC case definition, it has been difficult to definitively determine incidence, identify specific risk factors, and compare studies to evaluate the effectiveness of different therapeutic modalities. In this chapter, we will discuss the clinical characteristics of IBC, methods that have been developed to better define this disease, the controversy surrounding case definition and its associated implication, and the diagnostic criteria established in a consensus statement released by a panel of international experts on IBC.

Keywords Locally advanced breast cancer • Inflammatory breast cancer • Clinical definition • Diagnostic criteria • T4d disease • Dermal lymphatic invasion

S. Dawood, F.A.C.P., M.R.C.P. (UK), M.P.H., C.P.H. (✉)
Department of Medical Oncology, Department of Health and Medical Services,
Dubai Hospital, P.O. Box 8179, Dubai, UAE
e-mail: shaheenah_d@yahoo.com

V. Valero, M.D.
Department of Breast Medical Oncology, The University of Texas MD Anderson Cancer Center,
1515 Holcombe Boulevard, Houston, TX 77030, USA
e-mail: vvalero@mdanderson.org

N.T. Ueno and M. Cristofanilli (eds.), *Inflammatory Breast Cancer: An Update*,
DOI 10.1007/978-94-007-3907-9_3, © Springer Science+Business Media B.V. 2012

3.1 Introduction

An estimated 207,090 women in the United States were diagnosed with breast cancer in 2010, and approximately 39,840 deaths were attributed to this disease [1]. Among women who are diagnosed with breast cancer, approximately 2.5% are diagnosed with a subtype of locally advanced breast cancer (LABC) known as inflammatory breast cancer (IBC) [2]. This term was coined by Lee and Tannenbaum in 1924 [3] to describe a peculiar form of advanced breast cancer that was historically associated with a particularly grim prognosis. IBC follows an aggressive biological course that is typically associated with rapid onset of signs and symptoms. Because of its rapid course of progression, many patients present with an advanced stage of disease at diagnosis, with either regional nodal metastases or distant metastases that may also be attributed in part to delayed diagnosis. Before the advent of systemic chemotherapy, IBC was typically managed with surgery or radiation therapy alone or in combination; these approaches were associated with a 5-year actuarial overall survival rate of <5%, median survival of only 15 months [4], and local recurrence rate as high as 50% [5, 6]. A combination of both early diagnosis and aggressive early multidisciplinary management that includes pre-operative chemotherapy, surgery, and radiation therapy has transformed this once uniformly fatal disease into one that is now associated with 15-year survival rates of 20–30% [7, 8].

Despite significant advances made in the management of IBC, the outcome of women with this disease still remain inferior to those of women with non-IBC LABC [9]. The inferior prognosis can be attributed in part to biology and in part to the difficulty of accurately diagnosing this aggressive disease early. Early diagnosis of IBC has been an issue of controversy over the years, and several methods have been developed in an effort to accurately diagnose this rare disease. Because of a lack of consensus on IBC case definition, it has also been difficult to definitively determine incidence, identify specific risk factors, and compare studies to evaluate the effectiveness of different therapeutic modalities [10]. IBC is currently clinically diagnosed using a combination of information obtained from the patient's medical history, of the affected breast, and diagnostic confirmation of invasive carcinoma via core biopsy. To date, the most widely used case description of IBC is the definition set forth by the American Joint Committee on Cancer (AJCC), which defines IBC as "a clinicopathologic entity characterized by diffuse erythema and edema (peau d'orange) involving a third or more of the skin of the breast" and classifies IBC as T4d disease [11].

In this chapter, we will discuss the clinical characteristics of IBC, the methods that have been developed to better define this disease, the controversy surrounding case definition and its associated implication, and the diagnostic criteria established in a consensus statement released by an international multidisciplinary expert panel on IBC [12]. Two types of IBC, primary and secondary, are typically recognized. Primary IBC develops in a previously normal breast. Secondary IBC describes a situation in which a non-IBC acquires inflammatory features or when an inflammatory recurrence develops at the site of mastectomy for a non-IBC. In this chapter, "IBC" will refer to primary IBC.

3.2 Clinical Characteristics

The history of IBC dates back to as early as 1814, when Sir Charles Bell first described the clinical presentation of this disease as "a purple color on the skin over the tumor accompanied by shooting pain" [13]. However, Lee and Tannenbaum [3] did not propose the term "IBC" until 1924, at the suggestion of James Ewing; until then, the disease had been referred to by a variety of terms, including lactation cancer, carcinoma mastitoides, mastitis carcinomatosa, acute encephaloid cancer, acute mammary carcinoma, acute brawny cancer, acute scirrhous carcinoma, and carcinoma telangiectaticum [14]. In 1938, Taylor and Meltzer provided a classic description of IBC [15] that included the following: "The redness, which may vary from a faint blush to a flaming red, spreads diffusely over the breast, which becomes hot, pitted, and edematous, presenting an 'orange-skin' appearance. Meanwhile, the cancer spreads rapidly throughout the entire breast in the form of a diffuse, ill-defined induration. The breast may swell to two or three times its original volume within a few weeks." In 1956, Haagensen [16] set forth a set of diagnostic criteria derived from information attained from patients' medical history, physician examination, and core biopsy that is currently the cornerstone of diagnosing IBC.

3.2.1 History and Symptoms

A woman presenting with IBC typically has a history of rapid development of signs and symptoms of the affected breast. The affected breast rapidly enlarges in size, is warm and red, and may exhibit nipple changes. The rapid development (<6 months) of signs and symptoms distinguishes IBC from neglected LABC, which can at times have the same appearance. In general, women presenting with IBC tend to be younger than those who have LABC [17].

3.2.2 Physical Examination

Patients with IBC have diffuse erythema that often occupies at least one-third of the breast (Fig. 3.1). Initially, the skin overlying the breast has a pink or mottled pink hue that quickly changes to a dark red or purple. Examination also reveals edema caused by tumor blockage of the lymphatic system, which is associated with exaggerated hair follicle pits that give the characteristic orange peel appearance (peau d'orange) of the overlying skin. The edema results in an increase in breast size and weight, generalized induration of the affected breast, and, in some cases, wheals or ridging of the skin. Contrary to the historical descriptions of IBC, none of these changes are associated with pain. In about one-third of women, no discrete palpable mass is present. In approximately 55–85% of women, ipsilateral supraclavicular

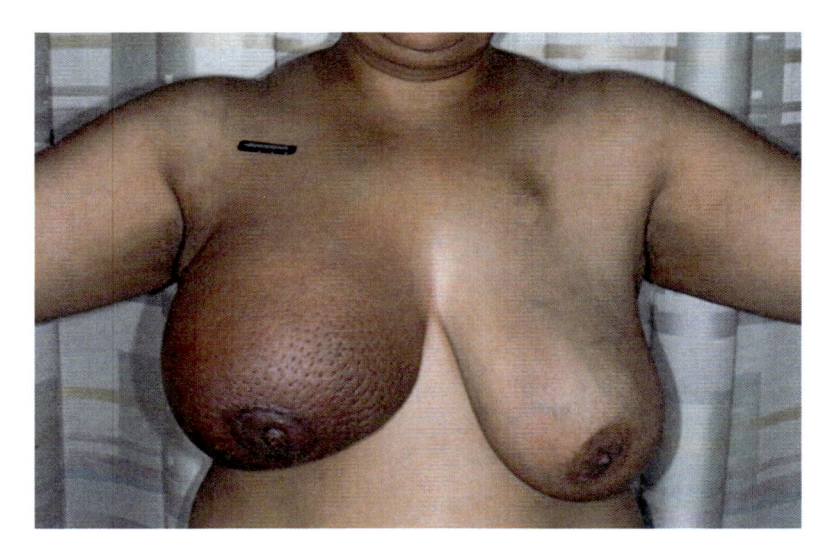

Fig. 3.1 Inflammatory carcinoma of the right breast. Breast shows erythema, peau d'orange skin, and overall increased size

and/or axillary lymph nodes may be palpable [17]. Physical examination may further reveal abnormalities of the nipple in the form of flattening, retraction, blistering, or crusting.

3.2.3 Differential Diagnosis

One reason for the delay in the diagnosis of IBC is a wide range of diseases that can mimic physical signs typically associated with IBC (Table 3.1). Various features from patients' medical history and physical examination may allow the physician to distinguish IBC from other conditions. The most frequent misdiagnosis is an infection cause, during which a woman presents with a history of having been treated with a prolonged course of antibiotics that has not abated the signs or symptoms. Acute mastitis and breast abscesses are the most common infectious cause of misdiagnosis. However, Acute mastitis or breast abscess tend to occur in lactating women. Postradiation dermatitis may be distinguished from IBC in that it typically shows a well-demarcated rather than diffuse area of erythema that occurs within the area of the radiation port and typically begins to develop 2–3 weeks after the beginning of radiation therapy. Malignancies such as lymphoma, leukemia, and sarcoma of the breast can mimic some or all of the clinical features associated with IBC but can be ruled out by tissue diagnosis. Other diagnoses such as generalized dermatitis or insect bites clear up fairly rapidly. When in doubt, it is reasonable to offer a course of antibiotics. However, when the signs and symptoms do not disappear after a week of treatment, a biopsy should then be strongly considered to prove or refute a diagnosis of IBC or any other malignancy.

Table 3.1 Differential diagnosis for inflammatory breast cancer

Classification	Differential diagnosis
Infectious causes	Lactational mastitis
	Breast abscess
	Tuberculosis
	Syphilis
	Other infections
Noninfectious causes	Lymphoma
	Leukemia
	Sarcoma
	Congestive heart failure
	Postradiation dermatitis
	Generalized dermatitis
	Duct ectasia

3.2.4   Findings on Imaging

Imaging plays a role in the diagnosis and assessment of IBC. IBC is clinically diagnosed, and imaging plays a key role in characterizing the tumor, assessing nodal basins and potential distant metastatic sites, and evaluating response to preoperative chemotherapy. In terms of initial diagnosis and assessment, mammography is still the standard imaging assessment method, and key characteristic findings include skin thickening and stromal coarsening and/or diffusely increased breast density, which may obscure the presence of malignant-type microcalcifications [18]. In some patients, a discrete mass or axillary lymphadenopathy may be detected as well. However, in general, the findings on mammography are largely quite subtle and as such may be deemed negative [19].

3.2.5   Role of Biopsy

Although the diagnosis of IBC relies heavily on clinical components such as medical history and physical examination, the diagnosis must be supported by confirmation of invasive carcinoma using a tissue sample obtained via a core biopsy of the affected breast. Examination of tissue obtained from a breast affected by IBC may also reveal dermal lymphatic invasion (DLI), a histologic hallmark of IBC during which numerous dilated dermal lymphatics are filled with tumor emboli that are usually retracted from the surrounding endothelial lining [20]. DLI results in lymphatic obstruction that is responsible for the clinical signs and symptoms observed in patients with IBC. Because of sampling heterogeneity, DLI is identified in only 75% of IBC tumors. Furthermore, obstruction of the dermal lymphatic system may also occur in other conditions, such as non-Hodgkin's lymphoma of the breast and non-IBC breast tumors [21]. As such, the presence of DLI is not currently required for the diagnosis of IBC.

3.2.6   Staging

As is the case when diagnosing any other type of breast cancer, a staging work-up to define the extent of disease is required. Radiological imaging studies are used to determine the presence of distant metastatic disease. After a full staging work-up, the AJCC tumor-node-metastasis (TNM) staging system is used to determine the stage of disease. All IBC tumors are classified as T4d, whereas N and M categories are designated according to pathological and radiological information attained at baseline. All nonmetastatic cases are classified as stage IIIb or IIIc, depending on the extent of nodal involvement (i.e., axillary alone versus axillary and infraclavicular and/or supraclavicular and/or internal mammary chain[s]). The presence of metastatic disease results in a stage IV designation.

3.3   Variability of Case Definition: An Ongoing Controversy

The predominant clinical criteria required to diagnosis IBC have been debated for over a century. The most important aspects of this debate have been the subjective nature of the clinical criteria and whether to include pathological features such as DLI in the diagnostic criteria. Restricting the definition to primarily clinical criteria is problematic because some population-based registries require the presence of DLI to assign the designation of IBC [2], and clinicians assigning the designation of IBC may not strictly follow the clinical criteria. Furthermore, data also indicate that outcomes can vary depending on the critieria used diagnose IBC [22, 23]. For example Lucas and Perez-Mesa [22] divided women with IBC into three groups: those with clinical and pathological features of IBC, those with only clinical features of IBC, and those whose tumors demonstrated only DLI without clinical features of IBC. The authors noted that the group with both clinical and pathological features of IBC and the group with only clinical features of IBC had a similar prognostic outcome (a 3-year survival rate of 20%) compared to the superior prognostic outcome observed in those whose tumors had only pathological features of IBC (a 3-year survival rate of 70%). Similarly, Amparo et al. [23] reported on two groups of women: one whose tumors exhibited clinical signs of IBC and another whose tumors exhibited the presence of DLI without clinical signs of IBC. The authors reported that the 5-year survival rate was significantly worse in the former group than in the latter group (25.6% vs. 51.6%).

The subjective nature of the clinical criteria and the use of variable case definitions of IBC in a number of studies have limited the comparison of results of studies specifically examining IBC, including those examining aspects of IBC epidemiology and therapy. Kim et al. [10] recently conducted a systematic review of the literature in an attempt to characterize the reporting of clinical criteria. The authors reported significant variability in the criteria used and thus in the reporting of IBC.

The authors noted that of 27 studies included in the review, 59% did not report the extent of breast involvement and 85% did not report or clearly define the time from the onset of symptoms to the diagnosis of disease.

It is clear that case definition of IBC is an important issue that has implications not only for comparing study results but also for enrollment in multicenter international trials examining various therapeutic modalities geared toward improving the prognostic outcome of IBC. Apart from the widely used gold standard definition of IBC established by the AJCC, several models have been developed to encompass the disease manifestations of IBC in an attempt to standardize reporting criteria. One model consists of the poussée evolutive criteria (PEV) developed by Denoix [24] at the Gustave-Roussy Institute, which describe a rapidly progressing breast cancer with inflammatory features. The PEV system classifies rapidly progressing breast tumors into four categories: PEV0 describes a tumor without inflammatory signs or an any observable increase in size over the previous 3 months; PEV1 describes a tumor without inflammatory signs but with an increase in size over the previous 3 months; PEV2 describes a tumor with inflammatory signs involving less than half the breast surface; and PEV3 describes a tumor with inflammatory signs involving more than half the breast. Tumors classified as PEV2 and PEV3 are considered to be consistent with IBC. The PEV2 and PEV3 categories have since been modified to include a time interval of ≤4 months, with regard to symptom onset thereby allowing for a distinction between IBC and neglected LABC [25]. The PEV system, however, is not widely used outside certain institutions.

3.4 Diagnostic Criteria: The Consensus Statement

The ambiguity surrounding the case definition of IBC is evident. In an effort to clarify and standardize the clinical definition of IBC and to improve the management of this disease, a group of international IBC experts met in 2008 to review all the published literature and establish the diagnostic criteria and management guidelines [12] (Table 3.2). The criteria are an extension of the AJCC definition of IBC but more clearly define the clinical aspects of the medical history and physical examination and emphasize the need for definitive evidence of invasive carcinoma from a core biopsy. The panel agreed that the time from the initial presentation of signs and symptoms to diagnosis should be less than 6 months in order to distinguish IBC from non-IBC LABC. The panel further agreed that as of now, pending further data, DLI is not required for the diagnosis of IBC and that IBC diagnosis remains a primarily clinical one. With a more definitive set of criteria outlined, oncologists may be better able to identify cases of IBC; such criteria would also facilitate enrollment into future clinical trials. Future studies may be able to define a molecular profile unique to IBC that will function as a molecular fingerprint for developing a more unambiguous method of diagnosis.

Table 3.2 Diagnostic criteria for inflammatory breast cancer established in the international expert panel consensus statement

Component	Criteria
Medical history	Rapid onset of breast erythema, edema and/or peau d'orange, and/or warmth of breast
	Possible history of mastitis that was unresponsive to at least 1 week of antibiotics
	History of no more than 6 months
Physical examination	Erythema occupying at least one-third of the breast
	Underlying palpable mass
	Palpable locoregional lymph nodes
	Nipple abnormalities (flattening, crusting, discharge, etc.)
Pathology	Pathological confirmation of invasive carcinoma from a core biopsy of the breast
	Dermal lymphovascular tumor emboli (may be present but not necessary for diagnosis)

References

1. Jemal A, Siegel R, Xu J, Ward E (2010) Cancer statistics, 2010. CA Cancer J Clin 60(5):277–300
2. Levine PH, Steinhorn SC, Ries LG, Aron JL (1985) Inflammatory breast cancer: the experience of the Surveillance, Epidemiology, and End Results (SEER) program. J Natl Cancer Inst 74:291–297
3. Lee BJ, Tannenbaum EN (1924) Inflammatory carcinoma of the breast. Surg Gynecol Obstet 39:580–595
4. Bozzetti F, Saccozzi R, De Lena M et al (1981) Inflammatory cancer of the breast: analysis of 114 cases. J Surg Oncol 18:355–361
5. Barker JL, Nelson AJ, Montague ED (1976) Inflammatory carcinoma of the breast. Radiology 121:173–176
6. Zucali R, Uslenghi C, Kenda R et al (1976) Natural history and survival of inoperable breast cancer treated with radiotherapy and radiotherapy followed by radical mastectomy. Cancer 37:1422–1431
7. Low J, Berman A, Steinber S et al (2004) Long term follow up for locally advanced and inflammatory breast cancer patients treated with multimodality therapy. J Clin Oncol 22:4065–4074
8. Ueno NT, Buzdar AU, Singletary SE et al (1997) Combined modality treatment of inflammatory breast carcinoma: twenty years of experience at M.D. Anderson Center. Cancer Chemother Pharmacol 40:321–329
9. Dawood S, Ueno NT, Valero V et al (2011) Differences in survival among women with stage III inflammatory and noninflammatory locally advanced breast cancer appear early: a large population-based study. Cancer 117(9):1819–1826
10. Kim T, Lau J, Erban J (2006) Lack of uniform diagnostic criteria for inflammatory breast cancer limits interpretation of treatment outcomes: a systematic review. Clin Breast Cancer 7:386–395
11. Edge SB, Byrd DR, Compton CC (eds) (2010) AJCC (American Joint Committee on Cancer) cancer staging manual, 7th edn. Springer, New York

12. Dawood S, Merajver SD, Viens P et al (2011) International expert panel on inflammatory breast cancer: consensus statement for standardized diagnosis and treatment. Ann Oncol 22(3):515–523
13. Bell C (1814) A system of operative surgery. Hale & Hosmer, Hartford
14. Anderson WF, Schairer C, Chen BE, Hance KW, Levine PH (2005–2006) Epidemiology of inflammatory breast cancer (IBC). Breast Dis 22:9–23
15. Taylor G, Meltzer A (1938) Inflammatory carcinoma of the breast. Am J Cancer 33:33–49
16. Haagensen CD (1956) Inflammatory carcinoma. Diseases of the breast. W.B. Saunders, Philadelphia, pp 488–498
17. Hance KW, Anderson WF, Devesa SS, Young HA, Levine PH (2005) Trends in inflammatory breast carcinoma incidence and survival: the surveillance, Epidemiology, and End Results program at the National Cancer Institute. J Natl Cancer Inst 97(13):966–975
18. Günhan-Bilgen I, Ustün EE, Memi A (2002) Inflammatory breast carcinoma: mammographic, ultrasonographic, clinical, and pathologic findings in 142 cases. Radiology 223(3):829–838
19. Kushwaha AC, Whitman GJ, Stelling CB, Cristofanilli M, Buzdar AU (2000) Primary inflammatory carcinoma of the breast: retrospective review of mammographic findings. AJR Am J Roentgenol 174(2):535–538
20. Bonnier P, Charpin C, Lejeune C et al (1995) Inflammatory carcinomas of the breast: a clinical, pathological, or a clinical and pathological definition? Int J Cancer 62(4):382–385
21. Singletary SE, Cristofanilli M (2008) Defining the clinical diagnosis of inflammatory breast cancer. Semin Oncol 35(1):7–10
22. Lucas FV, Perez-Mesa C (1978) Inflammatory carcinoma of the breast. Cancer 34:382–388
23. Amparo RS, Angel CD, Ana LH et al (2000) Inflammatory breast carcinoma: pathological or clinical entity? Breast Cancer Res Treat 64:269–273
24. Denoix P (1970) Treatment of malignant breast cancer. Recent Results Cancer Res 31:92–94
25. Attia-Sobol J, Ferrière JP, Curé H, Kwiatkowski F et al (1993) Treatment results, survival and prognostic factors in 109 inflammatory breast cancers: univariate and multivariate analysis. Eur J Cancer 29(8):1081–1088

Chapter 4
Inflammatory Breast Cancer Registry

Jie S. Willey and Naoto T. Ueno

Abstract The Morgan Welch Inflammatory Breast Cancer Research Program and Clinic at The University of Texas MD Anderson Cancer Center is spearheading development of an inflammatory breast cancer (IBC) registry. This registry includes clinical, epidemiological, and imaging data; serum and plasma samples; and tissue samples. Data and samples are collected from two patient cohorts: (1) patients with newly diagnosed IBC who have not received systemic therapy and (2) patients with previously diagnosed IBC who have received systemic therapy, but have tissues available for IBC registry. Data will be stored in an IBC registry specific database, and blood and tissue samples will be stored in central repositories. Each patient will be assigned a unique patient number that will be associated with that patient's data and samples; patient identifiers will not be included in the registry. Data in the database and stored blood and tissue samples will be available for institutional review board-approved research projects in the future.

Keywords Biospecimens • Inflammatory breast cancer • Blood • Tissue • Biopsy • Repository

List of Abbreviations

IBC   Inflammatory breast cancer

J.S. Willey, RN, MSN (✉)
Department of Breast Medical Oncology, Unit 1354, The University of Texas MD Anderson Cancer Center, 1515 Holcombe Blvd., Houston, TX 77030-4095, USA
e-mail: jwilley@mdanderson.org

N.T. Ueno, M.D., Ph.D., F.A.C.P.
Morgan Welch Inflammatory Breast Cancer Program and Clinic, Department of Breast Medical Oncology, The University of Texas, MD Anderson Cancer Center,
Unit 1354, Holcombe Blvd. 1515, Houston, TX, USA
e-mail: nueno@mdanderson.org

N.T. Ueno and M. Cristofanilli (eds.), *Inflammatory Breast Cancer: An Update*,   21
DOI 10.1007/978-94-007-3907-9_4, © Springer Science+Business Media B.V. 2012

4.1 Background

Biospecimens are critically important to cancer research because they contain a tremendous amount of information about the biological characteristics of cancer cells. Collections of a large number of biospecimens of a particular cancer type provide the statistical power needed to produce a comprehensive genomic profile of that type of cancer, information that is essential to understanding the disease and identifying the best targets for drug development.

In recent years, the use of more sophisticated technologies has been advocated to differentiate inflammatory breast cancer (IBC) from other types of breast cancer at the genomic and protein levels (e.g., gene profiling and proteomic analysis). These technologies have shown promise but also have produced contrasting results, which suggests that the peculiar clinical behavior of IBC could be related to the interaction between the host (microenvironment and immunological response) and tumor cells [1–3]. Therefore, the molecular diagnostic criteria are yet to be established. In order to improve understanding of the biological features and molecular characteristics of IBC, identify diagnostic and prognostic markers for this disease, and develop targeted therapies based on enhanced knowledge of the biology of IBC, it is crucial to establish an IBC registry through prospective collection of clinical, epidemiological, and imaging data, serum and plasma samples, and tissue samples.

To date, in the United States and around world, very few breast cancer registries specifically focus on IBC. Because of the rarity of the disease, only small numbers of patients with IBC are seen in any single institution [4]. It has been very difficult to develop large-scale prospective clinical trials for patients with IBC, and therefore much of the information about this disease is based on retrospective studies. To increase IBC sample collection and collect the samples in a central location to facilitate their use in future biological studies, it is imperative to develop a network of collaborators who are able to provide retrospectively and prospectively collected samples from patients with IBC.

To address the need for a centralized repository of a large collection of blood and tissue samples from patients with IBC, the Morgan Welch Inflammatory Breast Cancer Research Program and Clinic at The University of Texas MD Anderson Cancer Center is spearheading development of the IBC registry.

4.2 Study Plan

This is a multicenter IBC registry. The Morgan Welch Inflammatory Breast Cancer Research Program and Clinic will coordinate all aspects of the IBC registry. All other participating centers will obtain approval from their institutional review board for the IBC registry protocol, and all patients eligible for inclusion in the study will provide written informed consent for participation and will be registered in the human subjects study registration systems in their participating centers. A unique patient number will be assigned to each patient. It is expected that minimum of 450 patients will be enrolled in this prospective study.

Two cohorts will be included in the IBC registry. Cohort I will consist of patients with newly diagnosed IBC who have not received systemic therapy. From these patients, participating centers will prospectively collect clinical and epidemiological data; imaging data; tumor tissue (including samples of primary tumor, ipsilateral nodal metastases, and/or distant metastasis [if applicable]) obtained prior to primary systemic therapy and mastectomy plus axillary dissection (if applicable); and samples of serum, plasma, and whole blood.

Cohort II will consist of patients with previously diagnosed IBC who have received systemic therapies, and have tissue available for IBC registry. From these patients, participating centers will collect clinical and epidemiological data; imaging data (if available); paraffin tissue blocks or unstained slides of tumor tissue (including samples of primary tumor, ipsilateral nodal metastases, and/or distant metastasis [if applicable]) obtained prior to primary systemic therapy and mastectomy and/or axillary dissection, and samples of serum, plasma, and whole blood.

4.2.1 Patient Selection

For inclusion in the study, patients must have a clinical diagnosis of primary IBC according to AJCC definition and have a histological diagnosis of invasive breast cancer. Patients are either newly diagnosed IBC (Cohort I) or have received systemic therapies and have tissue or unstained slides at the time of initial diagnosis of IBC available (cohort II).

4.2.2 Demographic and Clinical Information

Demographic and clinical information to be collected for each patient will include age, gender, height, weight, race/ethnic background, month and year of initial IBC diagnosis, stage at initial IBC diagnosis, hormonal status, and HER2 status.

4.2.3 IBC Questionnaire

Patients will be asked to participate in an interview. The principal investigator at each participating institution or his or her designee will conduct the interview. During the interview, the patient will be asked about sociodemographic characteristics, history of tobacco and alcohol use, occupational history, family history, including the status of blood related siblings, biological children, and siblings of patient parents, and personal medical history. The personal medical history will include a reproductive history, including questions about previous pregnancies, live births, spontaneous abortions, and induced abortions, menstrual and breast health history. Every completed questionnaire will be linked to the unique patient number to protect the confidentiality of the information.

A database was created specifically for the IBC registry by the Department of Epidemiology at MD Anderson Cancer Center. The unique patient number will be used for data entry and sample collection. No patient identifiers will be used for data entry. Only approved personnel will be given access to the database.

4.2.4   Photographs of Breasts

For all patients in cohort I, baseline digital photographs of the breasts will be obtained. These photographs will include (1) photographs of both breasts, (2) close-up front view photographs of the affected breast, and (3) close-up lateral view photographs of involved skin around breast (if applicable). For patients in cohort II, if digital photographs from baseline are available, they will be included in the registry. All photographs will be encrypted and sent electronically to MD Anderson for future evaluation and analysis.

4.2.5   Imaging Data

For patients in cohort I, imaging data, particularly magnetic resonance imaging and positron emission tomography/computed tomography images of the involved breast, will be collected at baseline as part of standard of care. For patients in cohort II, if imaging data from baseline are available, reports will be collected and included in the study.

4.2.6   Blood Specimens

Using approved, standardized methods and supplies, trained phlebotomists will draw 30 ml of blood from each patient. Serum and plasma will be collected. Cell separation, cell counting, and cryopreservation of peripheral blood mononuclear cells will be conducted in centers where appropriate equipment and technology are available. Blood samples will be collected at study entry, before mastectomy plus axillary dissection (if applicable), and before radiation therapy (if applicable).

4.2.7   Tissue Specimens

4.2.7.1   Cohort I

For newly diagnosed patients (cohort I), the following tissue specimens will be obtained before systemic therapy as part of standard care for patients with IBC. In addition to specimens collected for diagnostic purpose, additional samples will be collected specifically for the IBC registry.

- Skin punch biopsy specimens: Up to four skin punch biopsy specimens will be obtained from the lesions on the affected breast.
- Tumor core biopsy specimens: Up to four core biopsy specimens will be obtained from the primary tumor under ultrasonographic guidance provided by a radiologist.
- Lymph node biopsy specimens (if applicable): During ultrasonographically guided core biopsy, if lymph nodes are clinically palpable, core biopsy or fine-needle aspiration of the lymph nodes will be performed. Paraffin blocks of core biopsy specimens, cell blocks of fine-needle aspiration specimens, or up to 20 unstained slides from each representative block will be collected.
- Biopsy specimens of locoregional and/or distant metastases (if applicable): Paraffin blocks of core biopsy specimens or cell blocks of fine-needle aspiration specimens or up to 20 unstained slides per block will be collected.
- Surgical specimens from mastectomy plus axillary dissection (if applicable): After systemic therapy, patients will undergo mastectomy plus axillary dissection (if applicable).

4.2.7.2   Cohort II

For IBC patients who had their initial biopsies performed and have paraffin blocks or unstained slides available for tissue banking (cohort II), paraffin blocks or up to 20 unstained slides from each representative block from skin punch biopsy, tumor core biopsy, lymph node biopsy, or biopsy of locoregional and/or distant metastases will be collected, if applicable. Paraffin blocks will be maintained in the IBC Laboratory at MD Anderson, or, if the original institution prefers, the blocks will be cut by a technician at the IBC Laboratory and the remaining portions of the blocks will be returned to the original institution.

4.2.8   Sample Shipping and Storage

All plasma, serum, and tissue samples from collaborating institutions will be stored at each institution. Samples will be shipped to MD Anderson Cancer Center upon request according to the instructions for Shipping of Biological Infectious Human Exempt Specimens Category B and specific guidelines stipulated by the United

States Government Pipeline and Hazardous Materials Safety Administration. Upon receiving samples, the research staff at IBC laboratory at MD Anderson Cancer Center will organize the samples, verify the sample information, document the source, and record the samples on freezer log-in sheets. The central location for tissue samples will be the IBC laboratory at MD Anderson Cancer Center. Tissues prepared in the paraffin blocks embedded in Tissue-Tek® embedding rings and cassettes will be stored in impact-resistant plastic cabinets. The central location for plasma and serum samples will be the Cryogene Lab, a state-of-the-science facility located in the Texas Medical Center in Houston that specializes in sample processing and secure storage of biological specimens. The Cryogene Lab utilizes the latest freezer technology, continuous monitoring systems, and a computer software to fulfill the storage requirements.

4.2.9 Use of Samples for Research

The blood and tissue samples in the IBC registry will be available for research projects in the future. All requests to the IBC registry for use of patient samples must include a copy of the submitted or approved institutional review board-approved protocol and informed consent or waiver of the requirement for informed consent. A steering committee composed of members of participating Institution will review the proposal and select the project approved for access to the research specimens. Participants will have appropriate representation in the resulting manuscript(s) based on the contribution to the project. In order to facilitate the participation of centers located in countries with strict regulations for specimens shipping we have discussed the possibility to expand the concept of the IBC registry to the creation of a "virtual" IBC registry allowing the participating centers to retain the specimens collected in their Institution and make it available to the other members of the team. Additionally, it is hoped that with the increased availability of sophisticated diagnostic technologies future sharing of genomic and proteomic data could further expand the capabilities of IBC investigations and allow to expedite research for the benefit of our patients.

References

1. Wu M, Wu ZF, Kumar-Sinha C, Chinnaiyan A, Merajver SD (2004) RhoC induces differential expression of genes involved in invasion and metastasis in MCF10A breast cells. Breast Cancer Res Treat 84:3–12
2. Bertucci F, Finetti P, Rougemont J et al (2004) Gene expression profiling for molecular characterization of inflammatory breast cancer and prediction of response to chemotherapy. Cancer Res 64:8558–8565
3. Bertucci F, Finetti P, Rougemont J et al (2005) Gene expression profiling identifies molecular subtypes of inflammatory breast cancer. Cancer Res 65:2170–2178
4. Dawood S, Cristofanilli M (2011) Inflammatory breast cancer: what progress have we made? Oncology 25:264–270

Chapter 5
Pathology: Histomorphometrical Features of IBC – Angiogenesis, Lymphangiogenesis, and Tumor Emboli

Sanford H. Barsky and Fredika M. Robertson

Keywords Lymphovascular invasion • Tumor emboli • Lymphangiogenesis • E-cadherin • E-cadherin fragments • Gamma secretase • p120 catenin • EIF4GI • Spheroidgenesis

5.1 Introduction

Inflammatory breast cancer (IBC) is a form of human breast cancer that, unfortunately, has not benefited from the recent advances that have been made for the more common forms of breast cancer. For example the greatest advances that have benefited patients with breast cancer made over the past decade have been the recognition that breast conserving therapy (lumpectomy with radiation therapy) can be as effective as total mastectomy in certain situations; that axillary-sparing sentinel node dissection can be as informative as full axillary dissection, again, in certain situations; that, mammographic screening in postmenopausal women can be effective at detecting disease while it is organ confined and hence curable, reducing the age-adjusted mortality from breast cancer; that tamoxifen treatment in both an adjuvant setting and a chemopreventive setting can effectively treat and/or reduce the occurrence of estrogen positive breast cancer; that the major susceptibility genes for

S.H. Barsky, M.D. (✉)
Molecular Pathology and Laboratory Services, The University of Nevada School of Medicine, Reno, NV, USA

The Nevada Cancer Institute, Las Vegas, NV, USA
e-mail: sbarsky@medicine.nevada.edu

F.M. Robertson, Ph.D.
The Department of Experimental Therapeutics, The University of Texas MD Anderson Cancer Center, Houston, TX, USA

The Morgan Welch Inflammatory Breast Cancer Research Program, The University of Texas MD Anderson Cancer Center, Houston, TX, USA

N.T. Ueno and M. Cristofanilli (eds.), *Inflammatory Breast Cancer: An Update*, DOI 10.1007/978-94-007-3907-9_5, © Springer Science+Business Media B.V. 2012

breast cancer, *BRCA1* and *BRCA2*, increase breast cancer risk and mandate more aggressive surveillance and therapy; and that Her-2/neu status effectively stratifies patients with Her-2/neu positive breast cancers and triggers the use of Herceptin (Trastuzumab) which can be effective. Unfortunately none of these advances have directly benefited patients with IBC.

This is because IBC presents with florid lymphovascular invasion (LVI) or lymphovascular tumor emboli very early in its natural history. Lymphovascular emboli are clumps of tumor cells within lymphovascular spaces. These emboli escape breast confinement very early and form distant metastasis. IBC often presents only with these lymphovascular emboli and not with a dominant mass within the breast. Because of these lymphovascular emboli, and the disease's penchant for spreading within the breast, breast-conserving surgery is not an option; moreover, IBC metastasizes to the axillary lymph nodes with great regularity, the presumption is that the axillary lymph nodes are always involved and hence selective sentinel lymph node biopsy has no role in the management of IBC. The peculiar clinical presentation of IBC without a palpable mass and diffuse skin involvement secondary to lymphovascular emboli the disease demonstrates diffuse and escape organ confinement quickly, therefore mammographic screening is not effective in detecting early IBC.

In comparison to non-IBC cases, the majority of IBC are ER negative and BRCA1 and BRCA2, suggesting minimal impact for standard prevention methods including tamoxifen chemoprevention. Although a significant number of cases of IBC overexpress Her-2/neu and therefore theoretically can benefit from Trastuzumab [Herceptin®] and/or lapatinib [Tykerb®] treatment, the overall survival of IBC has not improved significantly even with this or related therapies. Higher incidence of Her2/neu gene amplification in IBC reported by several groups and availability of HER-2-targeted agents like trastuzumab and lapatinib however, have created opportunities to study the impact of targeted therapy alone or in combination with chemotherapeutic agents on response rate and overall outcome in IBC.

Although primary IBC may be relatively infrequent, its importance can not be overstated. It causes a disproportionate number of deaths from breast cancer and its defining signature, the lymphovascular embolus, is expressed to varying degrees by a large number of common non-IBC breast cancers. Following neoadjuvant chemotherapy for the advanced primary breast cancer, the residual disease often exhibits florid LVI. When the common forms of non-IBC breast cancer recur or relapse, the recurrence is characterized by florid LVI. Virtually everyone who dies of metastatic breast cancer, dies with the disease showing LVI [1]. All of these manifestations might be aptly termed secondary IBC. If we include secondary IBC in our definition, then IBC becomes a very common type of human breast cancer.

As has been mentioned, the signature of both primary as well as secondary IBC is the lymphovascular tumor embolus and this signature explains most of the clinicopathological aspects of the disease. For example, the disease does not benefit from early detection strategies. Because there often is no dominant mass, breast self-examination, breast physical examination by a physician and mammographic screening all fail. The typical presentation of IBC is a tender and reddened breast. These symptoms are due to the obstruction of lymphovascular drainage due to the tumor emboli. Inflammatory conditions of the breast such as bacterial mastitis mimic this clinical presentation and women who present with these symptoms are often given a trial of antibiotics. When the condition worsens or at least does not improve with antibiotics, a biopsy is performed which may indicate the presence of dermal lymphovascular emboli and then the diagnosis of IBC is confirmed. Women at this point are often angry at their family physician for not diagnosing the disease initially but do not realize that even if the disease had been diagnosed at first presentation, this would not have made a difference. When the breast turns red from IBC, the disease is already advanced and the lymphovascular emboli which are present are numerous and have already escaped organ confinement. Although there are no inflammatory cells in IBC, the clinical manifestations strongly suggest that the symptoms of the disease may be a byproduct of inflammatory cytokines released by the tumor cell emboli themselves.

Recent studies with a human-murine xenograft model of IBC, MARY-X, have shed some light on the molecular mechanisms underlying the formation of the lymphovascular embolus responsible for LVI. For example the lymphovascular embolus of IBC overexpresses E-cadherin, an important cell attachment molecule involved in cell-cell adhesion. This adhesion molecule causes the cells of IBC to form a compact embolus. Interestingly the tumor embolus of IBC resembles the appearance of the human blastocyst, a tight clump of embryonal cells which implant in the uterus during gestation. The human blastocyst also overexpresses E-cadherin which explains its property of having cells in tight clusters. Its high cellular density results in its high efficiency in implanting into the uterine wall and growing into a fetus. Similarly the high cellular density of the tumor embolus results in its high efficiency at implanting at its metastatic site and growing into a metastasis. The lymphovascular embolus of IBC also overexpress MUC-1, another adhesion molecule which, when sialylated, contributes to tumor cell-endothelial cell adhesion. However the lymphovascular embolus of IBC lacks this sialylation and, as a result, is not strongly attached to the vascular endothelium. The result is that the lymphovascular embolus easily spreads or metastasizes. This can be triggered with mild physical maneuvers such as palpation. One might then question the wisdom of repetitive palpation during physical examination or compression mammography if lymphovascular emboli or IBC is suspected. The lymphovascular embolus of IBC is also resistant to chemotherapy and radiation therapy. Apparently the tight aggregation of tumor cells exerts important autocrine cytoprotective effects against cellular insults. Additional studies with the human xenograft model of IBC have shown that if the tumor emboli are disadhered by using an antibody to E-cadherin which neutralizes its adhesion properties, the individual cells liberated undergo a high degree of spontaneous cell death (or apoptosis). In addition disadhering the tumor cell embolus in this manner increases the susceptibility of the tumor cells to radiation and chemotherapy. Studies using lymphatic endothelium-specific markers, e.g. podoplanin have demonstrated that the vast majority of lymphovascular emboli are found within lymphatic vessels rather than blood vessels. This observation offers a potential explanation of why lymphovascular emboli in IBC are so resistant to chemotherapy. Chemotherapy is delivered intravenously and not intralymphatically. Therefore the mere concentration of drug reached within the lymphatics may not even approach a tumoricidal dose. Other potential explanations for the resistance of the tumor embolus of IBC to chemotherapy may be the inherent cytoprotective effects of high tumor density, the stem cell nature of the embryonal blastocyst-like structure and the inherent state of quiescence present within this structure. Still these are all hypotheses awaiting proof. It is our hope that new biological and pathological insights into the lympho-vascular embolus can be translated into a new therapeutic approach that may some day benefit patients with IBC.

5.2   Overview of the Studies of the Lymphovascular Embolus of IBC

The lymphovascular tumor embolus is an entity efficient at metastasis. Studies using a human xenograft model of inflammatory breast cancer (IBC), MARY-X, demonstrated the equivalence of xenograft-generated spheroids with lymphovascular emboli *in vivo* with both structures demonstrating E-cadherin overexpression and specific proteolytic processing. Western blot revealed full length E-cadherin (120 kDa) and four fragments: E-cad/NFT1 (100 kDa), E-cad/NFT2 (95 kDa), E-cad/NFT3 (85 kDa), E-cad/NFT4 (80 kDa). Compared to MARY-X, only E-cad/NFT1 was present in the spheroids. E-cad/NFT1 was produced by calpain, E-cad/NFT2 by γ-secretase and E-cad/NFT3 by a matrix metalloproteinase. E-cad/NFT1 retained the p120ctn binding site but lost both the β-catenin and α-binding sites, facilitating its disassembly from traditional cadherin-based adherens junctions (CAJs) and its 360° distribution around the embolus.

5.3   Significance of the Studies

The lymphovascular tumor embolus is a blastocyst-like structure resistant to che-motherapy, efficient at metastasis and overexpressing E-cadherin. Conventional dogma has regard E-cadherin as a metastasis-suppressor gene involved in epithelial-mesenchymal transition. However within the lymphovascular embolus E-cadherin and its proteolytic processing by calpain and other proteases play a dominant onco-genic rather than suppressive role in metastasis formation and tumor cell survival.

5.4   Highlights of These Studies

- MARY-X spheroidgenesis is an *in vitro* model of tumor emboli formation *in vivo*
- Emboli are characterized by E-cadherin overexpression and its proteolysis
- E-cad/NFT1 produced by calpain retained p120ctn but lost α, β-catenin sites
- Calpain-mediated proteolysis confers to E-cadherin an oncogenic role in metastasis

5.5 Details of the Studies

E-cadherin, an adhesion protein present in normal epithelial cells within lateral junctions (zona adherens), is thought, according to conventional dogma, to function as a tumor suppressor gene whose loss of expression by gene mutation, promoter methylation or promoter repression by snail/slug and other mediators of epithelial-mesenchymal transition (EMT) results in increased invasion and metastasis [2–4]. However our previous studies have demonstrated that within the lymphovascular embolus, E-cadherin is actually overexpressed [5–7].

The lymphovascular embolus is an enigmatic structural-functional entity that is efficient at metastatic dissemination, resistant to chemotherapy and responsible for tumor recurrences. Present studies using a unique human xenograft model of inflammatory breast cancer (IBC), MARY-X, a model which spontaneously exhibits florid lymphovascular emboli and widespread metastasis have demonstrated the equivalence of xenograft-generated spheroids *in vitro* with lymphovascular emboli laser-captured *in vivo* with both structures demonstrating E-cadherin overexpression. Because of this central role of E-cadherin within the lymphovascular embolus, a role based on its presence rather than its absence, we decided to examine this molecule more closely in the present study.

Since our previous studies had also demonstrated that the high levels of E-cadherin within the lymphovascular embolus were not primarily transcriptionally regulated [8], we focused on examining post-translational E-cadherin events in the present study.

5.5.1 MARY-X In Vitro Spheroidgenesis Provides Insights into Tumor Emboli Formation In Vivo

MARY-X manifests its IBC signature of lymphovascular emboli (Fig. 5.1a), exhibiting membrane E-cadherin immunoreactivity within podoplanin expressing lymphatic spaces (Fig. 5.1b). Mincing MARY-X in suspension culture initially gave rise to very loose crude cellular aggregates (Fig. 5.1c) in which increasing numbers of spheroids emerged at 8–12 h (Fig. 5.1d) and peaked at 12–24 h. Spheroids of different sizes could be purified to near homogeneity through filtration. Principal Component Analysis (PCA) revealed near identity of gene expression across the whole transcriptome between MARY-X spheroids and MARY-X emboli but not between the MARY-X spheroids/emboli and the MARY-X non-embolic areas (control) and the different HMEC batches which resembled each other (Fig. 5.1e). Of 54,676 genes depicted in different canonical pathways (phenylalanine metabolism), cAMP mediated signaling, histidine metabolism, wnt/β-catenin signaling, chemokine signaling, acute phase response signaling, and tyrosine metabolism, no two fold or greater gene expression differences were observed between the MARY-X spheroids (SP) and the lymphovascular emboli (LCM) emboli (Fig. 5.1f).

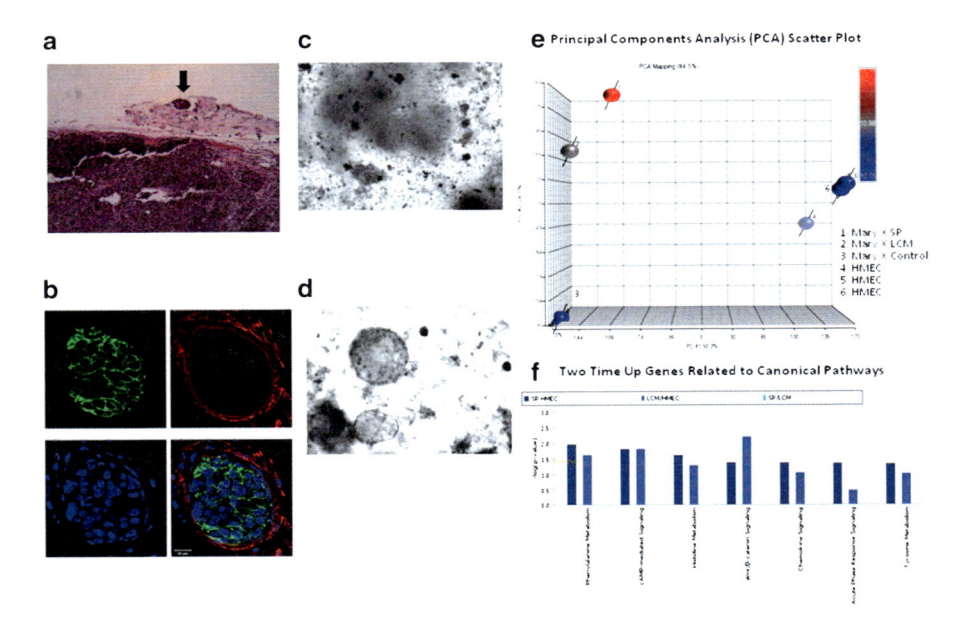

Fig. 5.1 MARY-X transitions to spheroids *in vitro*. (**a**) MARY-X consists of a multinodular mass in which a tumor embolus is observed (*arrow*). (**b**) Although the xenograft demonstrated significant E-cadherin positive emboli (*upper left panel*: *green* immunofluorescence) within podoplanin positive lymphatic channels (*upper right* and *lower right panels*: *red* immunofluorescence), the majority of the tumor consisted of non-embolic areas. (**c**) Mincing the extirpated xenograft gave rise to loose aggregates which gradually gave rise to emergent spheroids. (**d**) Prominent numbers of spheroids could be observed against a crude aggregate background at 8–12 h. (**e**) PCA scatter plot reveals minimal variation (strong identity) between MARY-X spheroids (*SP*) (*1*) and MARY-X lymphovascular emboli obtained by laser capture microdissection (*LCM*) (*2*) compared to non-embolic areas of MARY-X (*Control*) (*3*) and three separate batches of HMEC (*4*, *5*, *6*) which predictably bore strong identity to each other. (**f**) Of 54,676 genes expressed in the different canonical pathways so indicated, there were no two fold or greater differences between the MARY-X spheroids (*SP*) and the MARY-X emboli captured by laser capture microdissection (*LCM*). Significant differences were observed, however, between SP and HMEC and between LCM and HMEC

5.5.2 MARY-X In Vitro Spheroidgenesis Is Associated with Unique Proteolytic Processing of E-cadherin

During MARY-X *in vitro* spheroidgenesis, Western blot using two different anti-human E-cadherin antibodies, anti-ectodomain antibody, H108, that recognized the sequence surrounding amino acid residues 600–707 and anti-cytoplasmic antibody, 24E10, that recognized the sequence surrounding residues 780 showed the presence of full length E-cadherin (E-cad/FL) and a number of different E-cadherin fragments (Fig. 5.2a, b). With the anti-ectodomain antibody, H108, three E-cadherin fragments in addition to full length E-cadherin were detected (Fig. 5.2a). With the anti-cytoplasmic antibody, 24E10, only E-cad/FL and the E-cad/NTF1 were detected, showing that E-cad/NTF2, E-cad/NTF3 and E-cad/NTF4 truncated before

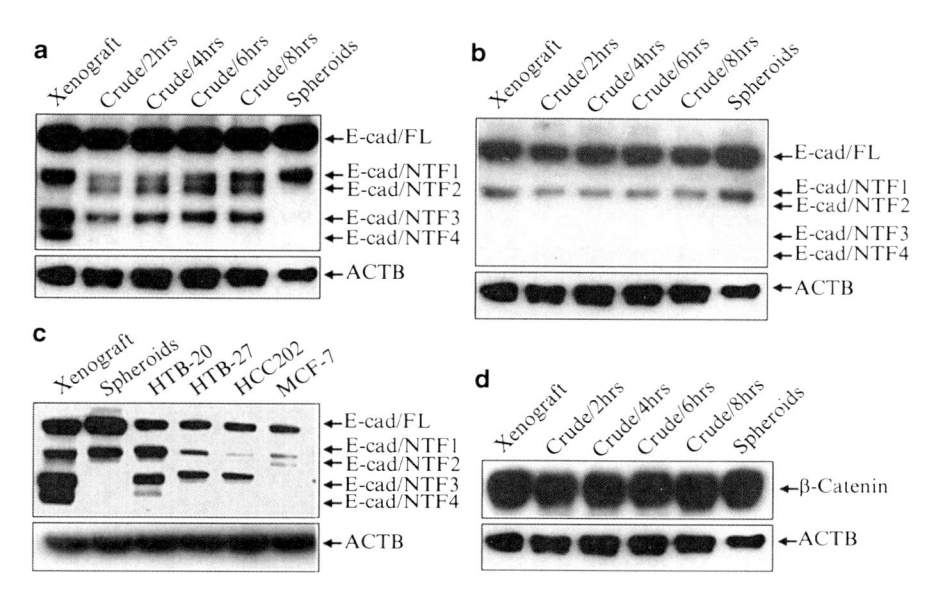

Fig. 5.2 MARY-X *in vitro* spheroidgenesis and E-cadherin proteolysis. (**a**) Western blot using anti-ectodomain E-cadherin antibody (H108) revealed full length E-cadherin (E-cad/FL), and a number of E-cadherin fragments (E-cad/NTF1-4), ranging in size from 100 kDa to 75 kDa. (**b**) Western blot using a second antibody, an anti-cytoplasmic domain further defined the domains contained within each of the fragments, recognizing E-cad/FL and E-cad/NTF1 but not recognizing E-cad/NTF2-4. (**c**) Western blot using H108 revealed the unique E-cadherin fragment pattern of MARY-X spheroids compared to both MARY-X as well as other human breast cancer cell lines. (**d**) Western blot using anti-β-catenin revealed no changes in β-catenin expression during MARY-X *in vitro* spheroidgenesis. ACTB served as housekeeping control for protein loading in all the western blots

residue 780 (Fig. 5.2b). The generation of the specific E-cadherin fragments was time dependent over the period of *in vitro* spheroidgenesis with both E-cad/FL and E-cad/NTF1 maximizing and E-cad/NTF2, E-cad/NTF3 and E-cad/NTF4 minimizing in the fully formed spheroids (Fig. 5.2a). Compared with other breast carcinoma cell lines, only MARY-X spontaneously formed spheroids and only the MARY-X spheroids exhibited the singular presence of E-cad/NTF1 and absence of E-cad/NTF2-4 (Fig. 5.2c). During MARY-X *in vitro* spheroidgenesis, Western blot revealed that β-catenin levels did not change (Fig. 5.2d).

5.5.3   The Unique Proteolytic Processing of E-cadherin During MARY-X In Vitro Spheroidgenesis Is Mediated by Specific Cellular Proteases

Experiments with different protease inhibitors suggested that the generation of each of the E-cadherin fragments was likely mediated by a specific intracellular protease.

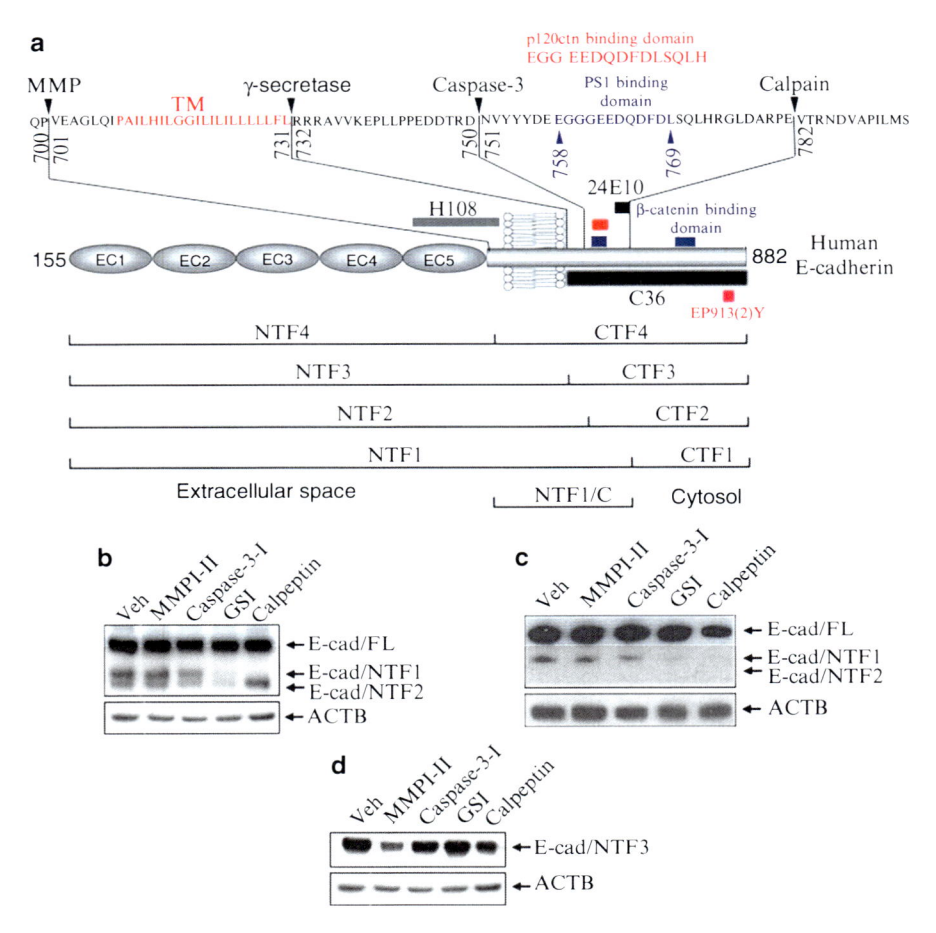

Fig. 5.3 Sites and enzymes involved in E-cadherin proteolysis. (**a**) Schematic adapted and modified by permission from Macmillan Publishers Ltd: The EMBO Journal 2002: 21: 1948–1956 of known protease cleavage domains on E-cadherin resulting in specific fragment generation and antibodies used to define these domains. EC1-5 denote the extracellular E-cadherin repeats, TM indicates transmembrane domains, H108, 24E10, C36 and EP913(2)Y (CDH1) are immunogenic regions recognized by the respective antibodies. PS1, p120ctn and β-catenin binding domains are also so indicated. (**b**) Western blot with H108 in protease inhibitor studies revealed that E-cad/NTF1 and E-cad/NTF2 were separately generated by different proteases, calpain and γ-secretase respectively. (**c**) Western blot with 24E10 confirmed the fidelity of the fragments in the same protease inhibitor studies. (**d**) Western blot with H108 revealed that E-cad/NTF3 was likely generated by matrix metalloproteinases. ACTB served as housekeeping control for protein loading in all the western blots

A map of E-cadherin depicts the cleavage sites and the different binding domains of E-cadherin in which the E-cadherin fragments generated can be reconciled with these protease inhibitor studies (Fig. 5.3a). Calpeptin, a calpain inhibitor, suppressed

E-cad/NTF1 whereas a γ-secretase inhibitor (GSI-I) suppressed E-cad/NTF2 (Fig. 5.3b) on Western blot studies using H108. GSI-I also suppressed E-cad/NTF1 (Fig. 5.3b) suggesting that this γ-secretase inhibitor also exhibited cross inhibition of calpain. Caspase-3 inhibitor III and matrix metalloproteinase inhibitor, MMP inhibitor II (MMPI-II), exerted no effects on the generation of either E-cad/NTF1 or E-cad/NTF2, suggesting that neither caspase 3 nor matrix metalloproteinases were proteolytically involved in the generation of these fragments. Western blot studies with 24E10 confirmed the identity of the E-cadherin fragments inhibited or not inhibited by the different protease inhibitors (Fig. 5.3c). MMPI-II, however, inhibited E-cad/NTF3 (Fig. 5.3d). Because E-cad/NTF4 was present only in MARY-X and remained absent during both early and late spheroidgenesis (Fig. 5.2a), its genesis in MARY-X could not be investigated with our *in vitro* protease inhibitor approaches.

5.5.4 *The Unique Proteolytic Processing of E-cadherin During MARY-X In Vitro Spheroidgenesis Is Further Supported by Correlative Levels of the Respective Proteases*

In late spheroidgenesis as compared to early spheroidgenesis, levels of calpain (both calpain I and calpain II) increased dramatically (Fig. 5.4a) whereas levels of γ-secretase activity decreased (Fig. 5.4b) and levels of caspase-3 activity also decreased (Fig. 5.4c). In the γ-secretase experiment the protein levels of the N-terminal fragment of presenilin-1 (PS1/NTF), the catalytic subunit of γ-secretase, which regulates γ-secretase cleavage of E-cadherin was used as a measurement of γ-secretase activity (Fig. 5.4b). In the caspase-3 experiment, levels of cleaved caspase-3 rather than full length caspase-3 was used as measurements of caspase-3 activity (Fig. 5.4c). The levels of calpain directly correlated with the levels of E-cad/NTF1 (Fig. 5.2a). The levels of both PS1/NTF and cleaved caspase-3 directly correlated with the levels of E-cad/NTF2 but by both its predicted size based on the cleavage map of E-cadherin (Fig. 5.3a) as well as its actual size on Western blot (Fig. 5.2a), E-cad/NTF2 was produced by γ-secretase and not caspase-3. Although E-cadherin contained a caspase-3 cleavage site, a specific E-cad/NT fragment corresponding to caspase-3 cleavage of E-cadherin could not be demonstrated during *in vitro* spheroidgenesis. In early and mid *in vitro* spheroidgenesis, both γ-secretase and caspase-3 increased (Fig. 5.4b, c) but within the fully formed MARY-X spheroids, the only protease which was dominant was calpain 1 and calpain 2 (Fig. 5.4a). In our initial gene expression profiling of MARY-X spheroids [6, 7], we found that only calpain 1 and calpain 2, among all other calpains, were increased in MARY-X spheroids compared to the other cell lines tested (data not shown). We also found that levels of calpastatin, the endogenous inhibitor of calpains was low in MARY-X spheroids (data not shown).

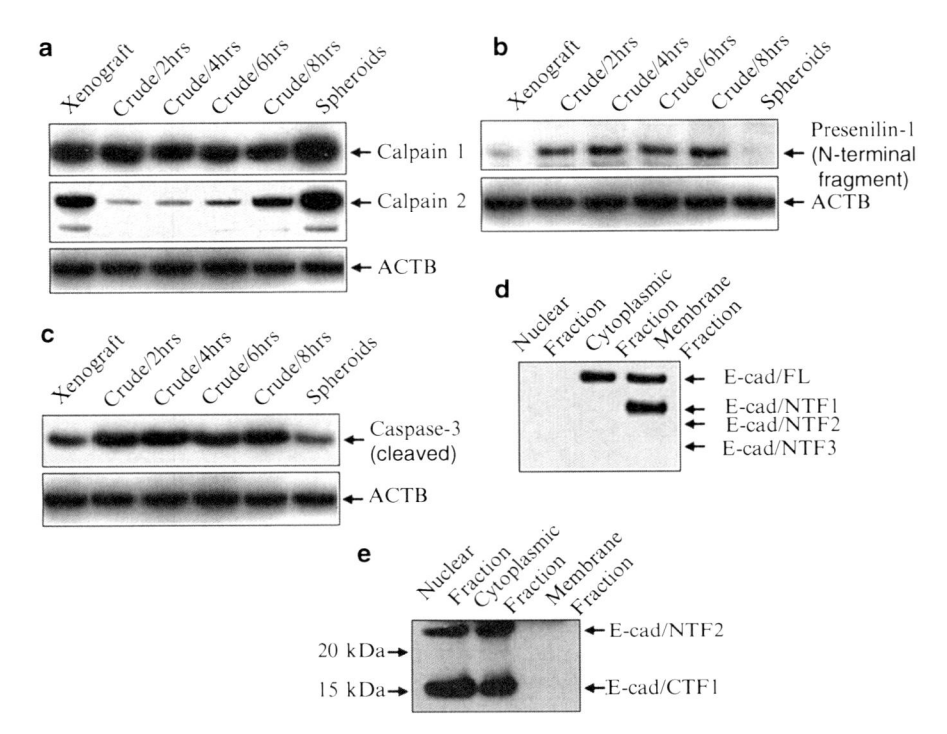

Fig. 5.4 Protease activities during MARY-X *in vitro* spheroidgenesis and localization of E-cad/NTF1-4 and E-cad/CTF1-4 in cellular subfractions. (**a**) Calpain 1 and calpain 2 both increased during spheroidgenesis peaking at the end point of well-formed spheroids. (**b**) γ-secretase (PS1/NTF) increased at early and mid spheroidgenesis then decreased at late spheroidgenesis. (**c**) Caspase-3 similarly increased at early and mid spheroidgenesis then decreased at late spheroidgenesis. ACTB served as housekeeping control for protein loading in all the western blots. (**d**) In late spheroidgenesis, western blot with H108 revealed that only E-cad/NTF1 localized to membrane. (**e**) In early to mid spheroidgenesis, western blot with C36 which recognized both E-cad/CTF1 as well as E-cad/CTF2 revealed that both E-cad/CTF1 and E-cad/CTF2 translocated to the nuclear fraction, suggesting the possibility that E-cad/CTF1 and/or E-cad/CTF2 may be transcription factors

5.5.5 E-cad/NTF1-3 and E-cad/CTF1-3 Differ in Their Subcellular Localization During In Vitro Spheroidgenesis

In late *in vitro* spheroidgenesis, E-cad/NTF1 is exclusively localized on the cellular membrane (Fig. 5.4d). According to the map of E-cadherin depicting the cleavage sites (Fig. 5.3a), E-cad/NTF1 retains the p120ctn binding site, but loses β- and α-catenin binding sites. In the membrane fraction, the amount of E-cad/NTF1 is greater than the amount of E-cad/FL although E-cad/FL is also present in the cytoplasmic fraction. Since the latter two molecules both contain the p120ctn binding site, which tether both molecules to the membrane, it follows that cytoplasmic E-cad/

FL is the likely source of membrane E-cad/FL, which, in turn is the likely source of E-cad/NTF1. Since in late spheroidgenesis, E-cad/NTF2 and E-cad/NTF3 are absent, none of these fragments was detected in any cellular subfraction (Fig. 5.4d). In early to mid spheroidgenesis, of the E-cad/CTF1-4 fragments, both E-cad/CTF1 as well as E-cad/CTF2 were present in the nuclear subfraction (Fig. 5.4e), raising the possibility that they were functioning as transcription factors.

5.5.6 Manipulation of the Levels of E-cad/NTF1 by Calpain Inhibition Both Induces Spheroid Disadherence and Prevents In Vitro Spheroidgenesis

Calpain inhibition with calpeptin on well-formed spheroids caused spheroid disadherence. Calpeptin blocked the production of E-cad/NTF1 without altering the levels of E-cad/FL in a dose dependent manner and a significant inhibition was obtained at 10–100 μM (Fig. 5.5a). Using 50 μM calpeptin in a time course experiment, its effects were noted at 2 h (Fig. 5.5b). Calpeptin also increased E-cad/NTF2 and E-cad/NTF3 over time (Fig. 5.5b). Calpeptin did not, however, alter the levels of calpain (data not shown). Calpeptin (50 μM) induced profound spheroid disadherence beginning at 6 h and peaking at 24 h (Fig. 5.5c). FITC-conjugated annexin V and propidium iodide (PI) was used to identify apoptosis (early and late) in the cells undergoing disadherence. At early disadherence at 6–8 h, no apoptosis could be detected but at 24 h, significant apoptosis which peaked at 48 h could be detected (Fig. 5.5d). Calpain inhibition with calpeptin (50 μM) fully inhibited MARY-X *in vitro* spheroidgenesis (Fig. 5.5e).

5.5.7 E-cad/NTF1 Contributes to In Vitro Spheroidgenesis and Increased Cellular Density

MARY-X spheroids form spontaneously and express only E-cad/FL and E-cad/NTF1 and not E-cad/NTF2-4 (Fig. 5.2a). Other human breast carcinoma cell lines (HTB20, HTB202, HTB27, MCF-7, MDA-MB-231, MDA-MB-468) do not spontaneously form spheroids but can be induced to form spheroids by growing them over soft agar. Induction of spheroidgenesis is uniformly accompanied by increased E-cad/NTF1 in all of the E-cadherin positive lines (Fig. 5.5f). Some of these lines, e.g. HTB20, like MARY-X spheroids, expressed sole E-cad/NTF1 whereas the other lines, e.g. MCF-7 also expressed E-cad/NTF2 and E-cad/NTF3 as well as E-cad/NTF1 (Fig. 5.5f). Both the density and compact appearance of the spheroids correlated with the E-cadherin fragment pattern. The presence of sole E-cad/NTF1 correlated with high density and compact rounded appearance whereas the co-presence of E-cad/NTF2 and E-cad/NTF3 with E-cad/NTF1 correlate with lower density and

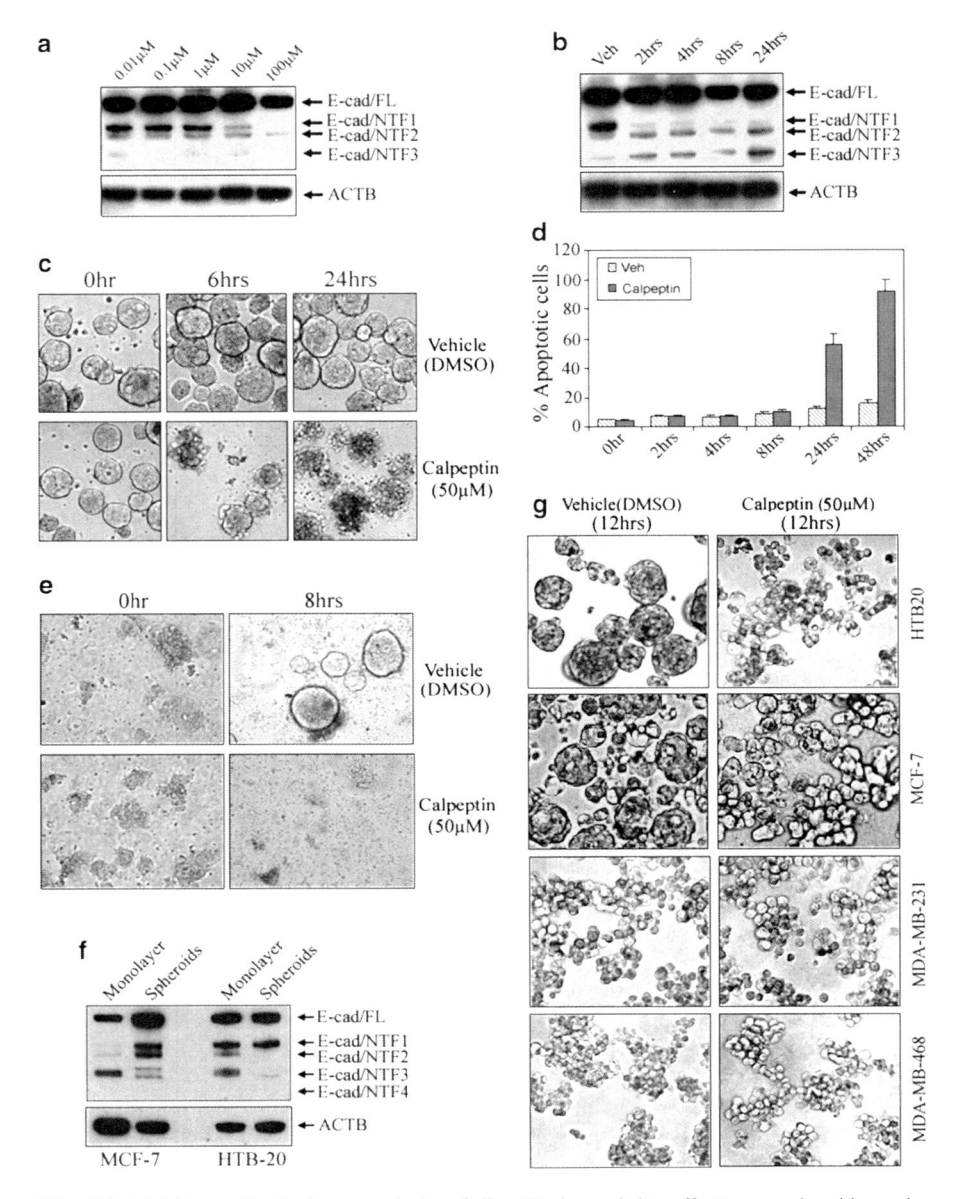

Fig. 5.5 Inhibition of calpain proteolysis of E-cadherin and its effects on spheroidgenesis. (**a**) MARY-X spheroids were treated with vehicle (DMSO) or with calpain inhibitor, calpeptin with the indicated concentrations for 2 h and there was a progressive inhibition of E-cad/NTF1 in a dose-dependent manner using H108 on Western blot. (**b**) MARY-X spheroids were treated with vehicle (DMSO) or calpeptin (50 μM) for the indicated times and there was a marked inhibition of E-cad/NTF1 as early as 2 h and an increase in E-cad/NTF2 and E-cad/NTF3 over time using H108 on Western blot. (**c**) MARY-X spheroids were treated with calpeptin (50 μM) for the indicated times and marked disadherence began at 6 h and was nearly complete by 24 h. (**d**) Total (early and late) apoptosis by staining with FITC-conjugated annexin V and propidium iodide (*PI*) is depicted as % apoptosis over 48 h with vehicle (DMSO) or calpeptin (50 μM). (**e**) Crude MARY-X aggregates were treated with vehicle (DMSO) or calpeptin (50 μM) for 8 h. Calpeptin prevented the formation of spheroids. (**f**) Presence of sole E-cad/NTF1 *v* E-cad/NTF1-4 in different cell lines with induction of spheroidgenesis determined whether calpeptin (50 μM) for 12 h caused complete *v* incomplete spheroid disadherence (**g**). ACTB served as housekeeping control for protein loading in all the western blots

loose irregular appearances (Fig. 5.5g). Treating these different aggregates with calpeptin (50 μM) for 12 h dramatically decreased E-cad/NTF1 when present and caused aggregate disadherence (Fig. 5.5g). The degree of disadherence (complete v incomplete) induced by calpeptin was a function of whether sole E-cad/NTF1 or E-cad/NTF1-3 were present. For example with the MARY-X spheroids and the HTB20, disadherence was complete; with MCF-7 disadherence was incomplete. The E-cadherin negative lines could also be induced to form spheroid-like aggregates but these exhibited very low density and were irregular in appearance (Fig. 5.5g). These latter lines, being E-cadherin negative, had no E-cad/NTF1. Treating these aggregates with calpeptin (50 μM) did not induce disadherence (Fig. 5.5g).

5.5.8 The Stability of In Vitro Spheroidgenesis Is Dependent on Ca²⁺

Ca^{2+}-depletion led to spheroid disadherence and this disadherence correlated with both a decrease of E-cad/NTF1 as well as E-cad/FL but the effects on E-cad/NTF1 were more dramatic as demonstrated with anti-E-cadherin antibody, H108 (Fig. 5.6a). Within 10 min E-cad/NTF1 decreased and nearly completely disappeared by 60 min (Fig. 5.6a). The media accompanying the disadhered spheroids showed an increase of E-cad/NTF3 over this same time period (Fig. 5.6b). This latter result indicated that Ca^{2+}-depletion increased the MMP product, E-cad/NTF3. Using anti-E-cadherin antibody, 24E10, that recognized the sequence surrounding residue 780 of human E-cadherin, identified a 35 kDa fragment, E-cad/CTF3 (Fig. 5.6c) as well as a 12 kDa fragment, E-cad/NTF1/C (Fig. 5.6d) in the cellular extracts from well-formed spheroids. E-cad/CTF3 and E-cad/NTF1/C were derived from the cleavages of E-cad/FL and E-cad/NTF1 respectively by MMP. Ca^{2+}-depletion also decreased calpain levels over a similar time course (Fig. 5.6e). Although previously it had been demonstrated that Ca^{2+}-depletion disrupted the extracellular E-cadherin antiparallel homodimers in EC1-5which contributed to MARY-X spheroid disadherence, the effects of Ca^{2+}-depletion were more pleiotropic: Ca^{2+}-depletion resulted in MMP-mediated cleavage of E-cad/NTF1 and E-cad/FL (Fig. 5.6a–d) with cleavage of E-cad/NTF1 being more immediate and more dramatic. This MMP-mediated cleavage of E-cad/NTF1 and E-cad/FL also contributed to spheroid disadherence.

5.5.9 In Vitro Spheroidgenesis Manifests Increased p120ctn, Bound E-cad/NTF1 and eIF4GI

The increases in E-cad/FL and E-cad/NTF1 which characterized in vitro spheroidgenesis (Fig. 5.2a, b) were accompanied by concomitant increased p120ctn (Fig. 5.7a), increased E-cadherin fragments associated with p120ctn (Fig. 5.7b) and increased eIF4GI (Fig. 5.7c). This suggested that eIF4GI, p120ctn, E-cad/FL and E-cad/NTF1

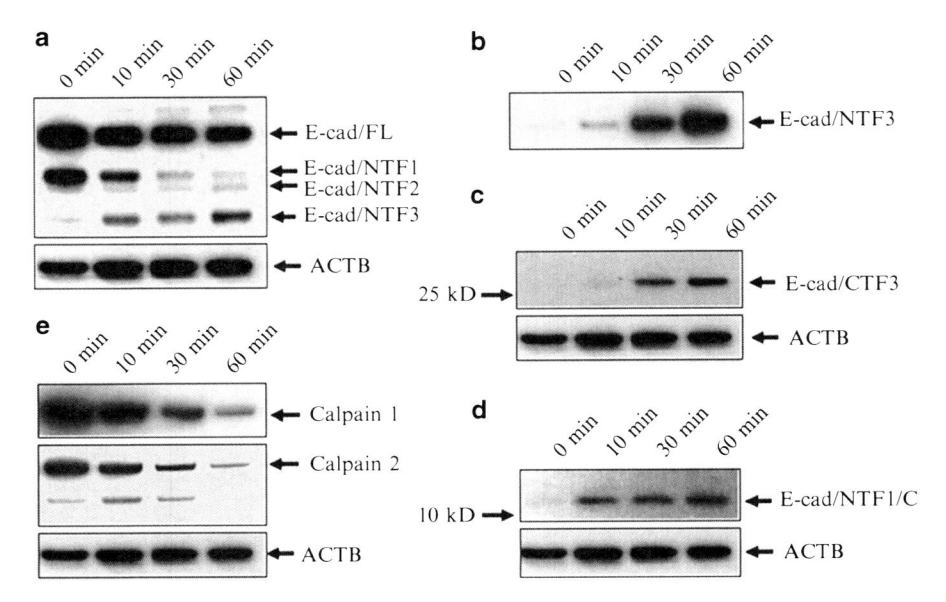

Fig. 5.6 Effects of Ca^{2+} depletion on E-cadherin proteolysis. (**a**) MARY-X spheroids were incubated in Ca^{2+}-free medium S-MEM. (**a**) Cell samples and medium samples were collected for the indicated times and studied by Western blot with H108, showing that Ca^{2+}-depletion resulted in a time-dependent decrease in E-cad/NTF1 in cells. (**b**) Analysis of cell medium revealed a time-dependent increase in E-cad/NTF3. (**c**) Western blot using 24E10 showed that E-cad/CTF3, the C-terminal fragment of E-cadherin resulting from MMP cleavage, correspondingly increased in cells with Ca^{2+}-depletion over time. (**d**) E-cad/NTF1/C, the C-terminal fragment of E-cad/NTF1 from MMP cleavage, also increased, but this increase was not as time-dependent. (**e**) Ca^{2+}-depletion resulted in a time-dependent decrease of both calpain 1 and calpain 2 in MARY-X spheroids. ACTB served as housekeeping control for protein loading in all the western blots

were working synergistically to contribute to the super adhesion state of the well-formed MARY-X spheroids. Interestingly p120ctn immunoprecipitation experiments of the well-formed spheroids showed that there was a relative increase in E-cad/NTF1 compared to E-cad/FL which was bound to p120ctn (Fig. 5.7b).

5.5.10 In Vitro Spheroidgenesis and In Vivo Emboli Formation Manifests a Unique and Enhanced Non-CAJ Membrane Distribution of E-cad/NTF1

Confocal microscopy with double and triple labeled immunofluorescence studies revealed a unique membrane distribution of E-cad/NTF1 in the native MARY-X spheroids and native MARY-X lymphovascular emboli (Fig. 5.8). In the MARY-X spheroids, green fluorochrome-conjugated 24E10 which recognized both E-cad/

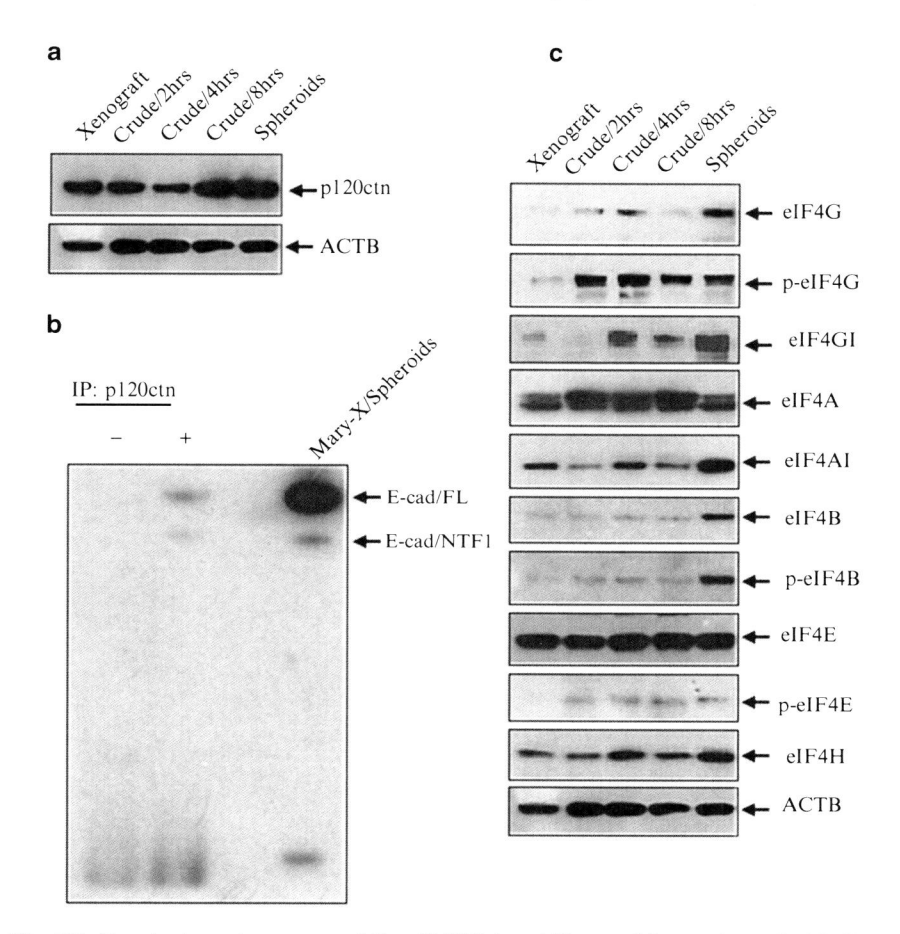

Fig. 5.7 Constitutive enhancement of E-cad/NTF1 by p120ctn and its regulators in MARY-X spheroids. (**a**) MARY-X well-formed spheroids express increased levels of p120ctn compared to its crude aggregate stages and MARY-X on Western blot using anti-p120ctn. (**b**) Immunoprecipitation of p120ctn in the well-formed MARY-X spheroids revealed a relative increase in E-cad/NTF1 compared to E-cad/FL bound to p120ctn. The C36 E-cadherin antibody was used in the Western blot following immunoprecipitation. (**c**) A study of a family of translational initiation factors, both phosphorylated and non-phosphorylated, revealed high and differential expression of eIF4GI in MARY-X spheroids compared to its crude aggregate stages and MARY-X. ACTB served as house-keeping control for protein loading in all the western blots

NTF1 and E-cad/FL compared with red fluorochrome-conjugated EP913(2)Y (CDH1) which recognized only E-cad/FL revealed a green spectral shift indicative of both the presence as well as the prominence of E-cad/NTF1 in the native (untreated) MARY-X spheroids compared to the spheroids treated with calpeptin (Fig. 5.8a). Calpeptin inhibits E-cad/NTF1 and so this green spectral shift due to E-cad/NTF1 would be abolished in the treated group. Similarly double labeled experiments using 24E10 compared with anti-β-catenin; and EP913(2)Y (CDH1)

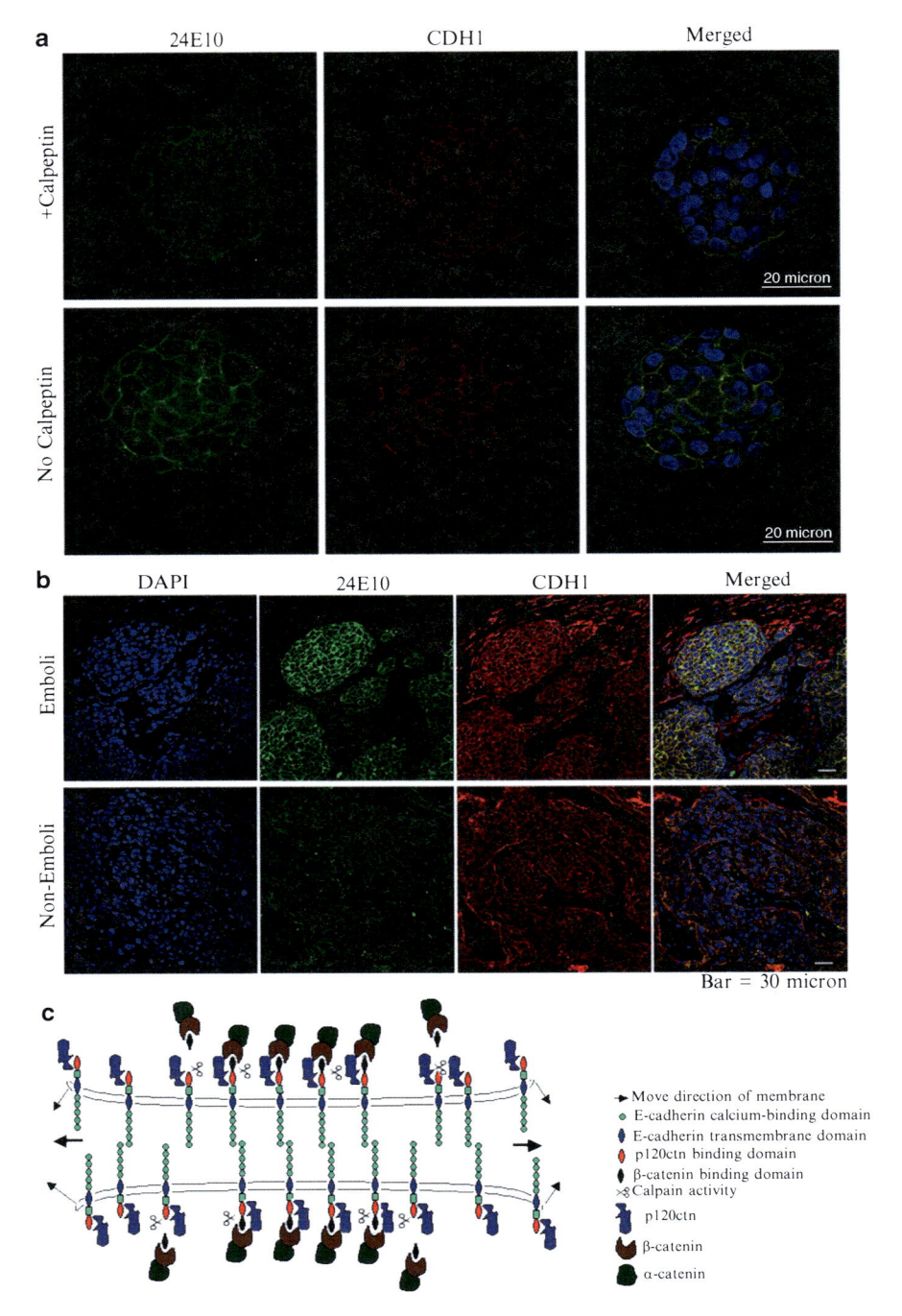

Fig. 5.8 Double and triple labeled immunofluorescence in both the MARY-X spheroids as well as the MARY-X lymphovascular emboli. (**a**) Green fluorochrome-conjugated 24E10 which recognized both E-cad/NTF1 and E-cad/FL illustrated more intense green signals in the absence of calpeptin (which inhibited E-cad/NTF1). Red fluorochrome-conjugated EP913(2)Y (CDH1)

compared with anti-β-catenin revealed a green spectral shift in only the 24E10/β-catenin comparisons and not the EP913(2)Y (CDH1)/β-catenin comparisons in the native (untreated) *v* calpeptin treated groups (data not shown). In the MARY-X lymphovascular emboli, a similar green spectral shift with triple labeled 24E10, EP913(2)Y (CDH1) and anti-murine podoplanin was observed in the lymphovascular emboli of MARY-X compared with the non-embolic areas (Fig. 5.8b). Similar triple labeled experiments using 24E10 compared with anti-β-catenin and EP913(2)Y (CDH1) compared with anti-β-catenin revealed a spectral shift in only the 24E10/β-catenin comparisons and not the EP913(2)Y (CDH1)/β-catenin comparisons in the lymphovascular emboli *v* non-embolic areas (data not shown). A schematic depicts the hypothesis that we are advancing in this study: that calpain-mediated cleavage of E-cadherin generates E-cad/NTF1 which is bound to p120ctn but not to α-, β-catenin and the actin cytoskeleton (Fig. 5.8c). E-cad/NTF1 therefore is not tethered to traditional CAJs and can redistribute itself along adjacent non-CAJ areas of the membrane.

5.6   Discussion of the Studies

In vitro models of tumor progression have shed mechanistic light on *in vivo* processes. Tumor invasion, for example, has been studied by using the Matrigel invasion chamber [9] or the chick allantoic membrane (CAM) [10]. Tumor angiogenesis has been studied using a modified Boyden chamber [11] and cellular transformation has been studied in monolayer culture [12]. To date there has not been an *in vitro* model of tumor emboli formation, despite the importance of this step of tumor progression. MARY-X *in vitro* spheroidgenesis sheds light on the *in vivo* step of tumor emboli formation.

Fig. 5.8 (continued) which recognized only E-cad/FL illustrated similar signals in both the presence and absence of calpeptin. The composite image (merged) revealed a green spectral shift indicative of both the presence as well as the prominence of E-cad/NTF1 in the native (untreated) MARY-X spheroids. (**b**) Green fluorochrome-conjugated 24E10 which recognized both E-cad/NTF1 and E-cad/FL illustrated more intense green signals in the lymphovascular emboli of MARY-X compared with the non-embolic areas. Red fluorochrome-conjugated EP913(2)Y (CDH1) which recognized only E-cad/FL illustrated similar signals in both the emboli as well as the non-embolic areas. The composite image (merged) superimposed on red-fluorchrome-conjugated anti-murine podoplanin which recognized lymphatic channels revealed a green spectral shift in the lymphovascular emboli indicative of both the presence as well as the prominence of E-cad/NTF1. (**c**) A schematic depicts the calpain-mediated cleavage of E-cadherin generating E-cad/NTF1 bound to p120ctn but not to β- or α-catenin nor the actin cytoskeleton. Therefore while E-cad/FL is tethered to the membrane in traditional CAJs, E-cad/NTF1 can redistribute itself along adjacent non-CAJ areas of the membrane contributing to more circumferential distribution and increased adhesion. DAPI was used as a blue nuclear counterstain in all experiments

It must be emphasized that most studies investigating a mechanism operating in humans employ at least several cell lines to control for possible idiosyncrasies and limitations inherent in a single cell line. In this study although there were other human IBC lines available including the SUM-149 and SUM-190 [13], these latter cell lines do not spontaneously form spheroids or exhibit lymphovascular emboli in mice. Therefore we could not use these other cell lines to study those molecules responsible for the phenotype they lack.

Our previous studies had demonstrated that E-cadherin is a key molecule involved in the generation of the lymphovascular embolus [5–7] and that E-cadherin is over-expressed not because of increased transcription but because of altered trafficking [8]. MARY-X spheroids have three unique features acting in tandem that distinguish them from MARY-X and the early and mid stages of MARY-X spheroidgenesis: (1) overexpressed E-cadherin; (2) high level of E-cad/NTF1 that is the cleavage product of E-cad/FL by calpains and (3) absent levels of E-cad/NTF2, E-cad/NTF3 and E-cad/NTF4.

The first unique feature of the MARY-X spheroids is their overexpression of E-cadherin. In normal epithelial cells, E-cadherin is located within the zona adherens, the lateral junctions between cells. In carcinomas which express E-cadherin, E-cadherin is located within cadherin-associated junctions (CAJs) which are found distributed 360° around the cell. E-cadherin normally is trafficked to and from the cell surface by multiple exocytic and endocytic pathways [14, 15]. However in a recent study [8] we have found that normal E-cadherin trafficking was altered within the MARY-X spheroids. We found Exoc5 to be upregulated and Hgs and Rab7 to be downregulated in the MARY-X spheroids. ExoC5 (Sec10 in *Drosophila*) is thought to jointly regulate trafficking of E-cadherin to the epithelial cell surface through interaction with ExoC6 (Sec15 in *Drosophila*), Exoc2 (Sec5 in *Drosophila*), GTP-bound Rab11 and β-catenin [15–18]. Therefore the increase of ExoC5 in MARY-X spheroids contributes to E-cadherin trafficking to the membrane. Hgs or Hrs, one of the master regulators that direct activated receptors toward lysosomes, has been shown to play an important role in the lysosomal targeting of E-cadherin [19]. Hgs contains an ubiquitin-interacting motif and is involved in the endosomal sorting of ubiquitinated membrane proteins, such as growth factor receptors and E-cadherin [20–22]. Ubiquitinated E-cadherin would normally be trafficked to the lysosome for degradation [19]. Hgs depletion has been associated with the up-regulation of E-cadherin and reduced β-catenin signaling [23]. The increased accumulation of E-cadherin observed in MARY-X spheroids and the lymphovascular tumor emboli most likely results from impaired E-cadherin degradation in lysosomes mediated, in part, by decreased Hgs. Rab7 is also thought to regulate E-cadherin trafficking from the cell surface to lysosomes and reduced Rab7 would be expected to decrease lyso-somal degradation [19, 24–26]. Rab7 functions in the endocytic pathway of mammalian cells by specifically regulating traffic from early to late endosomes. Interfering with Rab7 function inhibits this transport step, thereby blocking traffic from the cell surface to lysosomes and preventing lysosomal degradation [25, 26]. The increased accumulation of E-cadherin observed in MARY-X spheroids from impaired E-cadherin degradation in lysosomes most likely is also mediated by decreased Rab7.

The second unique feature of the MARY-X spheroids is the high level of E-cad/NTF1, the cleavage product of E-cad/FL by calpains. This second feature is dependent on the first feature because without a sufficient substrate for calpains, no E-cad/NTF1 could be produced. This second feature is also dependent on high levels of calpains. Calpains, a family of calcium-dependent thiol-proteases that proteolyze a wide variety of cytoskeletal, membrane-associated, and regulatory proteins, have previously been implicated as a regulator of the actin cytoskeleton and cell migration [27–32]. Inhibition of calpain reduces cell migration rates and invasiveness in some lines. Two major isoforms of calpain have been reported in mammals, calpain 1 (Mu-type) and calpain 2 (M-type). They differ in their calcium requirements for activation (~50 μM for calpain 1 and ~500 μM for calpain 2) and contain several calcium-binding sites [29]. Like other proteolytic cleavages of cytoskeletal E-cadherin mediated by matrix metalloproteinase (MMP), or caspase-3 or γ-secretase, the cleavage of cytoskeletal E-cadherin mediated by calpains cleaves the extracellular molecule away from the intracellular molecule and might be predicted to favor disadherence. However calpain cleavage produces a molecule (E-cad/NTF1) that retains the p120ctn binding domain and, in fact, is bound to p120ctn in immunoprecipitation studies.

The third unique feature of the MARY-X spheroids is absent levels of E-cad/NTF2, E-cad/NTF3 and E-cad/NTF4. This feature is accompanied by low levels of γ-secretase, caspase-3 and matrix metalloproteinase activities in the spheroids. This third feature operates synergistically with the first and second features in promoting adherence rather than disadherence. Certainly the disassembly of CAJs resulting from the proteolysis of E-cadherin from γ-secretase, caspase-3 or MMP [33–38] would be expected to disrupt cell-cell adhesion. Furthermore E-cad/NTF2, E-cad/NTF3 and E-cad/NTF4 each would lack the p120ctn binding domain and would not be tethered to the membrane yet would possess the extracellular domains able to form antiparallel homodimers with other E-cad/FL or E-cad/NTF1 molecules. E-cad/NTF2, E-cad/NTF3 and E-cad/NTF4 may well then be functioning in a dominant negative manner and compete against the adhesion effects of both E-cad/FL as well as E-cad/NTF1. Absent levels of E-cad/NTF2, E-cad/NTF3 and E-cad/NTF4 then would also favor adhesion. The low levels of the proteases that generate these fragments would also support adhesion because these proteases, if present, could cleave not only E-cad/FL but also E-cad/NTF1 which would cause disadherence. The first feature, overexpression of E-cadherin, contributes to the second feature, high levels of E-cad/NTF1 from high calpain activity. Similarly, the third feature, absent levels of E-cad/NTF2, E-cad/NTF3 and E-cad/NTF4 from low γ-secretase, caspase-3 and matrix metalloproteinase activities, also supports the second feature, high levels of E-cad/NTF1 from high calpain activity. All three features cause the spheroids of MARY-X and their *in vivo* counterpart of lymphovascular emboli to exhibit greater adhesion and greater cell density that that exhibited by any other cell line.

It must be remembered that E-cadherin is part of a macromolecular complex whose adhesive functions are not solely determined by the levels of E-cadherin and its fragments. In recent studies the levels of adhesion through E-cadherin were mediated by the levels of p120ctn [39, 40]. In other studies p120ctn kept E-cadherin confined to the membrane and retarded its endocytosis that led to its degradation [14, 41–43]. Furthermore, the knockdown of p120ctn using siRNAs reduced the levels of cadherin expression and cell adhesion [42]. The reconstitution of p120ctn in p120ctn-mutant cell lines restored both E-cadherin levels and cell–cell adhesion [44]. In MARY-X *in vitro* spheroidgenesis, p120ctn gradually increased and reached peak levels in the well-formed spheroids. P120ctn would promote adhesion because both E-cad/FL and E-cad/NTF1 contain p120ctn binding domains and p120ctn would be expected to retain both of these molecules in the membrane. The levels of p120ctn, in turn, are thought to be regulated by translation initiation factors, especially eIF4GI which target mRNAs with internal ribosome entry sites (IRESs) for increased translation [39, 40]. Increased eIF4GI directly increased p120ctn which, in turn, indirectly increased E-cadherin and adhesion. In MARY-X spheroids we observed high levels of eIF4GI. High levels of eIF4GI have also been observed in other IBC lines [39, 40]. Increased eIF4GI in MARY-X spheroids would also be expected to increase the presentation of E-cad/NTF1 on the membrane since it would directly increase p120ctn and increased p120ctn would enhance the presentations of E-cad/FL and E-cad/NTF1 on the membrane. Increased eIF4GI, increased p120ctn, increased E-cad/FL and increased E-cad/NTF1 all contribute to the unique superadhesion and super densities of MARY-X spheroids.

It must be also remembered that E-cadherin is part of a macromolecular complex whose functions are not solely limited to adhesion. It has been known for many years that β-catenin, normally part of the E-cadherin membrane complex, when present in excess or not properly phosphorylated by glycogen synthase kinase-3β, can translocate to the nucleus to become part of a heterodimeric transcription factor [45]. Each of the E-cadherin cleavage fragments produced during MARY-X *in vitro* spheroidgenesis have a NTF fragment and a corresponding CTF fragment. The E-cad/CTF2-4 fragments contain both p120ctn as well as β-catenin binding domains. The E-cad/CTF1 fragment lacks a p120ctn binding domain but contains the α,β-catenin binding domains. Any of these fragments when present in excess could escape tethering to the corresponding membrane catenin protein and be free to translocate to the nucleus and function as a transcription factor. We found evidence in the present study that both E-cad/CTF1 and E-cad/CTF2 translocate to the nucleus. Previously it had been reported that in HEK293 cells, E-cad/CTF2 regulated the p120-Kaiso-mediated signaling pathway in the nucleus [46].

It must also be remembered that E-cadherin is part of a macromolecular complex, termed cadherin-associated junctions (CAJs), whose main function is adhesion but whose assembly or disassembly is not solely determined by E-cadherin or its catenin partners. Calcium, for example, is an important regulator of CAJs. CAJs are thought to be the main mediators of Ca^{2+}-dependent cell-cell adhesion that is accomplished by homophilic protein-protein interactions between two cadherin molecules on the cell surface. Low concentration of Ca^{2+} or Ca^{2+} depletion led to

MARY-X spheroid disadherence. This disadherence has been thought to be the result of the disruption of Ca^{2+}-dependent homophilic interactions [47, 48]. Based on our data, however, we suggest that Ca^{2+} depletion causes spheroid disadherence through additional equally important mechanisms. Ca^{2+}-depletion leads to rapid inhibition of both calpain expression and activity. Ca^{2+}-depletion furthermore causes the cleavage of E-cadherin not by calpain but by other proteases including γ-secretase and MMP that lead to the rapid proteolysis of both E-cad/FL and E-cad/NTF1. All these effects were noted within minutes and could not possibly have been mediated at the level of transcription or translation. Ca^{2+}-depletion is known to be chaotropic [5–7] and we suggest that Ca^{2+}-depletion through chaotropic mechanisms induces spheroid disadherence by inactivating calpain and facilitating cleavages of E-cad/NTF1 and E-cad/FL by non-calpain mediated proteolysis. What the experiments of Ca^{2+}-depletion do not resolve is whether non-calpain mediated proteolysis is actually inhibited by calpain or directly stimulated by Ca^{2+}-depletion.

Our experiments with calpeptin, however, directly addressed this issue. Calpeptin inhibited the production of E-cad/NTF1 but stimulated the production of E-cad/NTF2 and E-cad/NTF3. By inference, calpain inhibition directly increased γ-secretase and MMP activities. Two possible mechanisms for this effect were suggested: One mechanism was stearic hindrance. The cleavage site on E-cadherin for calpain is at amino acid residue residues 782–787 [31], just 13 amino acid residues away from the PS1 binding of γ-secretase which is required for γ-secretase activity at amino acid residues 758–769. In early and mid MARY-X *in vitro* spheroidgenesis, where calpain levels are considerably lower, increased E-cad/NTF2, the product of γ-secretase is present. In late spheroidgenesis, increased calpains stearically interfere with γ-secretase (PS1/NTF) cleavage. and increased caspase-3 are present but there is no caspase-3 cleavage product. A second mechanism is direct calpain action on γ-secretase and MMP. Calpains are known to hydrophobically associate with plasma membranes in the presence of Ca^{2+} and cleave plasma membrane substrates [49, 50]. One membrane target is E-cadherin but other possible targets are membrane-associated proteases. Both γ-secretase and MMP exist in membrane-bound forms [51, 52] and calpain could cleave these proteases and inactivate them. The actions of calpain 1 and calpain 2 in supporting MARY-X spheroid super adherence and high density may not be limited to E-cadherin cleavage and generation of E-cad/NTF1 alone. This expansion of the actions of calpains directly address the question of why calpeptin causes disadherence while E-cad/FL is still present. Surely if the actions of calpeptin were solely limited to the inhibition of E-cad/NTF1 by calpain, then one might predict that the spheroids might loosen into less adherent structures like is observed in MCF-7 but not undergo full disadherence. Full disadherence suggests that calpeptin is inhibiting some other actions of calpain responsible for the superadhesion state uniquely exhibited by the spheroids of MARY-X.

The other E-cadherin fragments (E-cad/NTF2-4) do not contain the p120ctn binding site and do not localize to the membrane and would not be expected to contribute to adhesion between cells. In fact, as mentioned previously, they may exert "dominant negative" effects by competing for antiparallel homodimeric EC1-5 sites on adjacent E-cadherin molecules on neighboring cells. Remember that during MARY-X *in vitro* spheroidgenesis, only the end stage spheroids express high levels of E-cad/NTF1 and absent levels of E-cad/NTF2-4. Hence only the MARY-X spheroids are in a state of super-adhesion.

While the assembly of traditional CAJs generally favors adhesion and the disassembly generally favors non-adhesion, the disassembly of CAJs could under alternate circumstances paradoxically favor adhesion and this may be the case with the MARY-X spheroids and lymphovascular emboli *in vivo*. Calpain cleavage clearly disassembles the CAJ because calpain cleaves E-cadherin which is bound to the catenins and the underlying actin cytoskeleton. But calpain cleavage also generates E-cad/NTF1 which retains the p120ctn binding site and binds p120ctn. P120ctn, although localized to the membrane is not bound to β- and α- catenins nor the actin cytoskeleton and is therefore not tethered to CAJs. E-cad/NTF1 is a smaller molecule than E-cad/FL and is able to successfully compete with E-cad/FL for binding sites on p120ctn. This is why our p120ctn immunoprecipitation experiments showed enrichment of E-cad/NTF1. E-cad/NTF1, not being tethered to β- and α- catenins and the actin cytoskeleton, is also free to move out of the CAJs and distribute in non-CAJ p120ctn areas. Our immunofluorescent data in both the spheroids as well as lymphovascular emboli of MARY-X confirm that not only is E-cad/NTF1 present but plays a very prominent role in both spheroidgenesis as well as in the formation of the lymphovascular embolus. The migration of E-cad/NTF1 out of CAJs could contribute to the phenomenon of budding spheroidgenesis and budding emboli formation from pre-existing emboli (unpublished observations).

5.7 Conclusions

To achieve better therapies that result in an ultimate cure of IBC, we must target the lymphovascular embolus with embolus disadhering strategies that directly destroy the tumor cells and that make our chemotherapy and radiotherapy more effective. It is our hope that in the not too distant future, insights that we gain studying models of IBC can be translated into newer therapeutic approaches that can increase the number of long term survivors of IBC who can then join the advocacy ranks of women and baby boomers against this disease.

Acknowledgements We thank Dr. John J. Hasenau, Dr. Walter F. Mandeville, Patricia L. Atkins and Jared H. Smith of Laboratory Animal Medicine for their veterinarian and technical assistance with the maintenance of the MARY-X xenografts. This work was supported by the Department of Defense Breast Cancer Research Program Grants BC990959, BC024258, BC053405, the American Airlines-Susan G Komen for the Cure Promise Grant KG081287-02 and the University of Nevada Vasco A. Salvadorini Endowment.

Disclosure of Potential Conflicts of Interest

No potential conflicts of interest were disclosed.

References

1. Barsky SH (2006) Inflammatory breast cancer: Few survivors, fewer baby boomer advocates. Oncologistic 3:26–33
2. Berx G, Van Roy F (2001) The E-cadherin/catenin complex: an important gatekeeper in breast cancer tumorigenesis and malignant progression. Breast Cancer Res 3:289–293
3. Hajra KM, Chen DYS, Fearon ER (2002) The slug zinc-finger protein suppresses E-cadherin in breast cancer. Cancer Res 62:1613–1618
4. Lombaerts M, van Wezel T, Philippo K, Dierssen JWF, Zimmerman RME, Oosting J, van Eijk R, Eilers PH, van de Water B, Cornelisse CJ et al (2006) E-cadherin transcriptional down-regulation by promoter methylation but not mutation is related to epithelial-to mesenchymal transition in breast cancer cell lines. Br J Cancer 94:661–671
5. Tomlinson JS, Alpaugh ML, Barsky SH (2001) An intact overexpressed E-cadherin/α, β-catenin axis characterizes the lymphovascular emboli of inflammatory breast carcinoma. Cancer Res 61:5231–5241
6. Xiao Y, Ye Y, Yearsley K, Jones S, Barsky SH (2008) The lymphovascular embolus of inflammatory breast cancer expresses a stem cell-like phenotype. Am J Pathol 173:561–574
7. Xiao Y, Ye Y, Zou X, Jones S, Yearsley K, Shetuni B, Tellez J, Barsky SH (2010) The lymphovascular embolus of inflammatory breast cancer exhibits a notch 3 addiction. Oncogene 30:287–300, Epub ahead of print 20 January 2011
8. Ye Y, Tellez JD, Durazo M, Belcher M, Yearsley K, Barsky SH (2010) E-cadherin accumulation within the lymphovascular embolus of inflammatory breast cancer is due to altered trafficking. Anticancer Res 10:3903–3910
9. Albini A, Noonan DM (2010) The 'chemoinvasion' assay, 25 years and still going strong: the use of reconstituted basement membranes to study cell invasion and angiogenesis. Curr Opin Cell Biol 22:677–689
10. Quigley JP, Armstrong PB (1998) Tumor cell intravasation alu-cidated: the chick embryo opens the window. Cell 94:281–284
11. Nguyen M, Strubel NA, Bischoff J (1993) A role for sialyl Lewis-X/a glycoconjugates in capillary morphogenesis. Nature 365:267–269
12. Shih C, Weinberg RA (1982) Isolation of a transforming sequence from a human bladder carcinoma cell line. Cell 29:161–169
13. Robertson FM, Ogasawara MA, Ye Z, Chu K, Pickei R, Debeb BG, Woodward WA, Hittelman WN, Cristofanilli M, Barsky SH (2010) Imaging and analysis of 3D tumor spheroids enriched for a cancer stem cell phenotype. J Biomol Screen 15:820–829
14. Bryant D, Stow JL (2004) The ins and outs of E-cadherin trafficking. Trends Cell Biol 14:427–434
15. van IJzendoorn SC (2006) Recycling endosomes. J Cell Sci 119:1679–1681
16. Beronja S, Laprise P, Papoulas O, Pellikka M, Sisson J, Tepass U (2005) Essential function of *Drosophila* Sec6 in apical exocytosis of epithelial photoreceptor cells. J Cell Biol 169:635–646
17. Langevin J, Morgan MJ, Sibarita JB, Aresta S, Murthy M, Schwarz T, Camonis J, Bellaïche Y (2005) *Drosophila* exocyst components Sec5, Sec6, and Sec15 regulate DE-cadherin trafficking from recycling endosomes to the plasma membrane. Dev Cell 9:365–376
18. Zhang XM, Ellis S, Sriratana A, Mitchell CA, Rowe T (2004) Sec15 is an effector for the Rab11 GTPase in mammalian cells. J Biol Chem 279:43027–43034
19. Palacios F, Tushir JS, Fujita Y, D'Souza-Schorey C (2005) Lysosomal targeting of E-cadherin: a unique mechanism for the down-regulation of cell-cell adhesion during epithelial to mesenchymal transitions. Mol Cell Biol 25:389–402
20. Hammond DE, Carter S, McCullough J, Urbé S, Vande Woude G, Clague MJ (2003) Endosomal dynamics of Met determine signaling output. Mol Biol Cell 14:1346–1354
21. Kanazawa C, Morita E, Yamada M, Ishii N, Miura S, Asao H, Yoshimori T, Sugamura K (2003) Effects of deficiencies of STAMs and Hrs, mammalian class E Vps proteins, on receptor downregulation. Biochem Biophys Res Commun 309:848–856

22. Le Roy C, Wrana JL (2005) Clathrin- and non-clathrin-mediated endocytic regulation of cell signalling. Nat Rev Mol Cell Biol 6:112–126
23. Toyoshima M, Tanaka N, Aoki J, Tanaka Y, Murata K, Kyuuma M, Kobayashi H, Ishii N, Yaegashi N, Sugamura K (2007) Inhibition of tumor growth and metastasis by depletion of vesicular sorting protein hrs: its regulatory role on E-cadherin and β-catenin. Cancer Res 67:5162–5171
24. Edinger AL, Cinalli RM, Thompson CB (2003) Rab7 prevents growth factor-independent survival by inhibiting cell-autonomous nutrient transporter expression. Dev Cell 5:571–582
25. Feng Y, Press B, Wandinger-Ness A (1995) Rab 7: an important regulator of late endocytic membrane traffic. J Cell Biol 131:1435–1452
26. Vitelli R, Santillo M, Lattero D, Chiariello M, Bifulco M, Bruni CB, Bucci C (1997) Role of the small GTPase Rab 7 in the late endocytic pathway. J Biol Chem 272:4391–4397
27. Chun J, Prince A (2009) TLR2-induced calpain cleavage of epithelial junctional proteins facilitates leukocyte transmigration. Cell Host Microbe 5:47–58
28. Franco SJ, Huttenlocher A (2005) Regulating cell migration: calpains make the cut. J Cell Sci 118:3829–3838
29. Goll DE, Thompson VF, Li H, Wei W, Cong J (2003) The calpain system. Physiol Rev 83: 731–801
30. Lebart MC, Benyamin Y (2006) Calpain involvement in the remodeling of cytoskeletal anchorage complexes. FEBS J 273:3415–3426
31. Rios-Doria J, Day KC, Kuefer R, Rashid MG, Chinnaiyan AM, Rubin MA, Day ML (2003) The role of calpain in the proteolytic cleavage of E-cadherin in prostate and mammary epithelial cells. J Biol Chem 278:1372–1379
32. Wells A, Huttenlocher A, Lauffenburger DA (2005) Calpain proteases in cell adhesion and motility. Int Rev Cytol 245:1–16
33. Gumbiner BM (2000) Regulation of cadherin adhesive activity. J Cell Biol 148:339–404
34. Herren B, Levkau B, Raines EW, Ross R (1998) Cleavage of beta-catenin and plakoglobin and shedding of VE-cadherin during endothelial apoptosis: evidence for a role for caspases and metalloproteinases. Mol Biol Cell 9:1589–1601
35. Ito K, Okamoto I, Araki N, Kawano Y, Nakao M, Fujiyama S, Tomita K, Mimori T, Saya H (1999) Calcium influx triggers the sequential proteolysis of extracellular and cytoplasmic domains of E-cadherin, leading to loss of beta-catenin from cell-cell contacts. Oncogene 18:7080–7090
36. Marambaud P, Shioi J, Serban G, Georgakopoulos A, Sarner S, Nagy V, Baki L, Wen P, Efthimiopoulos S, Shao Z, Wisniewski T, Robakis NK (2002) A presenilin-1/gamma-secretase cleavage releases the E-cadherin intracellular domain and regulates disassembly of adherens junctions. EMBO J 21:1948–1956
37. Steinhusen U, Weiske J, Badock V, Tauber R, Bommert K, Huber O (2001) Cleavage and shedding of E-cadherin after induction of apoptosis. J Biol Chem 276:4972–4980
38. Vallorosi CJ, Day KC, Zhao X, Rashid MG, Rubin MA, Johnson KR, Wheelock MJ, Day ML (2000) Truncation of the beta-catenin binding of E-cadherin precedes epithelial apoptosis during prostate and mammary involution. J Biol Chem 113:3328–3334
39. Silvera D, Arju R, Darvishian F, Levine P, Zolfaghari L, Goldberg J, Hochman T, Formenti SC, Schneider RJ (2009) Essential role for elF4GI overexpression in the pathogenesis of inflammatory breast cancer. Nat Cell Biol 11:903–908
40. Silvera D, Schneider RJ (2009) Inflammatory breast cancer cells are constitutively adapted to hypoxia. Cell Cycle 8:3091–3096
41. Chen X, Kojima S, Borisy GG, Green KJ (2003) p120 catenin associates with kinesin and facilitates the transport of cadherin–catenin complexes to intercellular junctions. J Cell Biol 163:547–557
42. Davis MA, Ireton RC, Reynolds AB (2003) A core function for p120-catenin in cadherin turnover. J Cell Biol 163:525–534

43. Xiao K, Allison DF, Buckley KM, Kottke MD, Vincent PA, Faundez V, Kowalczyk AP (2003) Cellular levels of p120 catenin function as a set point for cadherin expression levels in micro-vascular endothelial cells. J Cell Biol 163:535–545
44. Ireton RC, Davis MA, van Hengel J, Mariner DJ, Barnes K, Thorenson MA, Anastasiadis PZ, Matrisian L, Bundy LM, Sealy L et al (2002) A novel role for p120 catenin in E-cadherin function. J Cell Biol 159:465–476
45. Behrens J, von Kries JP, Kühl M, Bruhn L, Wedlich D, Grosschedl R, Birchmeier W (1996) Functional interaction of beta-catenin with the transcription factor LEF-1. Nature 382:638–642
46. Ferber EC, Kajita M, Wadlow A, Tobiansky L, Niessen C, Ariga H, Daniel J, Fujita Y (2008) A role for the cleaved cytoplasmic domain of E-cadherin in the nucleus. J Biol Chem 283:12691–12700
47. Alattia JR, Ames JB, Porumb T, Tong KI, Meng YH, Ottensmeyer P, Kay CM, Ikura M (1997) Lateral self-assembly of E-cadherin directed by cooperative calcium binding. FEBS Lett 417:405–408
48. Koch AW, Pokutta S, Lustig A, Engel J (1997) Calcium binding and homoassociation of E-cadherin domains. Biochemistry 36:7697–7705
49. Gopalakrishna R, Barsky SH (1985) Quantitation of tissue calpain activity after isolation by hydrophobic chromatography. Anal Biochem 148:413–423
50. Gopalakrishna R, Barsky SH (1986) Hydrophobic association of calpains with subcellular organelles – compartmentalization of calpains and the endogenous inhibitor calpastatin in tissues. J Biol Chem 261:13936–13942
51. Messaritou G, East L, Roghi C, Isacke CM, Yarwood H (2009) Membrane type-1 matrix metalloproteinase activity is regulated by the endocytic collagen receptor Endo180. J Cell Sci 122:4042–4048
52. Wakabayashi T, De Strooper B (2008) Presenilins: members of the γ-secretase quartets, but part-time soloists too. Physiology (Bethesda) 23:194–204

Chapter 6
Imaging for the Diagnosis and Staging of IBC

Wei Tse Yang

Abstract The role of imaging in the diagnosis and assessment of inflammatory breast cancer (IBC) includes characterization of the known tumor, delineation of loco-regional disease extent in the ipsilateral and contralateral breasts and regional lymph node basins, diagnosis of distant metastases, and evaluation of response to neoadjuvant treatment. In this chapter, we review the role of conventional imaging modalities, including mammography and sonography, in the diagnosis and assessment of IBC. We also discuss the potential use of evolving imaging modalities, such as magnetic resonance imaging, positron emission tomography, and combined positron emission tomography and computed tomography, in patients diagnosed with IBC.

Keywords Breast • Ultrasound • Mammography • Magnetic resonance imaging (MRI) • Positron emission tomography- computed tomography (PET-CT) • Axillary lymph nodes • Internal mammary • Dermal lymphatics • Neoplasm

List of Abbreviations

CT	Computed tomography
IBC	Inflammatory breast cancer
MRI	Magnetic resonance imaging
PET	Positron emission tomography
LABC	Locally advanced breast cancer

W.T. Yang, M.D. (✉)
Department of Diagnostic Radiology, The University of Texas MD Anderson Cancer Center, 1515 Holcombe Boulevard, 77030 Houston, TX, USA
e-mail: wyang@mdanderson.org

N.T. Ueno and M. Cristofanilli (eds.), *Inflammatory Breast Cancer: An Update*,
DOI 10.1007/978-94-007-3907-9_6, © Springer Science+Business Media B.V. 2012

6.1 Introduction

Inflammatory breast cancer (IBC) is an uncommon and aggressive primary breast cancer, categorized by the American Joint Committee on Cancer as a T4d tumor [1–4]. The clinical presentation is typically rapid onset swelling and enlargement of the affected breast, accompanied by diffuse erythema, edema, local tenderness, and warmth of the affected breast. The time from the first symptom or sign to diagnosis is usually no longer than 3 months [5–7]. IBC can present with or without a palpable breast mass and is usually a poorly differentiated infiltrating ductal carcinoma. The prognosis of patients with IBC is poor because in most cases the disease has already micrometastasized at diagnosis. Histological diagnosis may be problematic because of the difficulty of defining an area for biopsy. Approximately 20% of patients with IBC have gross distant metastases at the time of diagnosis [8].

The main role of imaging in IBC is in diagnosis and staging, which includes identification of an abnormality in the breast for biopsy; staging of loco-regional disease in the ipsilateral breast, contralateral breast, and regional lymph node basins; diagnosis of distant metastases; and evaluation of response to neoadjuvant treatment. In this chapter, the role of mammography, sonography, magnetic resonance imaging (MRI), positron emission tomography (PET), and combined PET and computed tomography (PET-CT) in the assessment of IBC will be discussed.

6.2 Mammography

The primary imaging findings on mammography in patients with IBC are diffuse skin thickening, trabecular and stromal thickening, and diffuse increased breast density (Figs. 6.1a and 6.2a). Skin thickening is thought to reflect infiltration of the dermal lymphatics by tumor cells, although pathologic proof of dermal lymphatic involvement is not necessary for the diagnosis of IBC. The stromal and trabecular changes are presumed to be secondary to edema and obstruction of lymph vessels and capillaries. Increased breast size, breast density, trabecular thickening, and skin changes may be subtle and detected only when the affected breast is compared with the contralateral breast. IBC is generally a unilateral process [9].

Standard mammography findings in patients with IBC have previously been described [9–17]. The largest study to date describing the mammographic features of IBC was published in 2002 [12]. The higher percentage of bilateral cases reported in older studies of IBC [18, 19] likely reflects differences in case definition and the inclusion of patients with locally advanced breast cancer (LABC) in the older series. LABC is the major differential diagnosis to be considered in a patient with suspected IBC and can be excluded on the basis of clinical history. Additional, less common diagnoses to be considered in patients with mammographic findings suggestive of IBC include primary breast lymphoma and metastasis from an extramammary malignancy [20, 21].

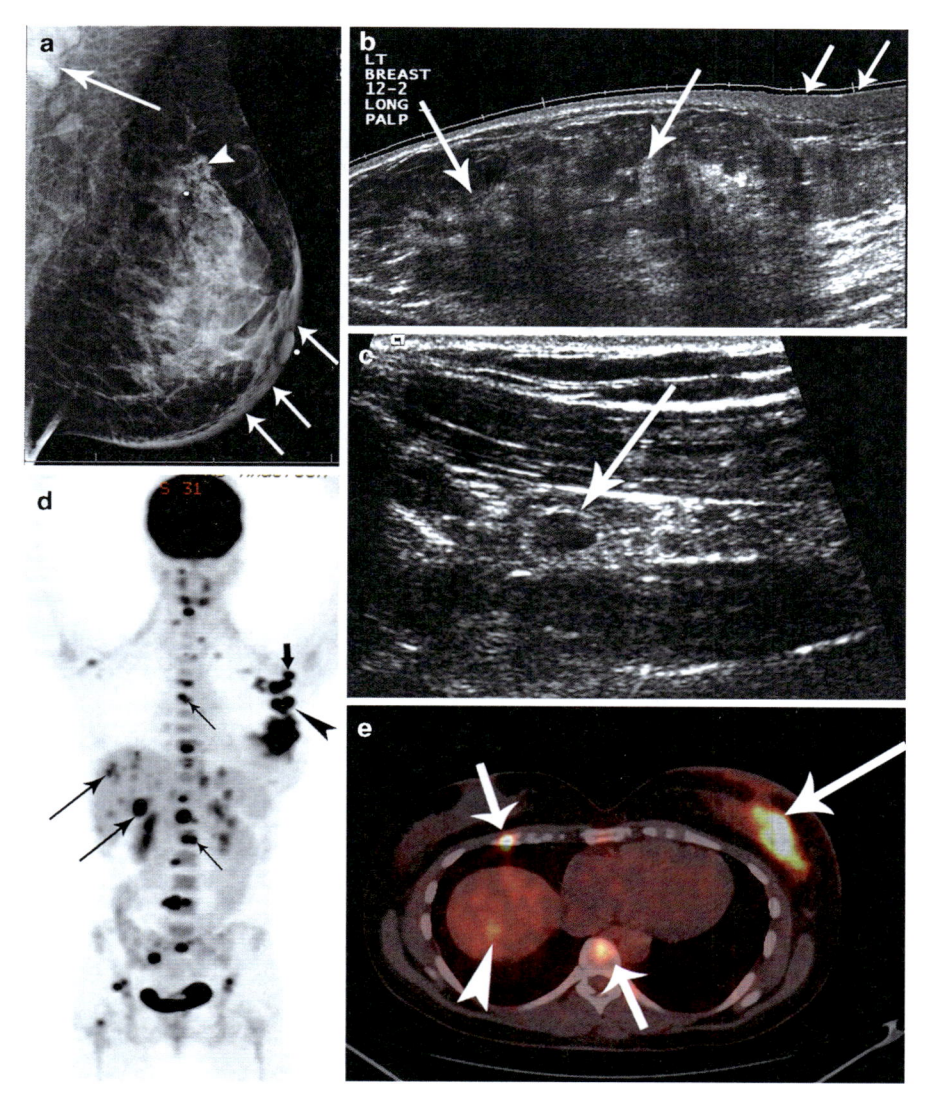

Fig. 6.1 Imaging findings in a 37-year-old woman with IBC. (**a**) Left mediolateral oblique mammogram shows global skin thickening (*short arrows*) with associated diffuse increased breast density and an area of architectural distortion with associated pleomorphic microcalcifications (*arrowhead*) in the left upper outer quadrant. Associated dense left axillary nodes are present (*long arrow*). Pathology review showed invasive ductal carcinoma. (**b**) Longitudinal extended-field-of-view ultrasound image shows global architectural distortion with marked posterior acoustic shadowing (*long arrows*) involving the entire lateral left breast. Note the associated skin thickening (*short arrows*). (**c**) Transverse ultrasound image shows a subcentimeter solid hypoechoic medial left infraclavicular node (*fat arrow*). Ultrasound-guided fine-needle aspiration biopsy showed metastatic carcinoma, confirming N3 disease per the American Joint Committee on Cancer criteria. (**d**) Coronal maximum intensity projection whole-body PET image shows multiple hypermetabolic masses in the left breast (*arrowhead*), hypermetabolic left axillary (*short thick arrow*) and infraclavicular adenopathy, increased uptake in the thoracic and lumbar spine (*short thin arrows*), and liver (*long thin arrows*). (**e**) Axial co-registered PET-CT image shows a hypermetabolic left breast mass (*long arrow*) and unsuspected FDG-avid foci in the right anterior rib and thoracic vertebrae (*short arrows*). Hypermetabolic liver lesions are poorly shown (*arrowhead*). The findings on staging PET-CT were consistent with disseminated metastases at diagnosis

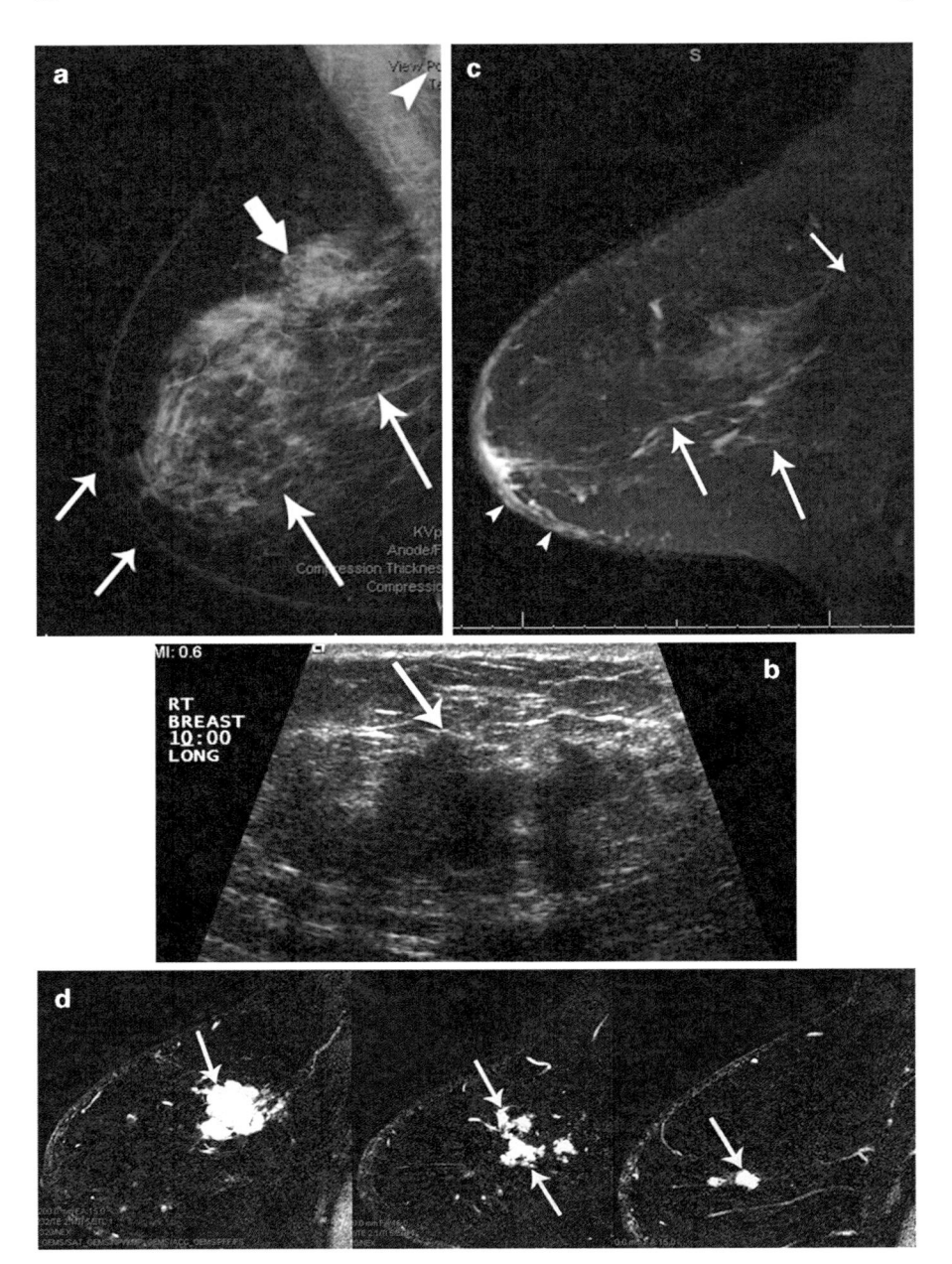

Fig. 6.2 Imaging findings in a 52-year-old woman with IBC. (**a**) Right mediolateral oblique mammogram shows global skin thickening (*short thin arrows*) and trabecular thickening (*long thin arrows*), an obscured mass in the right upper outer quadrant (*fat arrow*), and right axillary adenopathy (*arrowhead*). (**b**) Transverse gray-scale ultrasound image shows a solid irregular mass with indistinct margins (*arrow*). (**c**) Pre-contrast fat-suppressed T2-weighted image of the right breast demonstrates high signal intensity throughout the fibroglandular tissue (*long arrows*), skin (*arrowheads*),

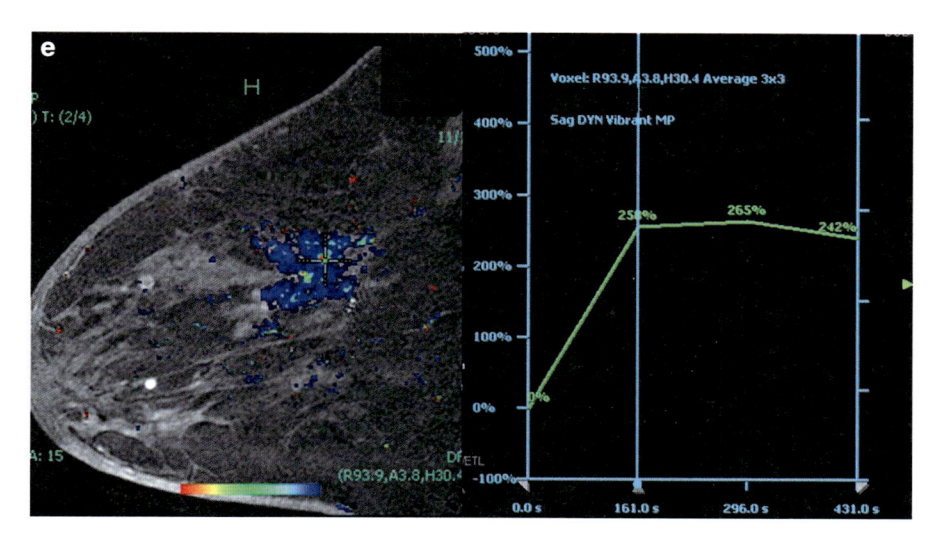

Fig. 6.2 (continued) which is markedly thickened, and pre-pectoral muscle region (*short arrow*), compatible with extensive edema. Biopsy showed invasive ductal carcinoma. (**d**) Contrast-enhanced T1-weighted fat-saturated gradient-recalled echo axial 3T image shows multiple enhancing masses involving the lateral right breast (*arrows*), marked global skin thickening, and heterogeneous skin enhancement. Pathology showed mixed invasive ductal and lobular carcinoma. (**e**) Sagittal contrast-enhanced T1-weighted subtracted image with parametric color coding shows an enhancing mass in the right upper outer quadrant. The time–signal intensity curve demonstrates rapid wash-in and delayed plateau kinetics

Although most patients with IBC present with a palpable mass, a dominant mass is not the most common finding on mammography. This may be related to the infiltrative nature of the tumor and because the overall increased breast density masks underlying masses (Fig. 6.1a). Patients' poor tolerance for compression secondary to the edema and swelling of the breast may also play a role. Calcifications are less common than in patients with locally advanced invasive ductal breast cancer [10, 13, 15], as are focal asymmetry and architectural distortion (Table 6.1). In a recent study of 80 patients with IBC, a mass or architectural distortion was the most common primary breast parenchymal feature [17]. Calcifications were noted in 41% of the patients in that study [17]. In a recent single-institution retrospective analysis, mammography was the least sensitive and least effective method of diagnosing IBC [17]. Mammography detected the lowest percentage of primary breast parenchymal lesions and the lowest percentage of cases of multicentric disease (43%). A recent analysis of nine mammography studies over 18 years showed associated axillary adenopathy in approximately 28% of patients with IBC [9]. Axillary adenopathy may be useful in differentiating IBC from other conditions with a similar appearance, such as radiation-induced changes.

Table 6.1 Mammography findings in patients with inflammatory breast cancer[a]

Year	Author and ref	No. of pts.	Palpable findings	Skin thickening	Trabecular thickening	Increased density	Focal asymmetry	Mass	Calcifi-cations	Arch distort.	AXLN	Nipple retract.
2000	Kushwaha [13]	26	–	24 (92)	16 (62)	21 (81)	13 (50)[b]	4 (15)	6 (23)	13 (50)[b]	15 (58)	–
2002	Belli [22]	10	–	10 (100)	10 (100)	10 (100)	–	2 (20)	–	–	–	–
2002	Gunhan-Bilgen [12]	142	88 (62)	119 (84)	115 (81)	53 (37)	87 (61)	23 (16)	80 (56)	–	34 (24)	61 (43)
2005	Caumo [14]	19	10 (56)	7 (37)	8 (42)	10 (53)	–	7 (37)	5 (26)	2 (11)	–	3 (16)
2005	Lee [16]	9	–	9 (100)	7 (78)	5 (56)	–	4 (44)	7 (78)	–	5 (56)	–
2008	Yang [17]	75	30 (40)	62 (83)	55 (73)	4 (5)	4 (5)	24 (32)	31 (41)	12 (16)	34 (45)	7 (9)
2008	Renz [23]	48	33 (69)	–	–	41 (85)	–	32 (67)	9 (19)	–	–	–

Arch. distort. architectural distortion, *AXLN* axillary lymphadenopathy, *pts.* patients, *retract.* retraction

[a]Values in table are number of patients (percentage) except where otherwise indicated

[b]Paper described architectural distortion or focal asymmetry in 13 patients (50%)

6.3 Sonography

The role of sonography in evaluating patients with a clinical diagnosis of IBC is to localize an abnormality for percutaneous biopsy [9]. Sonography successfully demonstrates a breast abnormality and skin thickening in up to 95% of cases of IBC [17] (Figs. 6.1b and 6.2b), and sonography detects a higher percentage of cases of multicentric or multifocal disease (72%) than does mammography [17] (Table 6.2). Sonography is an alternate imaging modality for affected breasts that are too painful and edematous to allow for adequate compression during mammography. Areas of heterogeneous breast tissue or parenchymal architectural distortion (Fig. 6.1b) can be targeted for biopsy in lieu of a focal mass, and biopsy of such areas yields a cancer diagnosis in virtually all cases [17]. When a mass is visible on sonography, it is most frequently an irregular hypoechoic mass with ill-defined margins and posterior acoustic shadowing (Fig. 6.2b). Skin thickening is characterized by blurring of the transducer, blurring of the skin, and more hypoechoic appearance of the dermal subcutaneous fat lines or, alternatively, by dilated lymphatic vessels (representing edema) surrounding the breast lobules. Edema and trabecular thickening are characterized by diffuse increased echogenicity of the breast and overlying subcutaneous tissue (Fig. 6.2b).

In our experience, sonography permits a more comprehensive evaluation of the regional nodal basins (including the axillary, infraclavicular, internal mammary, and supraclavicular basins) than does any other modality [17, 24, 25]. Previous series have reported axillary adenopathy in 22–56% of IBC patients (mean, 28%) [1, 3, 4, 9]. Supraclavicular, infraclavicular, or internal mammary nodal disease was diagnosed in at least 50% of patients on sonography (Fig. 6.1c) [17]. The findings on pretreatment nodal staging using sonography may affect loco-regional therapeutic planning, which is based on the extent of initial disease involvement [25].

6.4 Magnetic Resonance Imaging

MRI is a powerful breast imaging technique that does not involve the use of ionizing radiation, has superior sensitivity in the diagnosis of invasive breast cancer, and has the potential to characterize and quantify dynamic contrast agent enhancement in a region of interest. The major roles of MRI in breast cancer are in the diagnosis and staging of the disease and in the monitoring of response to neoadjuvant treatment.

Reports on MRI findings of IBC are scarce in the published literature [9, 16, 17, 22, 26, 27] (Table 6.3). Most of the published data describe MRI studies performed on a 1-Tesla or 1.5-Tesla unit. Skin thickening, skin enhancement, and enhancing tendrils of tumor mass extending to the skin have been described as characteristic MRI features of IBC [9]. In the same report, breast deformity, breast enlargement, and enlarged enhancing axillary nodes were also noted [9]. A discrete necrotic mass was noted in 38% of cases, and an infiltrative mass with a reticular dendritic pattern and extension to the pectoralis muscle was also common [9]. Tumor masses showed either wash-in with plateau or washout enhancement kinetics in this study [9].

Table 6.2 Sonography findings in patients with inflammatory breast cancer[a]

Year	Author	No. of patients	Mass	Skin thickening	Lymphatic dilatation	Posterior acoustic shadowing or architectural distortion	AXLN	Hypervascularity
2002	Belli [22]	10	5 (50)[b]	–	–		–	–
2002	Gunhan-Bilgen [12]	142	114 (80)	136 (96)	96 (68)	104 (73)	104 (73)	–
2005	Caumo [14]	16	9 (56)	7 (44)	2 (13)	–	11 (69)	–
2005	Lee [16]	9	7 (78)	–	5 (56)	–	5 (56)	5 (56)
2008	Yang [17]	76	54 (71)	72 (95)	–	18 (24)	71 (93)	56 (74)
2008	Renz [23]	48	36 (75)	–	–	41 (85)	–	–

AXLN axillary lymphadenopathy

[a]Values in table are number of patients (percentage) except where otherwise indicated

[b]Five patients had masses or nodules

Table 6.3 MRI findings in patients with inflammatory breast cancer[a]

Year	Author	No. of pts.	Skin thicken.	Skin enhance.	Breast edema	Breast mass	Arch. distort.	NME	Parench. enhance.	Kinetic curve			AXLN
										WI	PT	WO	
1997	Rieber [26]	10	9 (90)	–	9 (90)	1 (10)	–	–	9 (90)	–	–	–	–
2002	Belli [22]	10	–	–	–	2 (20)	–	5 (50)	10 (100)	9 (90)	–	10 (100)	–
2005	Chow [9]	26	26 (100)	26 (100)	–	11 (42)	–	–	–	3 (12)	12 (46)	10 (38)	23 (88)
2005	Lee [16]	9	9 (100)	7 (78)	–	2 (22)	–	–	2 (22)	–	–	–	–
2008	Yang [17]	33	32 (97)	31 (94)	18 (54)	23 (70)	20 (61)	10 (31)	–	32 (97)	b	b	29 (88)
2008	Renz [23]	48	40 (83)	–	33 (69)	40 (80)	–	8 (17)	–	41 (85)	11 (23)	33 (69)	–
2010	Carbognin [28]	14	8 (58)	2 (14)	9 (64)	5 (36)	8 (57)		9 (64)	–	2 (14)	12 (86)	–
2011	Girardi [29]	30	16 (53)	10 (33)	–	8 (27)	22 (73)		22 (73)	–	8 (27)	22 (73)	20 (67)

Arch. distort. architectural distortion, *AXLN* axillary lymphadenopathy, *distort.* distortion, *enhance.* enhancement, *NME* non-mass like enhancement, *parench.* parenchymal, *PT* plateau, *pts.* patients, *thicken.* thickening, *WI* wash-in, *WO* wash-out

[a]Values in table are number of patients (percentage) except where otherwise indicated

[b]Thirty-two patients had wash-out or plateau kinetics

The most frequent MRI findings in two recent studies describing IBC patients were multiple masses with irregular margins and heterogeneous internal enhancement pattern associated with a delayed washout or plateau kinetic curve [17, 27]. In studies to date on MRI in IBC, skin thickening and skin enhancement were seen in 90–100% of patients [9, 16, 17, 22, 27]. Chow et al. commented that breasts with greater skin thickening demonstrated skin enhancement more frequently than breasts with less skin thickening [9]. Similar findings were observed in a study by Le-Petross et al [27]. Over half of the patients had breast edema, which manifested as bright T2-weighted signal throughout the affected breast [17, 27] (Fig. 6.2c). Associated breast enlargement and asymmetric breast enhancement were also observed, compatible with the inflammatory process of this disease.

On MRI, the primary breast lesion may present as a mass-like or non-mass-like enhancement (Fig. 6.2d). Recent studies demonstrated that the rate of identification of a primary breast lesion was 100% with MRI (33 of 33), compared to 96% with PET-CT, 80% with mammography, and 95% with sonography [17]. These new results are most likely due to technical advances in MRI and suggest that MRI may presently be the imaging modality of choice for IBC.

Qualitative assessment of the primary breast lesion enhancement demonstrated a delayed washout or plateau kinetic pattern in the majority of tumors [9, 17, 22, 27]. Axillary involvement was identified in over 80% of patients [9, 17, 22, 27]. In our experience, the size and morphological characteristics of the lymph nodes are more useful in differentiating between benign and malignant lymph nodes than is kinetic assessment. This is because normal lymph nodes usually do enhance and often demonstrate a washout pattern.

The other diagnoses to be considered in patients with suspected IBC on MRI are non-puerperal mastitis, LABC, and primary breast lymphoma, all of which may result in skin thickening, diffuse breast enlargement, and diffuse increased mammographic density. More recent publications comparing the MRI features of IBC versus LABC suggest that the following variables may be useful in differentiating between these diseases: skin thickening, skin edema, and skin enhancement [23, 28, 29]. Additionally, non-mass-like enhancements were significantly more frequent in patients with IBC than in patients with LABC [29]. Other incidental MRI findings in a small study of 14 IBC patients were hypertrophy of the internal mammary artery (21%) and significant pre-pectoral edema (28–42%) [23, 28, 29]. IBC should be differentiated from LABC on the basis of clinical history [9, 30, 31]. MRI does not allow sufficient differentiation between mastitis and IBC [22, 26].

Despite being a powerful test in the diagnosis and staging of IBC, MRI is not suitable for all IBC patients. Gentle immobilization of both breasts in the prone position, single breast coil size, and the extended duration of the study (approximately 30 min) contribute to patient discomfort and lack of tolerance. Because of these factors, in some patients with IBC, it may not be possible to complete an MRI examination of the breast. Premedication with an anxiolytic may alleviate patient discomfort due to the prone position and pressure from the breast coil on the inflamed breast and chest.

A recent study in 19 patients evaluated the potential application of dynamic contrast-enhanced MRI as a tool for assessing changes in vascularity in patients with IBC treated with anti-angiogenic therapy [32]. MR-derived general pharmacokinetic parameters and region-of-interest selection within the tumor were important for the quantification of cancer response to therapy [32].

6.5 PET and PET-CT

18-Fluoro-deoxy-glucose (18-FDG)-PET imaging in breast cancer has met with varying degrees of success. Prospective studies on the current use of FDG-PET in primary breast cancer have focused primarily on patients with early or small-volume disease for whom there is a low probability of lymph node involvement, and these studies have shown limited value of FDG-PET in the evaluation of local lymph nodal disease [33–35]. These findings may not necessarily apply to patients with IBC, who frequently have extensive loco-regional disease. Appropriate delineation of disease extent is helpful for treatment planning, including radiotherapy and chemotherapy [17]. A single study on seven patients with IBC described increased uptake in enlarged breasts, with associated prominent skin uptake, and intense scattered foci [36]. Six patients (86%) had associated ipsilateral axillary adenopathy, one patient had infraclavicular and supraclavicular adenopathy, and one patient had bone metastases [36].

PET-CT is an emerging imaging method that is gaining wide clinical acceptance because of its ability to co-register anatomic and functional information on one image [37–39]. Mounting evidence indicates a role for PET-CT in the comprehensive staging of advanced breast cancer, particularly in the determination of ipsilateral multicentric, bilateral, and distant metastatic disease. A retrospective study on the role of PET-CT in 41 patients with IBC showed that PET-CT was accurate in demonstrating loco-regional disease and distant metastases [40]. Hypermetabolic skin uptake was noted in all 41 patients (100%)—in the affected breast in 40 patients (98%) and in the ipsilateral axillary nodes in 37 patients (90%) [40] (Fig. 6.1d–e). Distant metastases were documented in 20 patients (49%), 3 (17%) of whom were not known to have metastases prior to PET-CT. This rate of metastatic disease is higher than that reported for breast cancers in general and may reflect the aggressive nature of IBC. Such findings suggest that despite its cost, PET-CT should be considered in the initial staging of women diagnosed with IBC.

An important evolving application of PET-CT is assessment of response to neoadjuvant chemotherapy or endocrine therapy in patients with IBC or LABC [39, 41–45]. Given the new paradigm of treating breast cancer with targeted therapies, the ability to predict response early with a functional imaging tool is critically important. This will allow early cessation of potentially toxic and expensive therapeutic regimens that are predicted to have no benefit for individual patients.

6.6 Conclusion

In conclusion, mammography is the least sensitive imaging modality for diagnosis of a primary breast abnormality in the assessment of IBC. Sonography is useful in localizing areas for biopsy and histological confirmation of invasive cancer and also in the comprehensive evaluation and staging of the regional nodal basins (including axillary, infraclavicular, internal mammary, and supraclavicular). MRI demonstrates parenchymal breast abnormality in virtually all patients with IBC and provides the advantage of exquisite anatomical detail and functional information through kinetic evaluation. PET-CT is accurate in demonstrating loco-regional disease and distant metastases.

References

1. Levine PH, Steinhorn SC, Ries LG et al (1985) Inflammatory breast cancer: the experience of the Surveillance, Epidemiology, and End Results (SEER) program. J Natl Cancer Inst 74:291–297
2. Chang S, Parker SL, Pham T et al (1998) Inflammatory breast carcinoma incidence and survival: the Surveillance, Epidemiology, and End Results program of the National Cancer Institute, 1975–1992. Cancer 82:2366–2372
3. Hance KW, Anderson WF, Devesa SS et al (2005) Trends in inflammatory breast carcinoma incidence and survival: the Surveillance, Epidemiology, and End Results program at the National Cancer Institute. J Natl Cancer Inst 97:966–975
4. Greene FL, Page DL, Fleming ID et al (2002) American Joint Cancer Committee cancer staging manual, 6th edn. Springer, New York, pp 221–240
5. Lee B, Tannenbaum N (1924) Inflammatory carcinoma of the breast: a report of twenty-eight cases from the breast clinic of Memorial Hospital. Surg Gynecol Obstet 39:580–585
6. Jaiyesimi IA, Buzdar AU, Hortobagyi G (1992) Inflammatory breast cancer: a review. J Clin Oncol 10:1014–1024
7. Dirix LY, Dam PV, Prove A et al (2006) Inflammatory breast cancer: current understanding. Curr Opin Oncol 18:563–571
8. Wingo PA, Jamison PM, Young JL et al (2004) Population-based statistics for women diagnosed with inflammatory breast cancer (United States). Cancer Causes Control 15:321–328
9. Chow CK (2005) Imaging in inflammatory breast carcinoma. Breast Dis 22:45–54
10. Dershaw DD, Moore MP, Liberman L et al (1994) Inflammatory breast carcinoma: mammographic findings. Radiology 190:831–834
11. Droulias CA, Sewell CW, McSweeney MB et al (1976) Inflammatory carcinoma of the breast: a correlation of clinical, radiologic and pathologic findings. Ann Surg 184:217–222
12. Gunhan-Bilgen I, Ustun EE, Memis A (2002) Inflammatory breast carcinoma: mammographic, ultrasonographic, clinical, and pathologic findings in 142 cases. Radiology 223:829–838
13. Kushwaha AC, Whitman GJ, Stelling CB et al (2000) Primary inflammatory carcinoma of the breast: retrospective review of mammographic findings. AJR Am J Roentgenol 174:535–538
14. Caumo F, Gaioni MB, Bonetti F et al (2005) Occult inflammatory breast cancer: review of clinical, mammographic, US and pathologic signs. Radiol Med 109:308–320
15. Tardivon AA, Viala J, Corvellec Rudelli A et al (1997) Mammographic patterns of inflammatory breast carcinoma: a retrospective study of 92 cases. Eur J Radiol 24:124–130
16. Lee KW, Chung SY, Yang I et al (2005) Inflammatory breast cancer: imaging findings. Clin Imaging 29:22–25

17. Yang WT, Le-Petross HT, Macapinlac H et al (2008) Inflammatory breast cancer: PET/CT, MRI, mammography, and sonography findings. Breast Cancer Res Treat 109:417–426
18. Haagensen CD (1971) Diseases of the breast, 2nd edn. Saunders, Philadelphia, pp 576–584
19. Taylor GW, Meltzer A (1938) Inflammatory carcinoma of the breast. Am J Cancer 133:33–49
20. Yang WT, Lane DL, Le-Petross HT et al (2007) Breast lymphoma: imaging findings of 32 tumors in 27 patients. Radiology 245:692–702
21. Yang WT, Muttarak M, Ho L (2000) Nonmammary malignancies of the breast: ultrasound, CT, and MRI. Semin Ultrasound CT MR 21:375–394
22. Belli P, Costantini M, Romani M et al (2002) Role of magnetic resonance imaging in inflammatory carcinoma of the breast. Rays 27:299–305
23. Renz DM, Baltzer PA, Bottcher J et al (2008) Magnetic resonance imaging of inflammatory breast carcinoma and acute mastitis. A comparative study. Eur Radiol 18:2370–2380
24. Yang WT, Ahuja A, Tang A et al (1996) High resolution sonographic detection of axillary lymph node metastases in breast cancer. J Ultrasound Med 16:241–246
25. Vlastos G, Fornage BD, Mirza NQ et al (2000) The correlation of axillary ultrasonography with histologic breast cancer downstaging after induction chemotherapy. Am J Surg 179:446–452
26. Rieber A, Tomczak RJ, Mergo PJ et al (1997) MRI of the breast in the differential diagnosis of mastitis versus inflammatory carcinoma and follow-up. J Comput Assist Tomogr 21:128–132
27. Le-Petross HT, Cristofanilli C, Carkaci S et al (2011) MRI features of inflammatory breast cancer. AJR Am J Roentgenol 197: W769– W776
28. Carbognin G, Calciolari C, Girardi V et al (2010) Inflammatory breast cancer: MR imaging findings. Radiol Med 115:70–82
29. Girardi V, Carbognin G, Camera L et al (2011) Inflammatory breast carcinoma and locally advanced breast carcinoma: characterisation with MR imaging. Radiol Med 116:71–83
30. Walshe JM, Swain SM (2005) Clinical aspects of inflammatory breast cancer. Breast Dis 22:35–44
31. Anderson WF, Chu KC, Chang S (2003) Inflammatory breast carcinoma and noninflammatory locally advanced breast carcinoma: distinct clinicopathologic entities? J Clin Oncol 21:2254–2259
32. Thukral A, Thomasson DM, Chow CK et al (2007) Inflammatory breast cancer: dynamic contrast-enhanced MR in patients receiving bevacizumab – initial experience. Radiology 244:727–735
33. Wahl RL, Siegel BA, Coleman RE et al (2004) Prospective multicenter study of axillary nodal staging by positron emission tomography in breast cancer: a report of the staging breast cancer with PET study group. J Clin Oncol 2:277–285
34. Eubank WB, Mankoff DA (2005) Evolving role of positron emission tomography in breast cancer imaging. Semin Nucl Med 35:84–99
35. Osman MM, Cohade C, Nakamoto Y et al (2003) Clinically significant inaccurate localization of lesions with PET/CT: frequency in 300 patients. J Nucl Med 44:240–243
36. Baslaim MM, Bakheet SM, Bakheet R et al (2003) 18-Fluorodeoxyglucose-positron emission tomography in inflammatory breast cancer. World J Surg 27:1099–1104
37. Beyer T, Townsend DW, Brun T et al (2000) A combined PET/CT scanner for clinical oncology. J Nucl Med 41:1369–1379
38. Townsend DW, Beyer T (2002) A combined PET/CT scanner: the path to true image fusion. Br J Radiol 75(suppl):24–30
39. Fueger BJ, Weber WA, Quon A et al (2005) Performance of 2-deoxy-2-[F-18]fluoro-D-glucose positron emission tomography and integrated PET/CT in restaged breast cancer patients. Mol Imaging Biol 7:369–376
40. Carkaci S, Macapinlac HA, Cristofanilli M et al (2009) Retrospective study of 18F-FDG PET/CT in the diagnosis of inflammatory breast cancer: preliminary data. J Nucl Med 50:231–238
41. Rousseau C, Devillers A, Sagan C et al (2006) Monitoring of early response to neoadjuvant chemotherapy in stage II and III breast cancer by [18F] fluorodeoxyglucose positron emission tomography. J Clin Oncol 24:5366–5372

42. Larson SM, Erdi Y, Akhurst T et al (1999) Tumor treatment based on visual and quantitative changes in global tumor glycolysis using PET-FDG imaging: the visual response score and the change in total lesion glycolysis. Clin Positron Imaging 2:159–171
43. Krak NC, Hoekstra OS, Lammertsma AA (2004) Measuring response to chemotherapy in locally advanced breast cancer: methodological considerations. Eur J Nucl Med Mol Imaging 31(Suppl 1):S103–S111
44. Rosen EL, Eubank WB, Mankoff DA (2007) FDG PET, PET/CT, and breast cancer imaging. Radiographics 27(Suppl 1):S215–S229
45. Lim HS, Yoon W, Chung TW et al (2007) FDG PET/CT for the detection and evaluation of breast diseases: usefulness and limitations. Radiographics 27(Suppl 1):S197–S213

Chapter 7
Surgical Therapy for Inflammatory Breast Cancer

Sarah M. Gainer, Hideko Yamauchi, and Anthony Lucci

Abstract Surgical therapy for inflammatory breast cancer (IBC), the most aggressive and fatal form of breast cancer, continues to challenge surgeons. Surgical therapy should only be undertaken in patients with IBC who respond to neoadjuvant chemotherapy (NAC). The recommended definitive surgical treatment for IBC is modified radical mastectomy. Currently, breast conserving therapy, skin-sparing mastectomy, nipple-sparing mastectomy, sentinel lymph node biopsy, and immediate breast reconstruction are contraindicated for patients with IBC. Multimodality treatment, including surgery, is crucial for achieving optimal outcomes.

Keywords Inflammatory breast cancer • Surgery for inflammatory breast cancer • IBC • Modified radical mastectomy • MRM • Multimodal therapy for IBC • Axillary lymph node dissection • Chemotherapy response • Postmastectomy radiation • Local control for breast cancer

7.1 A Historical Perspective

In 1924, Lee and Tannebaum described 18 cases of inflammatory breast cancer (IBC). Three women in this series underwent radical mastectomy, and all three died of recurrent disease, prompting Lee and Tannebaum to recognize the "inefficiency of surgery" for IBC [1]. In 1951, Haagensen and Stout reported on a series of 29 patients

S.M. Gainer • A. Lucci
Surgical Oncology, The University of Texas MD Anderson Cancer Center,
1400 Pressler st, Unit 1484 Houston, TX 77030
e-mail: sgainer@mdanderson.org; alucci@mdanderson.org

H. Yamauchi (✉)
Breast Surgical Oncology, St Luke's International Hospital, 9-1,
Akashi-Cho, Chuo-ku, 104-8560, Japan
e-mail: hidekoyamauchi@mac.com

N.T. Ueno and M. Cristofanilli (eds.), *Inflammatory Breast Cancer: An Update*, 67
DOI 10.1007/978-94-007-3907-9_7, © Springer Science+Business Media B.V. 2012

with IBC treated with radical mastectomy alone. The mean survival time in these patients was 19 months, and all had died by 5 years [2]. In 1961, Barber et al. presented 53 cases of IBC. Of the 50 patients who underwent surgical therapy, two were treated with simple mastectomy, six were treated with radical mastectomy, and 42 were treated with radical mastectomy and postoperative radiation. The overall mean survival time was 25 months, and five patients were alive at 5 years. They concluded that this finding "would suggest that a more positive surgical attack on this highly malignant form of carcinoma [was] indicated" [3]. In 1981, Bozzetti et al. reported on a series of 114 patients with IBC. Eight patients underwent radical mastectomy alone, and only one was alive at 5 years, whereas 24 underwent radical mastectomy followed by radiation therapy, and seven were alive at 5 years [4]. These series had dismal results for patients treated with surgery alone and established that surgery in this setting yielded minimal survival benefit. In addition, local recurrence rates of approximately 50% were reported in patients treated with surgery alone [5, 6].

In the 1970s, doxorubicin-based chemotherapy was introduced. Shortly thereafter, oncologists began using chemotherapy in the neoadjuvant setting [7]. Neoadjuvant chemotherapy (NAC) was shown to improve overall survival time in patients with IBC, although local recurrence rates continued to be high [8–10]. Continued advancements in NAC regimens, including the introduction of taxanes and herceptin, have perpetuated improvements in both overall survival and local recurrence in patients with IBC [11–17]. The current recommendation of the panel at the First International Conference on IBC is a multimodality approach to treatment including NAC, modified radical mastectomy, and postoperative radiation therapy [18].

7.2 Selection of Surgical Candidates

Most patients with IBC have locoregional disease at diagnosis and are therefore initially considered inoperable. NAC is recommended for potentially shrinking the primary tumor and/or eradicating axillary disease, thereby rendering previously inoperable patients eligible for definitive surgical therapy. This approach has been reported to be successful in 86–95% of patients [11, 19, 20]. Kell and Morrow noted a trend toward increased use of mastectomy in multimodality treatment of IBC, despite a change in the use of surgery from an initial modality to a post-NAC modality [21].

Response to NAC should be monitored using both physical examination and radiographic imaging. Physical examination should be performed every 6–9 weeks during chemotherapy [22]. Imaging for assessment of response should be performed at the conclusion of chemotherapy and should be compared to baseline imaging. The panel at the First International Conference on IBC recommends using both mammography and ultrasonography to evaluate response to NAC. In addition, although data are limited, magnetic resonance imaging is recommended if parenchymal lesions are not detected on routine imaging or prior to enrollment in protocols examining the role of breast magnetic resonance imaging in patients with IBC [18]. Pictures of the affected breast are also required to determine the surgical field.

Patients who do not respond to NAC have lower rates of both local control and survival than patients who do respond [21]. Thus, definitive surgical therapy should be undertaken only in patients who respond to NAC, as there is no benefit from surgery in patients who have no significant response to NAC [22–25]. Thoms et al. showed that a partial response to NAC resulted in a lower local control rate (33%) following definitive surgical therapy than did a complete response (89%) [7]. Harris et al. examined mastectomy specimens for the degree of response to NAC and reported that 5- and 10-year overall survival rates were 52% and 31%, respectively, in patients with a partial response and 65% and 46%, respectively, in complete responders [26]. Surgical therapy is necessary for those with favorable response to NAC, because physical examination and imaging modalities underestimate the amount of residual disease in approximately 60% of patients with IBC [27, 28].

Surgical planning is important for optimizing outcomes. The surgical field must incorporate all involved skin. However, it is important to leave enough skin to ensure wound closure without tension, as tension may result in wound breakdown, which would delay the administration of radiation [29]. The current recommended definitive surgical treatment in patients who have responded to NAC is modified radical mastectomy [18].

7.3   Contraindicated Operations in Patients with IBC

Breast conserving therapy, skin-sparing mastectomy, and nipple-sparing mastectomy are contraindicated in patients with IBC. IBC is characterized by a diffuse pattern of extensive intraparenchymal lymphovascular invasion with tumor emboli. This diffuse pattern of disease involvement impedes obtaining negative margins, which is the primary oncologic principle in any patient with breast cancer [18]. Outcomes in patients with IBC are closely linked to margin status [30]. Consequently, use of breast conserving therapy, skin-sparing mastectomy, and nipple-sparing mastectomy are all oncologically inappropriate and thus contraindicated in patients with IBC.

7.4   Surgical Evaluation and Treatment of Axillary Disease in Patients with IBC

Although sentinel lymph node biopsy (SLNB) is the standard of care for axillary lymph node evaluation in breast cancer, this technique is currently contraindicated in patients with IBC. IBC results in lymphatic blockage by tumor cells, thus hindering localization of the sentinel lymph node (SLN) with either blue dye or radioactive colloid. In addition, SLNB following NAC has been a debated topic. The National Surgical Adjuvant Breast and Bowel Project (NSABP) B-27 addressed the use of SLNB after NAC and concluded that SLNB is suitable for patients with operable breast cancer after NAC [31]. Classe et al. evaluated the use of SLNB after NAC in patients with advanced breast cancer. The detection rate, false-negative rate, and accuracy of SLN detection did not differ between patients treated with or without NAC [32]. Stearns et al. described the use of SLNB in women with locally advanced breast cancer, including IBC. The overall SLN detection rate was 85%, and concordance between SLNB and axillary lymph node dissection was 90%. The overall false-negative rate and negative predictive value were 14% and 73%, respectively. However, when patients with IBC were excluded from the analysis, the false-negative rate and negative predictive value were 6% and 88%, respectively. They concluded that axillary disease could not be reliably staged with SLNB after NAC in patients with IBC [33]. Currently, the standard of care for evaluation and treatment of axillary disease in patients with IBC is axillary lymph node dissection [18].

7.5   Issues Surrounding Reconstruction

Although postmastectomy reconstruction is an eventual option in patients with IBC, the timing of reconstruction is of utmost importance [34]. Postmastectomy radiation therapy is required for patients with IBC, and current recommendations include incorporating the supraclavicular and internal mammary lymph nodes as well as the chest wall and axilla (i.e., traditional four-field postmastectomy radiation therapy). Immediate reconstruction in these patients may limit the delivery of radiation, including radiation to the internal mammary nodes, and thus may negatively affect oncologic outcomes [35, 36]. In addition, postmastectomy radiation therapy may negatively affect cosmesis [37–39]. Therefore, delayed reconstruction is routinely recommended for patients with IBC.

7.6   Conclusion

As the treatment of IBC evolves, surgical therapy will continue to be an integral part of a multimodality treatment approach. In patients who have had complete resolution of inflammatory changes of the breast following NAC, the standard of care is modified radical mastectomy with adjuvant radiation therapy. Currently, breast conserving therapy, skin-sparing mastectomy, nipple-sparing mastectomy, SLNB, and immediate breast reconstruction are contraindicated.

References

1. Lee BJ, Tannenbaum NE (1924) Inflammatory carcinoma of the breast. Clin Radiol 39:580–595
2. Haagensen CD, Stout AP (1951) Carcinoma of the breast. III. Results of treatment. Ann Surg 134:151–170

3. Barber KW Jr, Dockerty MB, Clagett OT (1961) Inflammatory carcinoma of the breast. Surg Gynecol Obstet 112:406–410

4. Bozzetti F, Saccozzi R, De Lena M, Salvadori B (1981) Inflammatory cancer of the breast: analysis of 114 cases. J Surg Oncol 18:355–361

5. Barker JL, Nelson AJ, Montague ED (1976) Inflammatory carcinoma of the breast. Radiology 121:173–176

6. Zucali R, Uslenghi C, Kenda R, Bonadonna G (1976) Natural history and survival of inoperable breast cancer treated with radiotherapy and radiotherapy followed by radical mastectomy. Cancer 37:1422–1431

7. Thoms WW Jr, McNeese MD, Fletcher GH, Buzdar AU, Singletary SE, Oswald MJ (1989) Multimodal treatment for inflammatory breast cancer. Int J Radiat Oncol Biol Phys 17:739–745

8. Buzdar AU, Montague ED, Barker JL, Hortobagyi GN, Blumenschein GR (1981) Management of inflammatory carcinoma of breast with combined modality approach – an update. Cancer 47:2537–2542

9. Knight CD Jr, Martin JK Jr, Welch JS, Ingle JN, Gaffey TA, Martinez A (1986) Surgical considerations after chemotherapy and radiation therapy for inflammatory breast cancer. Surgery 99:385–391

10. Zylberberg B, Salat-Baroux J, Ravina JH, Dormont D, Amiel JP, Diebold P, Izrael V (1982) Initial chemoimmunotherapy in inflammatory carcinoma of the breast. Cancer 49:1537–1543

11. Cristofanilli M, Buzdar AU, Sneige N, Smith T, Wasaff B, Ibrahim N, Booser D, Rivera E, Murray JL, Valero V, Ueno N, Singletary ES, Hunt K, Strom E, McNeese M, Stelling C, Hortobagyi GN (2001) Paclitaxel in the multimodality treatment for inflammatory breast carcinoma. Cancer 92:1775–1782

12. Cristofanilli M, Gonzalez-Angulo AM, Buzdar AU, Kau SW, Frye DK, Hortobagyi GN (2004) Paclitaxel improves the prognosis in estrogen receptor negative inflammatory breast cancer: the M.D. Anderson Cancer Center experience. Clin Breast Cancer 4:415–419

13. Dawood S, Gonzalez-Angulo AM, Peintinger F, Broglio K, Symmans WF, Kau SW, Islam R, Hortobagyi GN, Buzdar AU (2007) Efficacy and safety of neoadjuvant trastuzumab combined with paclitaxel and epirubicin: a retrospective review of the M.D. Anderson experience. Cancer 110:1195–1200

14. Hurley J, Doliny P, Reis I, Silva O, Gomez-Fernandez C, Velez P, Pauletti G, Powell JE, Pegram MD, Slamon DJ (2006) Docetaxel, cisplatin, and trastuzumab as primary systemic therapy for human epidermal growth factor receptor 2-positive locally advanced breast cancer. J Clin Oncol 24:1831–1838

15. Van Pelt AE, Mohsin S, Elledge RM, Hilsenbeck SG, Gutierrez MC, Lucci A Jr, Kalidas M, Granchi T, Scott BG, Allred DC, Chang JC (2003) Neoadjuvant trastuzumab and docetaxel in breast cancer: preliminary results. Clin Breast Cancer 4:348–353

16. Limentani SA, Brufsky AM, Erban JK, Jahanzeb M, Lewis D (2003) Phase II study of neoadjuvant docetaxel, vinorelbine, and trastuzumab followed by surgery and adjuvant doxorubicin plus cyclophosphamide in women with human epidermal growth factor receptor 2 –overexpressing locally advanced breast cancer. J Clin Oncol 25:1232–1238

17. Burstein HJ, Harris LN, Gelman R, Lester SC, Nunes RA, Kaelin CM, Parker LM, Ellisen LW, Kuter I, Gadd MA, Christian RL, Kennedy PR, Borges VF, Bunnell CA, Younger J, Smith BL, Winer EP (2003) Preoperative therapy with trastuzumab and paclitaxel followed by sequential adjuvant doxorubicin/cyclophosphamide for HER2 overexpressing stage II or III breast cancer: a pilot study. J Clin Oncol 21:46–53

18. Dawood S, Merajver SD, Viens P, Vermeulen PB, Swain SM, Buchholz TA, Dirix LY, Levine PH, Lucci A, Krishnamurthy S, Robertson FM, Woodward WA, Yang WT, Ueno NT, Cristofanilli M (2011) International expert panel on inflammatory breast cancer: consensus statement for standardized diagnosis and treatment. Ann Oncol 22:515–523

19. Ueno NT, Buzdar AU, Singletary SE, Ames FC, McNeese MD, Holmes FA, Theriault RL, Strom EA, Wasaff BJ, Asmar L, Frye D, Hortobagyi GN (1997) Combined-modality treatment

of inflammatory breast carcinoma: twenty years of experience at M.D. Anderson Cancer Center. Cancer Chemother Pharmacol 40:321–329

20. Chevallier B, Roche H, Oliver JP, Chollet P, Hurteloup P (1993) Inflammatory breast cancer. Pilot study of intensive induction chemotherapy (FEC-HD) results in a high histologic response rate. Am J Clin Oncol 16:223–228

21. Kell MR, Morrow M (2005–2006) Surgical aspects of inflammatory breast cancer. Breast Dis 22:67–73

22. Kaufmann M, von Minckwitz G, Bear HD, Buzdar A, McGale P, Bonnefoi H, Colleoni M, Denkert C, Eiermann W, Jackesz R, Makris A, Miller W, Pierga JY, Semiglazov V, Schneeweiss A, Souchon R, Stearns V, Untch M, Loibl S (2007) Recommendations from an international expert panel on the use of neoadjuvant (primary) systemic treatment of operable breast cancer: new perspectives 2006. Ann Oncol 18:1927–1934

23. Arthur DW, Schmidt-Ullrich RK, Friedman RB, Wazer DE, Kachnic LA, Amir C, Bear HD, Hackney MH, Smith TJ, Lawrence W Jr (1999) Accelerated superfractionated radiotherapy for inflammatory breast carcinoma: complete response predicts outcome and allows for breast conservation. Int J Radiat Oncol Biol Phys 44:289–296

24. De Boer RH, Allum WH, Ebbs SR, Gui GP, Johnston SR, Sacks NP, Walsh G, Ashley S, Smith IE (2000) Multimodality therapy in inflammatory breast cancer: is there a place for surgery? Ann Oncol 11:1147–1153

25. Swain SM, Sorace RA, Bagley CS, Danforth DN Jr, Bader J, Wesley MN, Steinberg SM, Lippman ME (1987) Neoadjuvant chemotherapy in the combined modality approach of locally advanced nonmetastatic breast cancer. Cancer Res 47:3889–3894

26. Harris EE, Schultz D, Bertsch H, Fox K, Glick J, Solin LJ (2003) Ten-year outcome after combined modality therapy for inflammatory breast cancer. Int J Radiat Oncol Biol Phys 55:1200–1208

27. Hortobagyi G, Singletary S, Strom E (2000) Treatment of locally advanced and inflammatory breast cancer. Lippincott, Williams & Wilkins, Philadelphia

28. Vlastos G, Fornage BD, Mirza NQ, Bedi D, Lenert JT, Winchester DJ, Tolley SM, Ames FC, Ross MI, Feig BW, Hunt KK, Buzdar AU, Singletary SE (2000) The correlation of axillary ultrasonography with histologic breast cancer downstaging after induction chemotherapy. Am J Surg 179:446–452

29. Woodward WA, Cristofanilli M (2009) Inflammatory breast cancer. Semin Radiat Oncol 19:256–265

30. Curcio LD, Rupp E, Williams WL, Chu DZ, Clarke K, Odom-Maryon T, Ellenhorn JD, Somlo G, Wagman LD (1999) Beyond palliative mastectomy in inflammatory breast cancer – a reassessment of margin status. Ann Surg Oncol 6:249–254

31. Mamounas EP, Brown A, Anderson S, Smith R, Julian T, Miller B, Bear HD, Caldwell CB, Walker AP, Mikkelson WM, Stauffer JS, Robidoux A, Theoret H, Soran A, Fisher B, Wickerham DL, Wolmark N (2006) Sentinel node biopsy after neoadjuvant chemotherapy in breast cancer: results from national surgical adjuvant breast and bowel project protocol B-27. J Clin Oncol 23:2694–2702

32. Classe JM, Bordes V, Campion L, Mignotte H, Dravet F, Leveque J, Sagan C, Dupre PF, Body G, Giard S (2009) Sentinel lymph node biopsy after neoadjuvant chemotherapy for advanced breast cancer: results of ganglion sentinelle et chimiotherapie neoadjuvante, a French prospective multicentric study. J Clin Oncol 27:726–732

33. Stearns V, Ewing CA, Slack R, Penannen MF, Hayes DF, Tsangaris TN (2002) Sentinel lymphadenectomy after neoadjuvant chemotherapy for breast cancer may reliably represent the axilla except for inflammatory breast cancer. Ann Surg Oncol 9:235–242

34. Chin PL, Andersen JS, Somlo G, Chu DZ, Schwarz RE, Ellenhorn JD (2000) Esthetic reconstruction after mastectomy for inflammatory breast cancer: is it worthwhile? J Am Coll Surg 190:304–309

35. Schechter NR, Strom EA, Perkins GH, Arzu I, McNeese MD, Langstein HN, Kronowitz SJ, Meric-Bernstam F, Babiera G, Hunt KK, Hortobagyi GN, Buchholz TA (2005) Immediate breast reconstruction can impact postmastectomy irradiation. Am J Clin Oncol 28:485–494

36. Motwani SB, Strom EA, Schechter NR, Butler CE, Lee GK, Langstein HN, Kronowitz SJ, Meric-Bernstam F, Ibrahim NK, Buchholz TA (2006) The impact of immediate breast reconstruction on the technical delivery of postmastectomy radiotherapy. Int J Radiat Oncol Biol Phys 66:76–82
37. Behranwala KA, Dua RS, Ross GM, Ward A, A'hern R, Gui GP (2006) The influence of radiotherapy on capsule formation and aesthetic outcome after immediate breast reconstruction using biodimensional anatomical expander implants. J Plast Reconstr Aesthet Surg 59:1043–1051
38. Tran NV, Chang DW, Gupta A, Kroll SS, Robb GL (2001) Comparison of immediate and delayed free TRAM flap breast reconstruction in patients receiving postmastectomy radiation therapy. Plast Reconstr Surg 108:78–82
39. Rogers NE, Allen RJ (2002) Radiation effects on breast reconstruction with the deep inferior epigastric perforator flap. Plast Reconstr Surg 109:1919–1924; discussion 1925–1926

Chapter 8
Radiation Therapy for Inflammatory Breast Cancer

Thomas A. Buchholz, Ian Bristol, and Wendy Woodward

Abstract Radiation therapy has always played an important role in the multidisciplinary management of inflammatory breast cancer (IBC). Before chemotherapy became available, radiation therapy was often the sole treatment modality, and although short-term locoregional control could be achieved in 50% of patients, nearly all patients rapidly developed metastatic disease and died. Prognosis has improved, and radiation is now most commonly used as adjuvant treatment after neoadjuvant systemic chemotherapy and a modified radical mastectomy.

IBC remains the most therapeutically challenging breast cancer clinical subtype for radiation oncologists. Because the disease tends to track through dermal lymphatics and recur at treatment field margins, treatment field designs must be comprehensive and broad. IBC also requires high radiation dosages. Our institution utilizes an accelerated hyperfractionation schedule, which data suggest may benefit patients with the highest risk, including those who are young, have poor clinical or pathological response to neoadjuvant treatment, and have close or positive margins after mastectomy. In addition, the subgroup of patients with triple-negative IBC (i.e., disease that lacks receptors for estrogen, progesterone, and HER2/neu) also maintains relevant local-regional recurrence risks despite aggressive radiation treatments. Accordingly, new strategies to selectively enhance radiation effects for patients with triple-negative IBC are needed.

Keywords Radiation • Hyperfractionation • Local-regional control • Local-regional treatment • Dose escalation • Mastectomy • Neoadjuvant chemotherapy • Lymphedema • Fibrosis

T.A. Buchholz, M.D. (✉) • W. Woodward, M.D., Ph.D.
Department of Radiation Oncology, Unit 1202, The University of Texas
MD Anderson Cancer Center, 1515 Holcombe Blvd., Houston, TX 77030, USA
e-mail: tbuchhol@mdanderson.org

I. Bristol, M.D.
Division of Radiation Oncology, Spectrum Medical Group, 324 Gannett Drive,
Suite 200, South Portland, ME 04106

N.T. Ueno and M. Cristofanilli (eds.), *Inflammatory Breast Cancer: An Update*, 75
DOI 10.1007/978-94-007-3907-9_8, © Springer Science+Business Media B.V. 2012

8.1 Introduction

Inflammatory breast cancer (IBC) remains a challenge for all professions involved in its treatment. Rapid disease progression, resistance to chemotherapy and radiotherapy, and early distant dissemination are well-described hallmarks of IBC [1, 2]. However, advances have been achieved: whereas IBC was once a universally fatal disease, patients who receive aggressive multimodality therapy for disease that is confined to the local-regional areas at diagnosis are potentially curable. Fortunately, the majority of patients are in this population. A recent study of patients in the United States with IBC showed that approximately 70% had locoregional disease without distant metastases at initial diagnosis [3].

Curative treatment of IBC requires a carefully coordinated multidisciplinary team approach. Patients with IBC require chemotherapy, mastectomy, postmastectomy radiation therapy, and, when indicated, hormonal therapy and anti-HER2/neu treatments. The success of systemic therapies in reducing the risk of developing distant metastases has heightened the importance of eradicating local-regional disease, which has thereby increased the importance of radiation therapy. Numerous studies have indicated that obtaining locoregional control in patients with IBC increases survival rates [4–6]. In part, these results reflect the fact that locoregional recurrence in patients with IBC is invariably associated with distant dissemination and death from disease [7–9].

Radiation therapy for IBC has a long history. Before combination chemotherapy became available, IBC was almost uniformly fatal, and radiation as the sole modality of therapy was often considered the standard. Without effective systemic treatment, fewer than 5% of patients treated with surgery and/or radiotherapy survived past 5 years, and the expected median survival time for these patients was less than 15 months [1]. Local recurrence rates with surgery and/or radiotherapy were also high at approximately 50% [10, 11]. Many patients had local disease recurrences immediately after mastectomy, and accordingly, many considered IBC to represent inoperable disease; therefore, radiation as the sole treatment modality became the standard.

The introduction of doxorubicin-based chemotherapy improved the 5-year survival rates from nearly 0% to 30% to 40% [12, 13]. In addition, when it was introduced as neoadjuvant therapy, doxorubicin led to clinically significant responses in the majority of patients, which made mastectomy a feasible option for many patients who were not initially candidates for surgery. This benefit led to the reinclusion of mastectomy in the therapeutic strategy. Radiotherapy continued to play a major role in the overall treatment of IBC, in that locoregional recurrence rates after chemotherapy or surgery alone remained high.

IBC is noted for its propensity to progress rapidly, suggesting that this type of cancer has a high degree of tumor cell repopulation. Repopulation is known to contribute to local recurrence within radiation fields, in that the tumor cells that survive after a daily radiation treatment can repopulate to close to their original tumor burden before the next daily treatment. One strategy for overcoming the effects of repopulation is shortening the overall duration of the treatment course thereby reducing the time for repopulation. This strategy has been investigated in IBC treated with radiation administered twice a day rather than once a day in an effort to reduce the overall radiation treatment time. These locoregional treatment strategies have proven successful. Indeed, by combining neoadjuvant chemotherapy, mastectomy, and postmastectomy hyperfractionated radiation therapy, investigators have reported locoregional control rates of ~85% [4]. However, this approach also increases normal tissue toxicity, and further work has indentified predictive factors to help determine which subsets of patients with IBC are candidates for this more aggressive locoregional approach.

This chapter will review many of the advances in the locoregional management of IBC, with a particular focus on the role of radiation treatment. The relevant literature pertaining to these local treatment options will be reviewed as will radiation treatment techniques.

8.2 Role of Radiotherapy

Radiation has been a standard component of IBC treatment since the 1940s, at which time radiotherapy was used as the primary treatment modality [14, 15]. Because of the high incidence of distant metastases, radiation treatments during this era were primarily palliative and were associated with a 50% local recurrence rate and a 5-year survival rate of nearly 0% [10].

The first attempt to improve radiation treatment outcomes by altering the radiation fractionation schedule was conducted at The University of Texas MD Anderson Cancer Center. IBC was known to have the potential to proliferate rapidly [16], and investigators sought to circumvent this rapid tumor-cell growth rate by incorporating accelerated hyperfractionated radiotherapy into its definitive treatment [14]. In the treatment schedule investigated, two fractions of radiation were administered per day instead of one and the overall radiotherapy course was shortened from 7 weeks to a little more than 4 weeks. The initial report on this strategy suggested an improvement. Specifically, 69 patients treated between 1948 and 1972 with once-daily fractions to a total radiation dose of 50 Gy to the breast and draining lymphatics followed by a boost to 60–65 Gy over a 7-week course had a 46% local recurrence rate. In contrast, 11 patients treated in 1973 with twice-daily radiation to the breast and draining lymphatics to a total dose of 51–54 Gy delivered over 4 weeks, with a boost dose of 15–20 Gy (also administered twice daily) to the gross tumor, had only a 27% risk of locoregional recurrence. Mastectomy and chemotherapy, which are current standards of treatment, were not investigated in this small pilot study, but it provided proof of concept for this accelerated treatment schedule.

During the 1970s, doxorubicin-based chemotherapy was introduced as a regimen for the management of IBC. This regimen proved to be a major advancement, as chemotherapy was found to significantly reduce the risk of developing metastatic disease. However, many patients who underwent radiation therapy followed by adjuvant chemotherapy continued to have high rates of locoregional recurrence, even with twice-daily fractionation schedules [14]. Therefore, a new sequencing of therapies was investigated in the late 1970s [17]. Neoadjuvant chemotherapy was introduced, and high rates of tumor response were noted; thus, mastectomy became an appropriate treatment option for most patients. This proved to be a significant therapeutic advance in locoregional management. The initial MD Anderson experience with neoadjuvant doxorubicin consisted of 61 patients, 92% of whom were able to undergo mastectomy after neoadjuvant chemotherapy, whereas the remaining five (8%) patients required preoperative radiation therapy. Among the patients who underwent mastectomy, nine had pathologically positive margins and underwent immediate postoperative radiation therapy. The remaining 46 patients completed the planned course of adjuvant chemotherapy prior to beginning radiation therapy. Of these, 14 (30%) received radiotherapy delivered to the chest wall and draining lymphatics using standard daily fractionation to 50 Gy given over 5 weeks. The remaining 32 (70%) were treated with twice-daily fractionations to a total dose of 45 Gy delivered over 3 weeks. All patients received a boost to the chest wall to a maximum dose of 60 Gy. Six patients had local disease progression, and nine had distant disease spread prior to receiving radiation therapy.

This study revealed an overall 5-year disease-free survival rate of 27%, a marked improvement in outcome. Initial clinical response to chemotherapy was associated with improved 5-year actuarial disease-free survival rates (70% for complete responders versus 35% for the partial response group; all patients in the no-response group had disease recurrence within 34 months). The 5-year actuarial locoregional control rates were 89% in patients with a complete response, 68% in those with a partial response, 33% those with no response, and 58% overall.

The next study built on these results, and the investigators attempted to escalate the dose of hyperfractionated radiation by approximately 10% to address the continued high rates of recurrence following postmastectomy radiation therapy [4]. In this study, the twice-daily regimen was delivered in 34 fractions over 3.5 weeks to fields encompassing the chest wall and the supraclavicular, infraclavicular, and internal mammary lymph nodes to a total dose of 51 Gy. Subsequently, a 15-Gy boost was delivered to the chest wall at a dosage of 1.5 Gy twice daily over 5 days, yielding a total dose of 66 Gy. In a comparison of patients treated before 1986 (n=61) versus those treated after 1986 (n=54), a significant improvement in locoregional control rates was noted with the dose escalation, and a similar trend was noted in disease-free and overall survival rates. The locoregional control rates for those treated with 66 Gy versus 60 Gy were 84% versus 58% at 5 years and 77% versus 58% at 10 years, respectively (p=0.04).

Other investigators have also studied dose fractionation schedules and/or dose escalation and have come to similar conclusions [5, 18, 19]. Pisansky et al. reported a 26% local recurrence rate in 16 patients who received once-daily preoperative radiation to a dose of 50.4 Gy over 28 days and an 8% local recurrence rate in 13 patients who received twice-daily preoperative radiation to a dose of 44.2 Gy over 13 days [19]. In addition, Liauw and colleagues reported their experience with 61 patients with IBC and found that doses of postmastectomy radiation >60 Gy resulted in a lower risk of locoregional disease progression. Local control was also strongly predictive of longer cause-specific survival (p = 0.0003) [5].

Bristol et al. updated the MD Anderson protocol by using high-dose accelerated hyperfractionation after neoadjuvant chemotherapy and mastectomy. This series consisted of 256 patients with nonmetastatic IBC treated with neoadjuvant chemotherapy with a curative intent for subsequent mastectomy and postmastectomy radiation therapy. The 192 patients who were able to complete the planned course of treatment had much better outcomes than those who had early disease progression before undergoing surgery or completing radiation therapy. The dose escalation from 60 Gy to 66 Gy was found to improve local-regional control and the outcome of patients with any one of the following high-risk features: aged 45 years or younger, less than a partial response to neoadjuvant chemotherapy, or close or positive surgical margins. Identifying the patients who did not require dose escalation was important because the late toxicity rate associated with 66 Gy was much higher than that associated with 60 Gy (5-year rates of grade 3 or higher complications: 29% vs. 15%, respectively). These data provided the rationale for administering 60 Gy in older patients who achieve an excellent clinical and pathological response to neoadjuvant chemotherapy [20].

8.3   Biological Subtype and Local-Regional Outcome

Breast cancer is increasingly being recognized as a heterogeneous disease with molecular subtypes that are driven in part by the estrogen receptor (ER), progesterone receptor (PR), and HER2/neu signaling pathways. Few data, however, are available about the biological significance of ER and HER2/neu with respect to outcomes of locoregional treatment of IBC. Investigators from MD Anderson recently updated and reanalyzed data on a cohort of 316 patients with nonmetastatic IBC treated with curative intent between 1974 and 2008 who had known ER, PR, and HER2/neu status. In a Cox regression analysis, the triple-negative (i.e., disease that lacks ER, PR, and HER2/neu) phenotype was associated with lower rates of locoregional control and overall survival relative to phenotypes with the expression of any of the receptors. The 5-year rate of locoregional recurrence in patients with triple-negative disease was 39% despite aggressive treatment, and the 5-year rate of distant metastasis was 57%. These data indicate that new therapeutic strategies are needed for patients with triple-negative IBC [21].

8.4   Breast Conservation Versus Mastectomy

As previously indicated, the optimal reported outcomes for patients with IBC have come from aggressive trimodality treatment with neoadjuvant systemic therapy, mastectomy, and postmastectomy radiation therapy. Although some studies have questioned the value of mastectomy for patients with an excellent clinical response to neoadjuvant chemotherapy [22, 23], the vast majority of data supports its routine use because it improves local control and may improve survival [6, 7, 12, 24]. For example, Perez and colleagues [24] retrospectively reviewed the outcome of 179 patients with IBC treated with radiation alone or in combination with chemotherapy (n = 68), radiation plus mastectomy (n = 25), or trimodality therapy (n = 86). The 5-year local control rates for the three groups were 30%, 76%, and 79%, respectively. Similarly, Panades et al. [6] reported on 308 patients who underwent chemotherapy and found that the 10-year local-recurrence-free survival rate was significantly higher in patients who underwent mastectomy than in those who did not (~60% versus 34%, respectively; p = 0.0001). A multivariate analysis in which other potential prognostic factors were considered revealed that the use of mastectomy remained a significant factor for improved local-recurrence-free survival (p = 0.04).

The majority of studies that have assessed the efficacy of breast conservation in selected patients who have achieved a complete response to chemotherapy have revealed local control rates that are less than optimal [25–30]. A trial of breast conservation in patients with advanced disease, including IBC, who achieved a complete clinical response was conducted at the National Cancer Institute from 1976 to 1986 [30]. Of the 46 patients with IBC [25], 15 (33%) achieved a biopsy-proven complete response and were treated with definitive radiation alone. The remaining 31 patients with residual disease underwent mastectomy and radiation therapy. Surprisingly, the locoregional control rate was higher in the 31 patients with residual disease than in the 15 patients with negative biopsies (77% versus 60%, respectively), presumably because those with residual disease were treated with mastectomy rather than with a breast conservation approach. Other studies confirm these results. Brun and colleagues reported a 54% local failure rate with attempts at breast conservation, and Chevallier and colleagues reported a 61% local failure rate in patients treated with breast conservation after they had achieved a complete response to neoadjuvant chemotherapy [26, 27].

Taken together, these data strongly support the routine use of both mastectomy and radiation as locoregional therapy for patients with nonmetastatic IBC. Furthermore, this therapeutic strategy is critically important, because local recurrence of IBC is invariably fatal [7–9]. Mastectomy seems most critical for patients who have an excellent response to chemotherapy, because they are the patients most likely to be cured [20].

8.5 Radiotherapy Techniques

Optimal radiation treatment requires the delivery of a dose to the targeted regions that are at risk for locoregional recurrence while minimizing exposure to adjacent, uninvolved normal tissue. The radiation dose must be minimized to critical structures such as the heart and lungs. For patients treated after mastectomy, the target volumes include the chest wall and lymph nodes within the axillary, infraclavicular, supraclavicular, and internal mammary regions. A variety of field arranges can be used to achieve conformal dose delivery to the targeted region while sparing the dose to the heart and lungs. Treatment planning starts with patient immobilization in an optimal treatment position, which is typically supine on a 10- to 15-degree angle board with the ipsilateral arm abducted and externally rotated to move the arm away from the chest wall. After immobilization, a computed tomography (CT) simulation is performed and reference marks are placed. Fields are then designed virtually on the CT dataset. Contours can be digitized and should include targeted lymphatic regions such as the infraclavicular, supraclavicular, and internal mammary lymph nodes of the upper three intercostal spaces. Radiation doses are calculated and optimized using three-dimensional dose calculation algorithms. Optimization allows the dose to be modulated within the target volume to provide optimal dose homogeneity and minimize regions of hot spots and cold spots.

For patients with IBC, it is particularly important to design treatment fields that give broad coverage of the chest wall because IBC involves dermal lymphatics, which can lead to marginal recurrences at the radiation field borders. Multiple matching fields are required to provide this broad coverage with minimal dose to the heart and lungs. We recommend using a combination of medial electron fields that are matched to lateral photon tangent fields (Fig. 8.1). The electron field(s) can be divided to use various electron energies that allow for the dose to be delivered to deeper or more superficial targets, depending on the individual patient anatomy and the depth of targets and normal tissues. The electron field is angled and overlapped 3 mm with the tangent field to minimize the risk of under-dosing at the field junctions. Bolus is used during the first 2 weeks and as needed afterwards to ensure a brisk skin reaction. The supraclavicular fossa and axillary apex are treated in a matched photon field. We routinely contour the region of the level III axilla and the internal mammary lymph node region to assist in dosimetry planning.

For the accelerated hyperfractionation schedule, we prescribe a total dose to these fields of 51 Gy delivered in 34 fractions of 1.5 Gy that are given twice per day with a minimum 6-h interval between treatments. Subsequently, the chest wall is further boosted using two appositional electron fields to an additional 15 Gy, also at 1.5 Gy per fraction delivered twice daily over 5 days. Areas of involved lymph nodes that have not been resected also receive a boost dose of radiation to 10–16 Gy.

This treatment schedule is associated with short-term and long-term toxic effects. Because the dermal tissue is an important therapeutic target, skin-sparing techniques should be avoided. Correspondingly, most patients will experience a brisk erythema and desquamative changes in the skin over the chest wall. The degree of acute skin reaction has previously been found to correlate with locoregional recurrence [17]. Moist desquamation typically lasts 3–4 weeks, during which time patients may require analgesics. Late complications are a bigger concern, however, because they can negatively affect patients' long-term quality of life. Potential late complications include lymphedema, soft-tissue fibrosis, telangiectasia, and rib fractures.

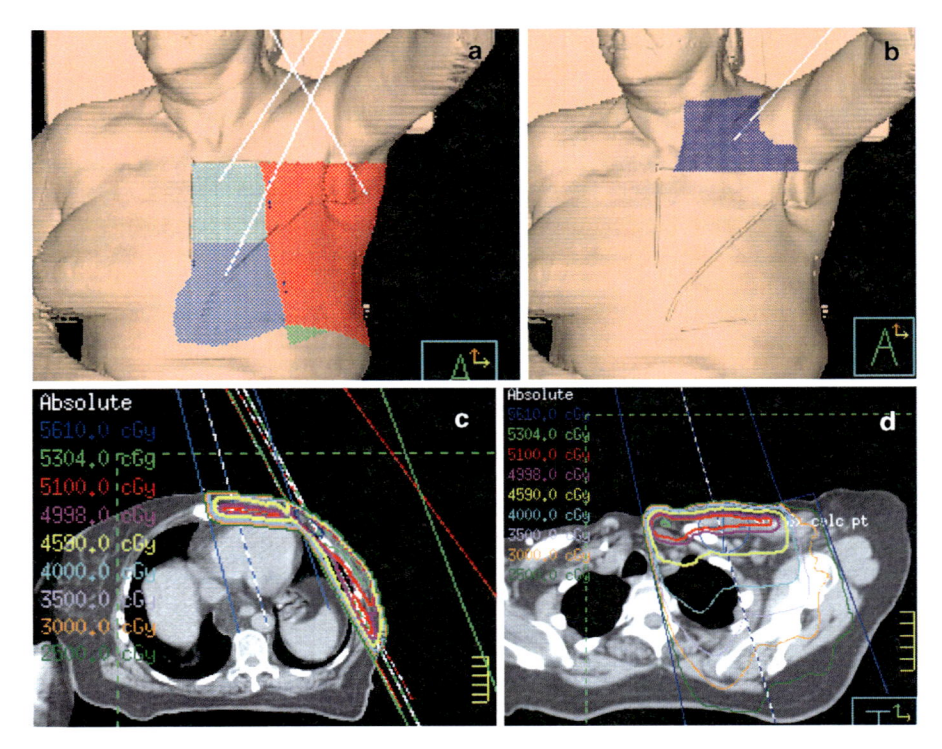

Fig. 8.1 (**a**) Skin rendering of radiation fields used to treat the chest wall and internal mammary lymph nodes of a patient with IBC. Two medial electron fields of different energies were used to treat the chest wall. The electron energies were determined to administer the dose deep enough to include the internal mammary lymph nodes in the upper interspaces but superficial enough to minimize exposure to the lungs and heart in the lower interspaces. These fields are matched to a lateral pair of tangent photon fields. (**b**) Skin rendering of the matched supraclavicular fossa photon fields for this patient. (**c**) Representative axial CT image of the fields from Fig. 8.1a. Note the very small volume of lung and heart receiving a high dose of radiation using this technique. (**d**) Representative axial CT image depicting the radiation beam targeting the supraclavicular field

8.6 Conclusions

Radiation remains a critical component of multimodality therapy for IBC. While the prognosis of IBC remains worse than that of noninflammatory breast cancer, the advances in treatment have offered patients the possibility of long-term survival and cure. Accordingly, patients who present with locoregional disease without distant metastases should be treated with curative intent. Optimally, this would include neoadjuvant systemic treatment, mastectomy, and postmastectomy radiation therapy with the consideration of an aggressive accelerated hyperfractionated schedule if the patient has high-risk features. Continued research is needed to develop new strategies to optimize systemic and locoregional treatment options for selected patients with IBC, such as those who respond poorly to initial neoadjuvant systemic treatments and those with triple-negative disease.

References

1. Bozzetti F, Saccozzi R, De Lena M, Salvadori B (1981) Inflammatory cancer of the breast: analysis of 114 cases. J Surg Oncol 18:355–361
2. Haagenson CD (1971) Diseases of the breast. WB Saunders Company, Philadelphia, pp 576–585
3. Wingo PA, Jamison PM, Young JL, Gargiullo P (2004) Population-based statistics for women diagnosed with inflammatory breast cancer (United States). Cancer Causes Control 15:321–328
4. Liao Z, Strom EA, Buzdar AU et al (2000) Locoregional irradiation for inflammatory breast cancer: effectiveness of dose escalation in decreasing recurrence. Int J Radiat Oncol Biol Phys 47:1191–1200
5. Liauw SL, Benda RK, Morris CG, Mendenhall NP (2004) Inflammatory breast carcinoma: outcomes with trimodality therapy for nonmetastatic disease. Cancer 100:920–928
6. Panades M, Olivotto IA, Speers CH et al (2005) Evolving treatment strategies for inflammatory breast cancer: a population-based survival analysis. J Clin Oncol 23:1941–1950
7. Fleming RY, Asmar L, Buzdar AU et al (1997) Effectiveness of mastectomy by response to induction chemotherapy for control in inflammatory breast carcinoma. Ann Surg Oncol 4:452–461
8. Hasbini A, Le Pechoux C, Roche B et al (2000) Alternating chemotherapy and hyperfractionated accelerated radiotherapy in non-metastatic inflammatory breast cancer. Cancer Radiother 4:265–273
9. Thomas F, Arriagada R, Spielmann M et al (1995) Pattern of failure in patients with inflammatory breast cancer treated by alternating radiotherapy and chemotherapy. Cancer 76:2286–2290
10. Barker JL, Nelson AJ, Montague ED (1976) Inflammatory carcinoma of the breast. Radiology 121:173–176
11. Zucali R, Uslenghi C, Kenda R, Bonadonna G (1976) Natural history and survival of inoperable breast cancer treated with radiotherapy and radiotherapy followed by radical mastectomy. Cancer 37:1422–1431
12. Fields JN, Perez CA, Kuske RR et al (1989) Inflammatory carcinoma of the breast: treatment results on 107 patients. Int J Radiat Oncol Biol Phys 17:249–255
13. Krutchik AN, Buzdar AU, Blumenschein GR et al (1979) Combined chemoimmunotherapy and radiation therapy of inflammatory breast carcinoma. J Surg Oncol 11:325–332
14. Barker JL, Montague ED, Peters LJ (1980) Clinical experience with irradiation of inflammatory carcinoma of the breast with and without elective chemotherapy. Cancer 45:625–629
15. Levine PH, Steinhorn SC, Ries LG, Aron JL (1985) Inflammatory breast cancer: the experience of the surveillance, epidemiology, and end results (SEER) program. J Natl Cancer Inst 74:291–297
16. Thames HD Jr, Peters LJ, Withers HR, Fletcher GH (1983) Accelerated fractionation vs hyperfractionation: rationales for several treatments per day. Int J Radiat Oncol Biol Phys 9:127–138
17. Thoms WW Jr, McNeese MD, Fletcher GH et al (1989) Multimodal treatment for inflammatory breast cancer. Int J Radiat Oncol Biol Phys 17:739–745
18. Chu AM, Cope O, Russo R et al (1980) Treatment of early stage breast cancer by limited surgery and radical irradiation. Int J Radiat Oncol Biol Phys 6:25–30
19. Pisansky TM, Schaid DJ, Loprinzi CL et al (1992) Inflammatory breast cancer: integration of irradiation, surgery, and chemotherapy. Am J Clin Oncol 15:376–387
20. Bristol IJ, Woodward WA, Strom EA et al (2008) Local-regional control of recurrent breast carcinoma after mastectomy: does hyperfractionated accelerated radiotherapy improve local control? Int J Radiat Oncol Biol Phys 72(2):474–484
21. Li J, Gonzalez-Angulo AM, Yu TK et al (2011) Triple-negative/basal subtype predicts poor overall survival and high locoregional relapse in inflammatory breast cancer. Oncologist 16(12):1675–1683

22. Arthur DW, Schmidt-Ullrich RK, Friedman RB et al (1999) Accelerated superfractionated radiotherapy for inflammatory breast carcinoma: complete response predicts outcome and allows for breast conservation. Int J Radiat Oncol Biol Phys 44:289–296
23. De Boer RH, Allum WH, Ebbs SR et al (2000) Multimodality therapy in inflammatory breast cancer: is there a place for surgery? Ann Oncol 11:1147–1153
24. Perez CA, Fields JN, Fracasso PM et al (1994) Management of locally advanced carcinoma of the breast. II. Inflammatory carcinoma. Cancer 74:466–476
25. Low JA, Berman AW, Steinberg SM et al (2004) Long-term follow-up for locally advanced and inflammatory breast cancer patients treated with multimodality therapy. J Clin Oncol 22:4067–4074
26. Brun B, Otmezguine Y, Feuilhade F et al (1988) Treatment of inflammatory breast cancer with combination chemotherapy and mastectomy versus breast conservation. Cancer 61:1096–1103
27. Chevallier B, Asselain B, Kunlin A et al (1987) Inflammatory breast cancer. Determination of prognostic factors by univariate and multivariate analysis. Cancer 60:897–902
28. Pierce LJ, Lippman M, Ben-Baruch N et al (1992) The effect of systemic therapy on local-regional control in locally advanced breast cancer. Int J Radiat Oncol Biol Phys 23:949–960
29. Swain SM, Lippman ME (1989) Treatment of patients with inflammatory breast cancer. Important Adv Oncol:129–150
30. Swain SM, Sorace RA, Bagley CS et al (1987) Neoadjuvant chemotherapy in the combined modality approach of locally advanced nonmetastatic breast cancer. Cancer Res 47:3889–3894

Chapter 9
Systemic and Targeted Therapy

Hideko Yamauchi, Teruo Yamauchi, Naoto T. Ueno, and Vicente Valero

Abstract Historically, single-modality therapy failed to control inflammatory breast cancer (IBC), a very aggressive and rare type of advanced breast cancer with poor prognosis. With the introduction of multimodality treatment (primary and adjuvant systemic therapy, surgery, and radiation therapy), the prognosis of inflammatory breast cancer (IBC) has significantly improved. Current standard treatment of IBC consists of primary systemic therapy, including trastuzumab for HER-2/*neu* overexpressing IBC, followed by surgery with mastectomy and complete axillary lymph node dissection, and subsequently radiation therapy.

Novel agents for systemic therapy have been investigated. Lapatinib, neratinib, pertuzumab, TDM-1, are the most promising targeted therapy in HER2-positive IBC. Molecular targets for vasculolymphatic processes—angiogenesis, lymphangiogenesis, and vasculogenesis—have shown greater potential in IBC than in non-IBC. Recent developments in molecular targeting toward WISP3 and RhoC GTPase may also be effective against IBC. Although loss of E-cadherin is a hallmark of invasive disease and epithelial-to-mesenchymal transition, paradoxically, E-cadherin is overexpressed in IBC. IBC's low incidence has limited the research on this aggressive disease, which points to the need for worldwide collaboration aimed at optimizing a more effective multidisciplinary approach to fight this disease.

H. Yamauchi
Department of Breast Surgical Oncology, St Luke's International Hospital, Tokyo, Japan

T. Yamauchi
Department of Medical Oncology, St Luke's International Hospital, Tokyo, Japan

N.T. Ueno M.D., Ph.D., F.A.C.P. • V. Valero (✉)
Morgan Welch Inflammatory Breast Cancer Program and Clinic, Department of Breast Medical Oncology, The University of Texas, MD Anderson Cancer Center, Unit 1354, Holcombe Blvd. 1515, Houston, TX, USA
e-mail: nueno@mdanderson.org; vvalero@mdanderson.org

N.T. Ueno and M. Cristofanilli (eds.), *Inflammatory Breast Cancer: An Update*,
DOI 10.1007/978-94-007-3907-9_9, © Springer Science+Business Media B.V. 2012

Keywords Chemotherapy • Targeted therapy • Systemic therapy • Taxanes • Anthracyclin

IBC, the most aggressive variant of breast cancer, is characterized by rapid onset and by skin involvement that is initially characterized as "inflammatory" based on the gross appearance of the involved breast. Prior to the advent of modern chemotherapy, treatment using surgery and/or radiation therapy failed to achieve long-term locoregional and systemic control of IBC. Multimodality treatment that includes systemic chemotherapy, surgery, and radiation therapy has led to improvement in prognosis; however, the 5-year progression-free survival rate for IBC patients is still only 30% [1], in part due to the rapid progression to advanced disease, which often occurred at presentation, and the inability to adequately control this disease with current therapy. Coordination of multidisciplinary therapeutic modalities, as well as multidisciplinary diagnostic modalities (radiological, pathologic, and molecular), results in optimal management of this entity. Research efforts have yielded progress in the design of new therapeutic approaches; nevertheless, the rareness of IBC has limited the development of defined targets, which are sorely needed.

In this section, we review optimal systemic therapy, including chemotherapy and target therapy approaches for both primary and metastatic IBC and summarize novel treatment concepts, including current ongoing clinical trials and candidate targets under evaluation in both primary and metastatic IBC.

9.1 Evolution of the Multimodality Approach

Before the era of chemotherapy, IBC was treated with surgery and/or radiation, and fewer than 5% of patients survived more than 5 years [2]. In the 1950s, 29 IBC patients treated with radical mastectomy had a mean overall survival of only 19 months, and few survived 5 years [3]. A poor outcome for patients treated with surgery alone was also reported, with 5-year survival rates of 0–10% [4]. Early efforts at the Joint Center for Radiation to treat IBC with definitive radiation therapy achieved 5-year relapse-free survival and overall survival rates of only 17% and 28%, respectively [5]. In studies published before the 1990s, surgery followed by radiation improved locoregional control but did not affect survival [6]. Meanwhile, in the 1970s, doxorubicin-based chemotherapy and the concept of neoadjuvant chemotherapy were introduced into the treatment of IBC. Prospective trials proved the efficacy of this strategy [7–10]. Subsequently, taxane-containing regimens were investigated for the treatment of IBC [11]. Together, these studies and changes in practice over the past two decades have led to the consensus that patients with primary IBC should receive systemic chemotherapy (including trastuzumab and hormonal therapy when indicated), followed by surgery, followed by radiation therapy.

9.1.1 Systemic Therapy

9.1.1.1 Anthracyclines

Initially one retrospective analysis showed the efficacy of anthracyclines regimens compared traditional regimen in 1995 [12]. Among 38 IBC patients, 28 received cyclophosphamide, methotrexate, and 5-fluorouracil (CMF)+- vincristine, prednisone (VP) and 10 patients received 5-fluorouracil, doxorubicin and cyclophosphamide (FAC). While the overall clinical response rate was 57% in CMF+- VP regimen, FAC achieved 100% of the overall response rate.

Following this report, at least four more studies indicate that anthracycline-containing primary systemic therapy resulted in improvement in progression-free and overall survival for patients with IBC. The efficacy of anthracycline-based chemotherapy in IBC was confirmed from pooled analysis of four prospective trials covering a 20-year period at MD Anderson Cancer Center [7]. Anthracycline-containing regimens were given as induction chemotherapy to 178 patients with IBC followed by local treatment with radiation with or without mastectomy. The overall response rate was 71% and the overall survival rates were 40% at 5 years, and 33% at 10 years.

One retrospective series from 54 IBC patients treated with CMF or FAC reported 52% of clinical complete response [13]. The 5-year and 10-year overall survival rates were 56% and 35%, respectively. They found that women with complete pathological response (pCR) had better overall survival and relapse-free survival rates compared with those without complete pathological response.

Treatment with either three cycles of CAF or CEF (cyclophosphamide, epirubicin, and 5-fluorouracil) followed by surgery, adjuvant therapy, and radiation therapy in a cohort study of 68 patients with IBC from two prospective randomized trials showed that overall survival rates were 44% at 5 years and 32% at 10 years [14].

In one prospective trail at the National Cancer Institute, 107 stage III breast cancer patients including 46 IBC treated with CAFM [15]. Overall response rate for IBC patients was 57% and 10-year OS was 26.7%. PCR was achieved 15 out of 46 IBC patients (33%).

9.1.1.2 Taxanes

The addition of taxanes, docetaxel and paclitaxel, into combination chemotherapy has showed efficacy in the primary systemic therapy of IBC same as in non-IBC cases. Initially, investigators from MD Anderson experienced that 7 of 16 patients who had crossover treatment from anthracycline-based induction chemotherapy to paclitaxel achieved a partial response and were able to undergo mastectomy among a series of 44 patients with IBC [16].

Following these results, the same investigators reviewed retrospectively 240 patients with IBC from six trials between 1973 and 2000. A cohort of 62 patients who received CAF followed by paclitaxel had a higher pCR rate than those from

Table 9.1 Anthracyclines

Author	Year	Type of study	No. of patients with IBC	Regimen	Results
Bauer [12]	1995	Retrospective	38	CMF+-VP	OR 57%
				FAC	OR 100%
Ueno [7]	1997	Pooled analysis of 4 prospective trials	178	Anthracyclines	OR 71% 5-year OS 40% 10-year OS 33%
Harris [13]	2003	Retrospective	54	CMF or CAF	OR 52% 5-year OS 56% 10-year OS 35%
Baldin [14]	2004	Pooled analysis of 2 prospective trials	68	CEF or CAF	OR 73.6% 5Y OS 44%
Low [15]	2004	Prospective	46	CAFM	OR 57% 10Y OS 26.7%

Table 9.2 Results of anthracycline-taxane based regimens in IBC

Author	Year	Type of study	No. of patients with IBC	Regimen	Results
Cristofanilli [16]	2001	Retrospective	16	FAC crossover P	OR 44%
Cristofanilli [11]	2004	Pooled analysis of 6 prospective trials	178	FAC	OR 74%, pCR 10%
			62	FAC + P	OR 82%, pCR 25%
Hennessy [17]	2006	Pooled analysis of 3 prospective trials	50	FAC	pCR in LN 16%
			11	FAC + P	pCR in LN 45%
Costa [18]	2010	Prospective trial	93	TAC or TAC followed by vinorelbine/ capecitabine	pCR 8.6%, OR 71%

Table 9.3 Response to primary systemic chemotherapy and outcomes

Author	Year	Type of study	No. of patients with IBC	Regimen	Results
Harris [13]	2003	Retrospective	54	CMF or CAF	pCR vs. residual disease 10Y OS 45% vs. 31%
Hennessy [17]	2006	Pooled analysis of 3 prospective trials	61	FAC or FAC + P	pCR in LN vs. residual disease 5Y OS 82.5 vs. 37.1% 5Y DFS 78.6 vs. 25.4%

178 patients with IBC who received CAF alone (25% versus 10%; $p = 0.012$). Median overall survival rate (54 months versus 32 months; $p = 0.03$), and progression-free survival rate (27 months versus 18 months; $p = 0.04$) were also better by adding paclitaxel [11].

Table 9.4 Trastuzumab

Author	Year	Type of study	No. of patients with IBC	Regimen	Results
Burstein [35]	2003	Prospective	40 stage 2&3 (6 IBC)	P + T Then AC as adj	CR 30% pCR 18%
Van Pelt [36]	2003	Prospective	22 LABC (9 IBC)	D + T	CR 77% pCR 40%
Hurley [37]	2006	Prospective	48 LABC	D + CDDP + T	pCR 17% 4-year OS 76%
Limentani [38]	2007	Prospective	31 LABC	D + V + T	CR 94% pCR 39%
Gianni [39]	2010	Prospective	63 IBC	AP + P + CMF vs. + T	pCR 19%, 3Y PFS 56% vs. pCR 38%, 3Y PFS 71%
Dawood [40]	2010	Retrospective	16	Chemotherapy + T	pCR 62.5% PR 37.5%

Table 9.5 Lapatinib

Author	Year	Type of study	No. of patients with IBC	Regimen	Results
Boussen [42]	2010	Prospective	42	P + L	CR 78.6% pCR 18.2%
Johnston [43]	2008	Prospective	45	L	CR in HER2 + 50% CR in HER2 − 7%

P paclitaxel, *L* Lapatinib, *CR* clinical response, *pCR* pathological complete response

From three trials for 175 IBC patients from 1987 to 2001, 61 patients who had cytology proved axillary lymph nodes metastasis were evaluated for the response of axillary lymph nodes from primary systemic chemotherapy. The addition of paclitaxel to FAC achieved better pathological response rate in axillary lymph nodes compared with FAC alone (45% versus 16%, respectively, p=0.01) [17]. These results indicated that the incorporation of taxanes resulted in a benefit for patients with IBC.

9.1.1.3 Response to Primary Chemotherapy and Outcomes

It is well known that in most of primary systemic chemotherapy studies, the better response to chemotherapy was correlated the better outcomes in breast cancer. However, we do not know whether response to primary therapy in IBC patients is poor compared with non-IBC since IBC patients are excluded from most of prospective clinical trials with non-IBC. Recently the German study group included 93 IBC patients in the GeparTrio trial, a large-scale, multicenter, randomized study of neoadjuvant therapy with six or eight cycles of docetaxel/doxorubicin/cyclophosphamide

Table 9.6 High-dose chemotherapy

Author	Year	Type of study	No. of patients with IBC	Regimen	Results
Schwartzberg [69]	1999	Prospective	56	Cyclophosphamide/thiotepa/carboplatin	3Y OS75% 3Y EFS 53%
Viens [20]	1999	Prospective	100	Sequential HDCT with cyclophosphamide/doxorubicin/5-fluorouracil	OR 90%, pCR 32% 3Y OS 70%
Arun [22]	1999	Prospective	24	Carboplatin/cyclophosphamide	2Y OS 73% 2Y DFS 71%
Yau [21]	2000	Prospective	21	FAC with high-dose cyclophosphamide/etoposide/cisplatin vs. FAC	4y OS 78%, 4Y DFS 45% vs. 4Y OS 58%, 4Y DFS 39%
Dazzi [70]	2001	Prospective	21	Mitoxantrone/thiotepa/cyclophosphamide	OR 95%
Bertucci [71]	2004	Retrospective	74	Cyclophosphamide/melphalan/methotrexate vs. anthracycline-based standard therapy	5Y OS 50% 5Y DFS 28% vs. 5Y OS 18% 5Y DFS 15%
Somlo [24]	2004	Retrospective	120	Dose-intense chemotherapy	5Y RFS 44% 5Y OS 64%
Cheng [19]	2004	Prospective	177LABC (18 IBC)	High-dose cyclophosphamide, carmustine, and thiotepa	5Y OS 36%
Veyret [25]	2006	Prospective	120	FEC-HD	pCR 14.7% 10Y DFS 35.7% 10Y OS 41.2%

LABC locally advanced breast cancer, *IBC* inflammatory breast cancer, *OR* overall response, *OS* Overall Survival, *RFS* relapse-free survival, *EFS* event-free survival, *FAC* 5-fluorouracil/doxorubicin/cyclophosphamide, *FEC* 5-fluorouracil/epirubicin/cyclophosphamide, *HD* high-dose

(TAC) or two cycles of TAC followed by four cycles of vinorelbine/capecitabine [18]. They observed pCR in 8.6% of IBC patients, with 11.3% of LABC patients and 17.7% of operable breast cancer patients. They concluded that response in IBC patients is not different compared with LABC and operable breast cancer once baseline risk factors were considered in the multivariable analysis.

Influences from response to primary therapy to outcomes were investigated in IBC patients. From three prospective trials, investigators at MD Anderson evaluated 61 IBC patients with cytologically confirmed axillary lymph node metastases treated with primary systemic anthracyclines and taxane-based chemotherapy. They observed significantly better outcomes in the group of patients who achieved a pCR in the axillary lymph nodes than in the patients with residual disease (5-year overall survival: 82.5% versus 37.1%, respectively; 5-year disease-free survival: 78.6% versus 25.4%, respectively) [17].

In a retrospective study of 54 IBC patients, patients who had pathological complete response with pCR had longer 10-year survival rates than patients with residual disease (45% versus 31%, respectively; $P = 0.09$) [13]. Thus, we can conclude that the response to primary systemic chemotherapy was the most important prognostic factor and plays an important initial role for patients with IBC.

9.1.2 High-Dose Chemotherapy

Several investigators have tried high-dose chemotherapy (HDCT) with autologous stem cell support to improve response in patients with IBC. In the prospective study, 177 high-risk breast cancer patients (18 with IBC) were treated with a high-dose cyclophosphamide, carmustine, and thiotepa (CBT) regimen plus autologous hematopoietic stem cell transplantation and patients with IBC had a 36% 5-year survival rate [19]. The results of the PEGASE 02 trial, in which 95 patients with IBC were treated with anthracycline-based, sequential HDCT, showed an objective response rate of 90%, a complete response rate of 80%, a pCR rate of 32%, and an estimated 3-year survival rate of 70% [20]. Other prospective studies also revealed the benefits for advanced breast cancer patients including IBC with 3–4 year OS more than 70% [21–23].

In a large cohort study, 120 patients with IBC received primary systemic chemotherapy with anthracyclines and/or taxanes followed by surgery and dose-intense chemotherapy using various regimens [24]. At 5 years, the relapse-free survival rate was 44%, and the overall survival rate was 64%.

The report from the French Adjuvant Study Group GETIS 02 Trial revealed the long-term result from patients with IBC who received high-dose FEC followed by a maintenance regimen. With median 10 years follow-up, DFS and OS achieved 35.7% and 41.2%, respectively [25].

HDCT has been shown encouraging results from data with better response than conventional chemotherapy in patients with IBC. However, the use of HDCT for IBC is still controversial due to more toxicity and worse quality of life.

9.1.3 Targeted Systemic Therapy

Targeted systemic therapy that addresses unique biological features of IBC is under investigation. Here, we will focus only on those targets that have already been suggested to be unique in IBC. However, a number of other potential molecular targets have been identified for the treatment of IBC [26]. It is also important to recognize that the novel and unique targets that drive IBC in a clinical setting have not yet been established. While HER-targeted therapy has been investigated largely on the basis of clinical hypotheses, recent extensive work with experimental models and molecular profiling has identified additional genes and pathways potentially involved in the development of IBC and/or responsible for the rapid progression of this disease.

The introduction of a multidisciplinary management approach to IBC (i.e., primary systemic chemotherapy followed by surgery and radiation therapy) has greatly improved the survival of patients with this disease. However, for the 70% of patients with IBC who present with distant metastatic disease [27], there is a strong need for novel approaches. Approaches that have been or are currently being evaluated for IBC include targeted systemic therapy and novel approaches to surgery and radiation therapy.

9.1.3.1 Therapy Targeting HER2 (Trastuzumab)

The introduction of targeted therapy combined with chemotherapy has been made great contributions for women with breast cancer. This benefit reached to IBC patients especially from HER2 targeted therapy since HER2 has been observed in increased frequency (36–60%) to be overexpressed and/or amplified in IBC [28–30] The first HER2 targeted therapy, trastuzumab has been shown effective in combination with chemotherapy for breast cancer in the neoadjuvant, adjuvant, and metastatic settings [31–34].

In a pilot study of the combination of paclitaxel and trastuzumab as a primary systemic chemotherapy, followed by surgery and adjuvant doxorubicin and cyclophosphamide chemotherapy, 40 women with stage 2 and 3 breast cancer (including 6 IBC) had complete clinical and pCR rates of 30% and 18%, respectively [35].

In a second study, 22 patients (9 patients with IBC) were treated with primary systemic docetaxel and trastuzumab [36]. The investigators noted 40% complete response and 77% objective clinical response rates.

One investigation in five prospective trials with primary systemic chemotherapy of the combination of docetaxel, cisplatin, and trastuzumab for 48 patients with HER2-positive LABC, including IBC In a study, LABC, including IBC, had a 17% pCR rate [37]. Four-year progression-free and overall survival rates were 100% among those who had a pathological response rate and 76% for the entire cohort.

A combination of docetaxel, vinorelbine, and trastuzumab were evaluated among 31 patients with HER2-amplified cancers, including IBC, and showed clinical and pCR rates of 94% and 39%, respectively [38].

The largest series of patients with IBC was reported from the NOAH (neoadjuvant trastuzumab) phase III trial. In 63 patients with HER2-positive IBC, a significantly higher pCR rate of 38% was noted in women who received doxorubicin, paclitaxel, and cyclophosphamide chemotherapy with trastuzumab, compared with a pCR rate of only 19% in women who received chemotherapy alone [39]. Three-year event free survival were also observed better among those who received trastuzumab-based regimen compared with chemotherapy alone. Furthermore, Dawood et al. reported the retrospective experience of a cohort of 16 HER2 positive - IBC patients who received primary systemic chemotherapy plus trastuzumab, investigators observed 62.5% pCR with 37.5% partial response [40].

Further study is warranted in a large cohort of patients with HER-2 neu amplified IBC to find the most effective combination of chemotherapy and trastuzumab in IBC.

9.1.3.2 Therapy Targeting HER2 (Lapatinib)

Lapatinib is an oral and dual tyrosine kinase inhibitor for EGFR and HER2 tyrosine kinases. HER2 overexpression was observed frequently in IBC. Furthermore, there was a report that EGFR expression is associated with poor prognosis in IBC [41]. Preclinical Clinical trials have shown that lapatinib is effective for patients with HER2-positive breast cancer and lapatinib has been investigated also in preclinical setting.

Results from a phase II trial of lapatinib and paclitaxel as primary systemic therapy in 42 patients with newly diagnosed IBC showed that 78.6% of the HER2-positive patients had a clinical response with 18.2% of pCR [42].

Data from a phase II trial of lapatinib monotherapy for heavily treated patients with IBC [43], the response rate was 50% among the 30 patients with HER2-positive tumors but only 7% among the 15 patients with HER2-negative, EGFR-positive tumors.

Currently, A randomized phase I/II trial of docetaxel and lapatinib as primary systemic therapy in patients with HER2-positive LABC, IBC, or resectable breast cancer is conducting by the European Organization for Research and Treatment of Cancer [44]. At M. D. Anderson, a phase II study of primary systemic lapatinib plus chemotherapy (sequential FEC and paclitaxel) in patients with HER2-positive IBC is in progress.

Combination with other drugs has been investigated in preclinical setting. The class 1 histone deacetylases (HDAC) inhibitor SNDX-275 showed activity in IBC cell models and synergistic effect with lapatinib at MD Anderson.

9.1.3.3 Therapy Targeting Vasculolymphatic Pathways—Angiogenesis, Lymphangiogenesis, and Vasculogenesis

Angiogenesis is the formation of new vessels from preexisting vessels that is necessary process for tumor growth and metastasis. Angiogenesis-related genes are upregulated [45] and microvessel count is significantly increased in IBC tumor samples compared with non-IBC tumor samples (51% versus 14%; $P=0.0031$) [46].

Bevacizumab, a human anti-VEGF monoclonal antibody, was evaluated for clinical activity in neoadjuvant therapy combined with doxorubicin and docetaxel in 21 previously untreated patients with locally advanced breast cancer, 20 of whom had IBC [47]. The studies revealed higher response rate (ORR 67%). Correlative biomarker study showed a significant decrease in the level of phosphorylated VEGF receptor-2 (VEGFR-2) in tumor cells, which suggests that anti-VEGF therapy have not only antiangiogenic effect but may also a direct antitumoral effect through VEGFR-2 [48].

Semaxanib (SU5416), a small-molecule inhibitor of VEGFR-2, was investigated in a phase I trial in combination with doxorubicin in 18 patients with IBC. Decreased tumor blood flow was observed using DCE(spell it) MRI. However, the study was aborted because of a significant decrease in cardiac function occurred in 22% of the patients (4 out of 18 patients) [49].

Pazopanib, an oral multi-targeted tyrosine kinase inhibitor of angiogenesis, is also under investigation in a phase III clinical trial in combination with lapatinib [50].

Lymphangiogenesis is the formation of a new lymph vessel network, which can lead to tumor cell dissemination, and promote tumor spread [51]. IBC tumor samples showed greater lymphatic endothelial cell proliferation compared with non-IBC tumor samples [52]. There have been also observed higher expression of lymphangiogenic factors (VEGF-C, VEGF-D, VEGFR-3, Prox-1, and fibroblast growth factor-2) in IBC tumor samples than in non-IBC tumor samples [53]. Targeting the VEGF-C/VEGF-D/VEGFR-3 signaling system would be an attractive therapy for IBC.

Vasculogenesis is the formation of new vascular channels due to *de novo* production of endothelial cells by tumor cells [54]. Clinically, higher vasculogenesis in tumor samples is related to a significantly higher rate of hematogenous metastasis and a worse 5-year survival rate [55]. Xenograft animal models of human IBC have been extensively studied to examine if targeting vasculogenesis would be a potential therapeutic approach. In a human IBC xenograft of WIBC-9, blocking vasculogenesis pathways showed growth inhibition of WIBC-9. This effect was more prominent in the WIBC-9 xenograft than in a non-IBC xenograft [56, 57]. However, whether vasculogenesis is a unique feature of IBC remains to be confirmed.

9.1.3.4   Therapy Targeting Overexpression of RhoC GTPase and Loss of WISP3

Overexpression of RhoC is observed significantly higher rate in IBC tumor samples in comparison with non-IBC samples (90% versus 38%). Loss of WISP3 is also seen in much higher rate in IBC samples versus non-IBC samples (80% versus 20%). Moreover, alterations of both RhoC and WISP3 are seen in 91% of IBC samples and 0% of non-IBC samples [58]. Overexpression of RhoC and loss of WISP3 jointly work to promote aggressiveness of IBC and in vivo study suggested that RhoC expression is modulated by WISP3 loss [59]. RhoC is a small GTPase that plays an important role for regulation of cytoskeleton [60]. Farnesyltransferase inhibitor to modulate RhoC expression [61, 62] has been investigated in preclinical and clinical setting.

9.1.3.5 Therapy Targeting Overexpression of E-Cadherin

E-cadherin is a transmembrane glycoprotein on the cell surface and regulates cell-cell adhesion; decreased E-cadherin expression was observed when cancer progressed and metastasized, especially when cells underwent epithelial-to-mesenchymal transition [63–67]. IBC cells, which are aggressively metastatic, paradoxically overexpress E-cadherin. E-cadherin has been investigated as a potential target for IBC treatment. In IBC xenograft models, targeting E-cadherin demonstrated dissolution of pulmonary lymphovascular emboli and reduction of tumorigenicity [64]. A gene called eIF4G has been recently discovered that may be related to the role of E-cadherin in IBC and may serve as a target for IBC treatment [68]. Overexpression of this gene was observed more frequently in IBC tumors than in normal and non-IBC cells. E-cadherin and related genes offer promise for further investigations related to the unique features of IBC.

9.1.4 Systemic Therapy for Metastatic Disease

It is very difficult to define standard treatment unique to metastatic IBC due to lack of both clinical and molecular definition of metastatic IBC. One area of controversy is whether patients with newly diagnosed metastatic IBC should undergo local resection. As standard care, locoregional management of metastatic disease is challenging and plays a limited role. There is some anecdotal evidence that debulking the primary tumor will improve overall survival duration. Whether this concept truly applies for IBC is completely unknown. Therefore, we generally recommend that patients with metastatic IBC undergo systemic therapy first and receive local therapy (radiation and/or surgery) for palliative purposes. A prospective study is needed to address whether local therapy is indicated in the IBC setting. Because IBC has a general tendency to progress rapidly and may not respond to many of the standard treatments, it is recommended that early phase I clinical trial consultation be obtained. Otherwise similar kind of treatment regimens would be offered to both groups of patients, while the biology of IBC might be unique and different [26].

9.2 Summary

In summary, the addition of anthracycline and taxane, either concomitant or sequential, primary systemic therapy is associated with a clinical pCR 10–40%, 5-year and OS 40–60%. The addition of trastuzumab to systemic anthracycline and taxane systemic chemotherapy leads to better response.

IBC is essentially a systemic disease at the time of presentation. Therefore, local treatment has a limited role in cure of this disease, though it is essential for locoregional control of the disease. Although there are not many novel advances in surgery and radiation treatment, there are many potential therapies for systemic treatment. To achieve further advances, researchers in IBC have been making enormous efforts to find clues to the cells' behavior.

Building on these preclinical and clinical efforts, we must enter the next era with international and specialized collaboration. Due to the rareness of the disease, a registry should be established for collecting clinical data and tissue worldwide. Because IBC is difficult to diagnose, it is essential to enlighten clinicians worldwide as to the existence of this disease. With greater awareness and continued investigation comes optimism that a cure for IBC will be found.

References

1. Gonzalez-Angulo AM, Hennessy BT, Broglio K et al (2007) Trends for inflammatory breast cancer: is survival improving? Oncologist 12:904–912
2. Bozzetti F, Saccozzi R, De Lena M et al (1981) Inflammatory cancer of the breast: analysis of 114 cases. J Surg Oncol 18:355–361
3. Haagensen CD, Stout AP (1951) Carcinoma of the breast. III. Results of treatment, 1935–1942. Ann Surg 134:151–172
4. Kell MR, Morrow M (2005) Surgical aspects of inflammatory breast cancer. Breast Dis 22:67–73
5. Lamb CC, Eberlein TJ, Parker LM et al (1991) Results of radical radiotherapy for inflammatory breast cancer. Am J Surg 162:236–242
6. Jaiyesimi IA, Buzdar AU, Hortobagyi G (1992) Inflammatory breast cancer: a review. J Clin Oncol 10:1014–1024
7. Ueno NT, Buzdar AU, Singletary SE et al (1997) Combined-modality treatment of inflammatory breast carcinoma: twenty years of experience at M. D. Anderson Cancer Center. Cancer Chemother Pharmacol 40:321–329
8. Koh EH, Buzdar AU, Ames FC et al (1990) Inflammatory carcinoma of the breast: results of a combined-modality approach–M. D. Anderson Cancer Center experience. Cancer Chemother Pharmacol 27:94–100
9. Singletary SE, Ames FC, Buzdar AU (1994) Management of inflammatory breast cancer. World J Surg 18:87–92
10. Buzdar AU, Singletary SE, Booser DJ et al (1995) Combined modality treatment of stage III and inflammatory breast cancer. M. D. Anderson Cancer Center experience. Surg Oncol Clin N Am 4:715–734
11. Cristofanilli M, Gonzalez-Angulo AM, Buzdar AU et al (2004) Paclitaxel improves the prognosis in estrogen receptor negative inflammatory breast cancer: the M. D. Anderson Cancer Center experience. Clin Breast Cancer 4:415–419
12. Bauer RL, Busch E, Levine E et al (1995) Therapy for inflammatory breast cancer: impact of doxorubicin-based therapy. Ann Surg Oncol 2:288–294
13. Harris EE, Schultz D, Bertsch H et al (2003) Ten-year outcome after combined modality therapy for inflammatory breast cancer. Int J Radiat Oncol Biol Phys 55:1200–1208
14. Baldini E, Gardin G, Evagelista G et al (2004) Long-term results of combined-modality therapy for inflammatory breast carcinoma. Clin Breast Cancer 5:358–363

15. Low JA, Berman AW, Steinberg SM et al (2004) Long-term follow-up for locally advanced and inflammatory breast cancer patients treated with multimodality therapy. J Clin Oncol 22:4067–4074

16. Cristofanilli M, Buzdar AU, Sneige N et al (2001) Paclitaxel in the multimodality treatment for inflammatory breast carcinoma. Cancer 92:1775–1782

17. Hennessy BT, Gonzalez-Angulo AM, Hortobagyi GN et al (2006) Disease-free and overall survival after pathologic complete disease remission of cytologically proven inflammatory breast carcinoma axillary lymph node metastases after primary systemic chemotherapy. Cancer 106:1000–1006

18. Costa SD, Loibl S, Kaufmann M et al (2010) Neoadjuvant chemotherapy shows similar response in patients with inflammatory or locally advanced breast cancer when compared with operable breast cancer: a secondary analysis of the GeparTrio trial data. J Clin Oncol 28:83–91

19. Cheng YC, Rondon G, Yang Y et al (2004) The use of high-dose cyclophosphamide, carmustine, and thiotepa plus autologous hematopoietic stem cell transplantation as consolidation therapy for high-risk primary breast cancer after primary surgery or neoadjuvant chemotherapy. Biol Blood Marrow Transplant 10:794–804

20. Viens P, Palangie T, Janvier M et al (1999) First-line high-dose sequential chemotherapy with rG-CSF and repeated blood stem cell transplantation in untreated inflammatory breast cancer: toxicity and response (PEGASE 02 trial). Br J Cancer 81:449–456

21. Yau JC, Gertler SZ, Hanson J et al (2000) A phase III study of high-dose intensification without hematopoietic progenitor cells support for patients with high-risk primary breast carcinoma. Am J Clin Oncol 23:292–296

22. Arun B, Slack R, Gehan E et al (1999) Survival after autologous hematopoietic stem cell transplantation for patients with inflammatory breast carcinoma. Cancer 85:93–99

23. Schwartzberg L, Weaver C, Lewkow L et al (1999) High-dose chemotherapy with peripheral blood stem cell support for stage IIIB inflammatory carcinoma of the breast. Bone Marrow Transplant 24:981–987

24. Somlo G, Frankel P, Chow W et al (2004) Prognostic indicators and survival in patients with stage IIIB inflammatory breast carcinoma after dose-intense chemotherapy. J Clin Oncol 22:1839–1848

25. Veyret C, Levy C, Chollet P et al (2006) Inflammatory breast cancer outcome with epirubicin-based induction and maintenance chemotherapy: ten-year results from the French Adjuvant Study Group GETIS 02 trial. Cancer 107:2535–2544

26. Yamauchi H, Cristofanilli M, Nakamura S et al (2009) Molecular targets for treatment of inflammatory breast cancer. Nat Rev Clin Oncol 6:387–394

27. Gonzalez-Angulo AM, Guarneri V, Gong Y et al (2006) Downregulation of the cyclin-dependent kinase inhibitor p27kip1 might correlate with poor disease-free and overall survival in inflammatory breast cancer. Clin Breast Cancer 7:326–330

28. Guerin M, Gabillot M, Mathieu MC et al (1989) Structure and expression of c-erbB-2 and EGF receptor genes in inflammatory and non-inflammatory breast cancer: prognostic significance. Int J Cancer 43:201–208

29. Guerin M, Sheng ZM, Andrieu N et al (1990) Strong association between c-myb and oestrogen-receptor expression in human breast cancer. Oncogene 5:131–135

30. Parton M, Dowsett M, Ashley S et al (2004) High incidence of HER-2 positivity in inflammatory breast cancer. Breast 13:97–103

31. Buzdar AU, Ibrahim NK, Francis D et al (2005) Significantly higher pathologic complete remission rate after neoadjuvant therapy with trastuzumab, paclitaxel, and epirubicin chemotherapy: results of a randomized trial in human epidermal growth factor receptor 2-positive operable breast cancer. J Clin Oncol 23:3676–3685

32. Slamon DJ, Leyland-Jones B, Shak S et al (2001) Use of chemotherapy plus a monoclonal antibody against HER2 for metastatic breast cancer that overexpresses HER2. N Engl J Med 344:783–792

33. Romond EH, Perez EA, Bryant J et al (2005) Trastuzumab plus adjuvant chemotherapy for operable HER2-positive breast cancer. N Engl J Med 353:1673–1684
34. Piccart-Gebhart MJ, Procter M, Leyland-Jones B et al (2005) Trastuzumab after adjuvant chemotherapy in HER2-positive breast cancer. N Engl J Med 353:1659–1672
35. Burstein HJ, Harris LN, Gelman R et al (2003) Preoperative therapy with trastuzumab and paclitaxel followed by sequential adjuvant doxorubicin/cyclophosphamide for HER2 overexpressing stage II or III breast cancer: a pilot study. J Clin Oncol 21:46–53
36. Van Pelt AE, Mohsin S, Elledge RM et al (2003) Neoadjuvant trastuzumab and docetaxel in breast cancer: preliminary results. Clin Breast Cancer 4:348–353
37. Hurley J, Doliny P, Reis I et al (2006) Docetaxel, cisplatin, and trastuzumab as primary systemic therapy for human epidermal growth factor receptor 2-positive locally advanced breast cancer. J Clin Oncol 24:1831–1838
38. Limentani SA, Brufsky AM, Erban JK et al (2007) Phase II study of neoadjuvant docetaxel, vinorelbine, and trastuzumab followed by surgery and adjuvant doxorubicin plus cyclophosphamide in women with human epidermal growth factor receptor 2-overexpressing locally advanced breast cancer. J Clin Oncol 25:1232–1238
39. Gianni L, Eiermann W, Semiglazov V et al (2010) Neoadjuvant chemotherapy with trastuzumab followed by adjuvant trastuzumab versus neoadjuvant chemotherapy alone, in patients with HER2-positive locally advanced breast cancer (the NOAH trial): a randomised controlled superiority trial with a parallel HER2-negative cohort. Lancet 375:377–384
40. Dawood S, Gong Y, Broglio K, et al (2010) Trastuzumab in primary inflammatory breast cancer (IBC): high pathological response rates and improved outcome. Breast J 16(5):529–532
41. Cabioglu N, Gong Y, Islam R et al (2007) Expression of growth factor and chemokine receptors: new insights in the biology of inflammatory breast cancer. Ann Oncol 18:1021–1029
42. Boussen H, Cristofanilli M, Zaks T et al (2010) Phase II study to evaluate the efficacy and safety of neoadjuvant lapatinib plus paclitaxel in patients with inflammatory breast cancer. J Clin Oncol 28:3248–3255
43. Johnston S, Trudeau M, Kaufman B et al (2008) Phase II study of predictive biomarker profiles for response targeting human epidermal growth factor receptor 2 (HER-2) in advanced inflammatory breast cancer with lapatinib monotherapy. J Clin Oncol 26(7):1066–1072
44. Geyer CE, Forster J, Lindquist D et al (2006) Lapatinib plus capecitabine for HER2-positive advanced breast cancer. N Engl J Med 355:2733–2743
45. Bieche I, Lerebours F, Tozlu S et al (2004) Molecular profiling of inflammatory breast cancer: identification of a poor-prognosis gene expression signature. Clin Cancer Res 10:6789–6795
46. McCarthy NJ, Yang X, Linnoila IR et al (2002) Microvessel density, expression of estrogen receptor alpha, MIB-1, p53, and c-erbB-2 in inflammatory breast cancer. Clin Cancer Res 8:3857–3862
47. Wedam SB, Low JA, Yang SX et al (2006) Antiangiogenic and antitumor effects of bevacizumab in patients with inflammatory and locally advanced breast cancer. J Clin Oncol 24:769–777
48. Weigand M, Hantel P, Kreienberg R et al (2005) Autocrine vascular endothelial growth factor signalling in breast cancer. Evidence from cell lines and primary breast cancer cultures in vitro. Angiogenesis 8:197–204
49. Overmoyer B, Fu P, Hoppel C et al (2007) Inflammatory breast cancer as a model disease to study tumor angiogenesis: results of a phase IB trial of combination SU5416 and doxorubicin. Clin Cancer Res 13:5862–5868
50. http://www.clinicaltrials.gov/ct2/show/NCT00558103: A randomized, multicenter, Phase III study comparing the combination of Pazopanib and Lapatinib versus Lapatinib monotherapy in patients with ErbB2 over-expressing inflammatory breast cancer
51. Achen MG, Mann GB, Stacker SA (2006) Targeting lymphangiogenesis to prevent tumour metastasis. Br J Cancer 94:1355–1360
52. Van der Auwera I, Van den Eynden GG, Colpaert CG et al (2005) Tumor lymphangiogenesis in inflammatory breast carcinoma: a histomorphometric study. Clin Cancer Res 11:7637–7642

53. Van der Auwera I, Van Laere SJ, Van den Eynden GG et al (2004) Increased angiogenesis and lymphangiogenesis in inflammatory versus noninflammatory breast cancer by real-time reverse transcriptase-PCR gene expression quantification. Clin Cancer Res 10:7965–7971

54. Shirakawa K, Kobayashi H, Sobajima J et al (2003) Inflammatory breast cancer: vasculogenic mimicry and its hemodynamics of an inflammatory breast cancer xenograft model. Breast Cancer Res 5:136–139

55. Shirakawa K, Wakasugi H, Heike Y et al (2002) Vasculogenic mimicry and pseudo-comedo formation in breast cancer. Int J Cancer 99:821–828

56. Shirakawa K, Shibuya M, Heike Y et al (2002) Tumor-infiltrating endothelial cells and endothelial precursor cells in inflammatory breast cancer. Int J Cancer 99:344–351

57. Shirakawa K, Tsuda H, Heike Y et al (2001) Absence of endothelial cells, central necrosis, and fibrosis are associated with aggressive inflammatory breast cancer. Cancer Res 61:445–451

58. van Golen KL, Davies S, Wu ZF et al (1999) A novel putative low-affinity insulin-like growth factor-binding protein, LIBC (lost in inflammatory breast cancer), and RhoC GTPase correlate with the inflammatory breast cancer phenotype. Clin Cancer Res 5:2511–2519

59. Kleer CG, Zhang Y, Pan Q et al (2004) WISP3 and RhoC guanosine triphosphatase cooperate in the development of inflammatory breast cancer. Breast Cancer Res 6:R110–R115

60. Hall A (1998) Rho GTPases and the actin cytoskeleton. Science 279:509–514

61. Rowinsky EK, Windle JJ, Von Hoff DD (1999) Ras protein farnesyltransferase: a strategic target for anticancer therapeutic development. J Clin Oncol 17:3631–3652

62. Cohen LH, Pieterman E, van Leeuwen RE et al (2000) Inhibitors of prenylation of Ras and other G-proteins and their application as therapeutics. Biochem Pharmacol 60:1061–1068

63. Colpaert CG, Vermeulen PB, Benoy I et al (2003) Inflammatory breast cancer shows angiogenesis with high endothelial proliferation rate and strong E-cadherin expression. Br J Cancer 88:718–725

64. Tomlinson JS, Alpaugh ML, Barsky SH (2001) An intact overexpressed E-cadherin/alpha, beta-catenin axis characterizes the lymphovascular emboli of inflammatory breast carcinoma. Cancer Res 61:5231–5241

65. Kleer CG, van Golen KL, Braun T et al (2001) Persistent E-cadherin expression in inflammatory breast cancer. Mod Pathol 14:458–464

66. Charafe-Jauffret E, Tarpin C, Bardou VJ et al (2004) Immunophenotypic analysis of inflammatory breast cancers: identification of an 'inflammatory signature'. J Pathol 202:265–273

67. Nguyen DM, Sam K, Tsimelzon A et al (2006) Molecular heterogeneity of inflammatory breast cancer: a hyperproliferative phenotype. Clin Cancer Res 12:5047–5054

68. Silvera D, Arju R, Darvishian F et al (2009) Essential role for eIF4GI overexpression in the pathogenesis of inflammatory breast cancer. Nat Cell Biol 11:903–908

69. Schwartzberg LS, Weaver CH, Campos L et al (1999) High-dose chemotherapy with peripheral blood stem cell support for operable locally advanced noninflammatory carcinoma of the breast. Breast J 5:238–245

70. Dazzi C, Cariello A, Rosti G et al (2001) Neoadjuvant high dose chemotherapy plus peripheral blood progenitor cells in inflammatory breast cancer: a multicenter phase II pilot study. Haematologica 86:523–529

71. Bertucci F, Tarpin C, Charafe-Jauffret E et al (2004) Multivariate analysis of survival in inflammatory breast cancer: impact of intensity of chemotherapy in multimodality treatment. Bone Marrow Transplant 33:913–920

Chapter 10
Inflammatory Breast Cancer: Chemotherapy of Metastatic Disease

Anthony Gonçalves and Patrice Viens

Abstract Metastatic disease is frequently observed in inflammatory breast cancer (IBC). IBC with synchronous metastases are generally treated similarly to non-metastatic disease, including optimal primary systemic treatment and, in case of favorable response, appropriate loco-regional treatment. Although evidences accumulate for considering IBC as a unique clinical, pathological and molecular entity, current treatment of secondary metastatic IBC follows the general recommendation of metastatic breast cancer management. Metastatic breast cancer (MBC) is considered to be incurable, but has a highly heterogeneous outcome. Quality of life and patient choices are important parameters in therapeutic decision. Specific treatment is based on standard molecular typing including ER, PR and HER2 expression. Chemotherapy is the major therapeutic option for hormone-insensitive and/or rapidly growing inflammatory MBC. Main classes of therapeutic compounds remains anthracyclines and taxanes. Issues such as monochemotherapy vs. polychemotherapy, optimal duration, optimal schedule of administration, place of high-dose chemotherapy are not clearly solved. Anti-metabolites, such as gemcitabine and capecitabine, as well as various antimicrotubules agents (vinorelbine and the most recently registered compounds ixabepilone and eribulin) may be used in anthracyclines and/or taxane-resistant disease. Cytotoxics must be combined to anti-HER-2 agents (such as trastuzumab or lapatinib) in HER2-positive inflammatory MBC, whereas the impact of adding bevacizumab to chemotherapy in HER2-negative disease was recently challenged. Development of specific, molecularly-driven, clinical trials is warranted for inflammatory MBC.

A. Gonçalves • P. Viens (✉)
Département d'Oncologie Médicale, Institut Paoli-Calmettes,
232 Bd Sainte-Marguerite, 13009 Marseille, France

Centre de Recherche en Cancérologie de Marseille, U1068 INSERM, UMR7258 CNRS,
Aix-Marseille Université
e-mail: goncalvesa@marseille.fnclcc.fr; viensp@marseille.fnclcc.fr

N.T. Ueno and M. Cristofanilli (eds.), *Inflammatory Breast Cancer: An Update*,
DOI 10.1007/978-94-007-3907-9_10, © Springer Science+Business Media B.V. 2012

Keywords Inflammatory breast cancer • Chemotherapy • Anthracyclines • Taxanes • Capecitabine • Vinorelbine • HER2 • Trastuzumab • Lapatinib • Bevacizumab • Monochemotherapy • Polychemotherapy • Metastasis

10.1 Introduction

Patients with inflammatory breast cancer (IBC) have a poor prognosis with 5-year survival rates of 30–40%, which are clearly inferior to the average rates for patients with non-IBC [1–3]. Mortality is essentially due to metastatic disease, which is clinically detectable on diagnosis in 30% of cases, and occurs in up to 70% in the outcome of initially non-metastatic patients [4]. Management of synchronous metastatic disease is generally the same as non-metastatic disease and includes primary systemic cytotoxic-based therapies, as described in a previous chapter. One area of controversy is whether patients with newly diagnosed metastatic IBC should undergo local resection. As standard care, locoregional management of metastatic disease is challenging and plays a limited role. Yet, there are some anecdotal evidences that debulking the primary tumor will prolong overall survival. Whether this concept truly applies for IBC is completely unknown. Therefore, it is generally recommended that patients with metastatic IBC undergo systemic therapy first and then local therapy (radiation and/or surgery) for palliative purposes. A prospective study is needed to address whether local therapy is indicated in the IBC setting and its impact on prolongation of disease control [5].

There are currently no standard IBC-specific treatments for patients with secondary metastatic disease [5]; therefore, enrollment in available clinical trials, including those of novel targeted therapies, is strongly recommended for IBC patient. Outside clinical trials, therapeutic management follows the same guidelines as in non-IBC metastatic disease. Metastatic breast cancer (MBC) patients are thought to be incurable and their overall survival has been recently reported to be 18–36 months, depending on the nature of the metastases and tumor biology [6–9]. Thus, the primary goals of therapy are restoration of quality of life, reduction of tumor-related symptoms, and maintenance of the patient's social environment and quality of life, as well as quantitatively increasing overall survival. In MBC, specific treatment must be initiated as soon as possible when diagnosis is obtained, with the aim of differing the occurrence of specific symptoms [10]. Currently, there are numerous specific therapeutic tools that can be used in MBC: several generations of endocrine therapies (surgical or chemical castration, tamoxifen, aromatase inhibitors, anti-estrogens), various cytotoxic compounds with distinct mechanisms of action (anthracyclines, taxanes, antimetabolites, vincas, alkylating agents) and, most recently, novel molecular targeted therapies (trastuzumab, lapatinib and bevacizumab). For a given patient, parameters allowing making a choice between these options include:

- Molecular phenotype: HER2 overexpression (by immunohistochemistry) and/or amplification (Fluorescence or Chromogenic in situ hybridization, FISH or CISH) and hormonal receptivity (Estrogen receptor, ER and Progesterone receptor, PR)

Table 10.1 Prognostic factors of metastatic disease

	Good-prognosis	Poor-prognosis
Performance status	Good	Poor
Nature of metastatic sites	Bones, soft tissue	Viscera
Number of metastatic sites	Oligometastatic	>1
ER/PR	Positive	Negative
Disease-free interval	>2 years	<2 years
Adjuvant chemotherapy	No	yes
CTC count (CellSearch system)	<5/7.5 ml	≥5 or more
HER2 status [a]	Negative [a]	Positive [a]

[a] Probably not true on trastuzumab era (see [15])

must be known. Since it was recently shown that both protein expression level may change in the course of metastasization, determination of receptor status should always be carried out when recurrence occurs, if reasonably possible [11–13].

- Duration of disease-free interval from diagnosis of primary
- Nature and tolerance of previously administered cytotoxic treatments
- Number and site of metastatic lesions, and their life-threatening potential ; recently, circulating tumor cells (CTC) dosage was shown to have independent prognostic value in MBC [14]; however, a small-sized study performed in 42 inflammatory MBC found a lower level of CTC positivity and did not reveal a significant prognostic impact in this cohort.
- Patient symptoms, performance status, menopausal status, comorbidities; expected side effects and patient preferences.

Some of these parameters may be combined to evaluate the prognosis of the disease and are summarized in Table 10.1.

Today, the particular aspects of HER2-positive disease and the impact of HER2-targeted therapies is so striking, that this molecular parameter represents the major point to stratify therapeutic options in MBC. This is particularly true in IBC, where the prevalence of HER2 positivity is known to be higher than in non-IBC [16, 17]. In HER2-negative disease, endocrine treatment remains the first-line therapy of choice for all patients with metastatic breast cancer, positive hormone receptor status and whose disease presents good-prognosis features (long disease-free interval, non-visceral metastases, limited number of metastatic sites, no or little symptoms). However, several reports have established that the majority of IBC tumors are ER and PgR negative [18]; in addition, virtually all patients with hormone sensitive disease will ultimately experience resistance to endocrine treatments. In these two latter settings, cytotoxic treatments are the only therapeutic option. In addition, HER2-, ER-, PR-negative disease (triple-negative) are increasingly recognized as a very poor-prognosis population, for which chemotherapy is the only validated therapeutic option, with a very limited activity in the metastatic setting [19, 20]. In HER2-positive disease, even though combinations of hormone therapy and trastuzumab or lapatinib have demonstrated superior efficacy over endocrine treatment alone in patients with both HER2 and hormone receptor positive status [21, 22], the combination of chemotherapy with anti-HER2 agents remains the standard of care for all patients. Thus, whatever the molecular status of tumors, all inflammatory MBC will have to receive cytotoxic chemotherapy during the course of the disease.

10.2 Chemotherapy for HER2-negative Inflammatory MBC

Importantly, although current management of MBC is strongly directed by HER2 status, most of the data available on the relative efficacy of various cytotoxic compounds come from studies performed in patient population which were not characterized for HER2 status. Most active cytotoxic molecules in MBC include anthracyclines (doxorubicin, epirubicin) and taxanes (docetaxel, paclitaxel). These compounds represent the basis for first-line treatments, either as single agent or in combination. Due to the lack of validated pathological or molecular factors predictive for efficacy, cytotoxics to be used are selected according to the nature of previously administered agents, as well as the demonstrated or expected sensitivity to these agents (Table 10.2). This latter point can be anticipated from the previously documented objective response and the disease-free interval following previous use of the drugs.

10.2.1 Patients with No or Little Previous Exposure to Anthracyclines and Taxanes

Of note, in metastatic IBC, the lack of previous exposure to anthracyclines is a situation almost impossible, since virtually all non-metastatic IBC have to receive anthracycline-based (and for most of them since 2000, anthracyclines plus taxanes)

Table 10.2 Chemotherapy options for HER2-negative inflammatory MBC

Pre-treatment history	Options
Previously untreated (synchronous metastases)	Anthracyclines-taxanes combination
	Anthracyclines or taxanes monotherapy followed by alternative regimen on progression
Previous exposure to anthracyclines	Taxanes monotherapy
	Taxanes + antimetabolites
	Taxanes-anthracyclines
	Paclitaxel-bevacizumab[a]
Previous exposure to anthracyclines and taxanes	Antimetabolites
	Vinorelbine
	Ixabepilone or ixabepilone-capecitabine[b]
	Eribulin
	Taxanes/anthracyclines reintroduction may be considered
	Alkylators

[a] This option is still registered by EMEA but its removal was proposed by FDA on December, 2010
[b] Not registered by EMEA, FDA-approved only

as primary systemic treatment. Thus, only IBC with synchronous metastases may be anthracycline-naïve. In those patients systemic treatment is usually the same as in non-metastatic IBC with anthracyclines plus taxanes concomitant or sequential combination. An alternative may be single-agent chemotherapy.

In previously untreated MBC patients, monotherapy using taxanes vs. anthracy-clines were compared in randomized trials. In a study enrolling 326 untreated MBC patients, docetaxel 100 mg/m² induced a higher response rate (RR) than doxorubicin 75 mg/m², (47.8% vs. 33.3%; $p = 0.008$) and had a more favorable toxicity profile. However, there were no differences in time to progression (TTP) (6 vs. 4.8 months) and overall survival (OS) (15 vs. 14 months) between the two arms [23]. In a three-arm study comparing paclitaxel, doxorubicin and combination of both, there were no differences in terms of response and time to progression between paclitaxel 175 mg/m² and doxorubicin 60 mg/m², when used as single-agents every 3 weeks. Combination provided higher RR and progression-free survival (PFS), but no OS advantage, since cross-over to the alternative regimen was planned in both single-agent arms [24]. In another study enrolling 331 untreated patients, 3-weekly single-agent doxorubicin (75 mg/m²) demonstrated a clear advantage compared to 3-weekly paclitaxel (200 mg/m²) in terms of RR (41% vs. 25%; p=0.003) and PFS (7.5 vs. 3.9 months; p<0.001). Again a cross-over with sequential use of the drug not received initially was planned and no difference in term of OS was observed [25]. Of note, several studies have suggested that weekly paclitaxel (80–90 mg/m²) is superior to 3-weekly paclitaxel [26–28].

Anthracyclines plus taxanes combinations were compared to taxane-free, anthacycline-based polychemotherapy, in MBC with no or little previous exposure to anthracyclines. Thus, a total of 267 MBC were randomized between AT (doxo-rubicine 50 mg/m²+paclitaxel 175 mg/m², every 3 weeks) vs. FAC 60 (5FU 500 mg/m², doxorubicin 60 mg/m² and cyclophosphamide 500 mg/m², every 3 weeks). A significant advantage was shown for AT in terms of RR (68% and 55%, respectively, p = 0.032), TTP (8.3 vs. 6.2 months, p = 0.034) and OS (23.3 vs. 18.3 months, p = 0.013). However, nearly 75% of patients in the FAC arm did not receive paclitaxel after progression [29]. Of note, toxicity profiles were differ-ent, with grade 3–4 neutropenia, arthralgia/myalgia, peripheral neuropathy and diarrhea more frequent in AT arm, and nausea/vomiting more common in FAC arm. Other randomized trials have evaluated paclitaxel-doxorubicin or epirubicin combination vs. cyclophosphamide-doxorubicin or epirubicin and did not reveal any significant differences in term of efficacy [30, 31]. As of docetaxel, several trials compared epirubicin or doxorubicin plus docetaxel (+/− cyclophosphamide) vs. epirubicin or doxorubicin plus cyclophosphamide (± 5FU) [32–34]. All of these trials showed an improvement of the RR in the docetaxel arm, and two of them demonstrated an increase in PFS. OS was increased in one trial. A recent meta-analysis examined the impact of taxanes when incorporated to first-line treatment of MBC patients with no or little exposure to anthracyclines in the adjuvant setting [35]: in combination with anthracyclines, taxanes were associated with higher RR and TTP, compared to anthracyclines-based, taxane-free polychemotherapy. There was no detectable effect on OS, whereas neutropenia and febrile neutropenia incidence were higher in taxane-treated patients.

To reduce the incidence of cardiac toxicity induced by anthracyclines, new formulations including liposome-encapsulated anthracyclines have been developed. In a phase III randomized trial, pegylated liposomal doxorubicin HCL (PLD, caelyx®) was shown to provide similar efficacy results as conventional doxorubicin, but with less cardiotoxicity. It induced less hair loss, nausea, vomiting and cardiac adverse effects (HR 3.16; $p < 0.001$), while hand–foot syndrome and stomatitis were more frequent with the pegylated liposomal doxorubicin [36]. Similarly, another non-pegylated liposome-encapsulated doxorubicin (liposomal doxorubicin, myocet®) was combined to cyclophosphamide and compared to conventional AC. Again, efficacy was comparable in term of RR, PFS and OS, but severe neutropenia and cardiotoxicity were reduced in the liposome arm. Thus, these anthracyclines compounds may represent an alternative to conventional doxorubicin [37].

10.2.2 Chemotherapy and Patients with Previous Exposure to Anthracyclines

In this setting, taxanes, notably docetaxel, are the best options. In phase II studies evaluating docetaxel monotherapy in MBC patients previously treated with anthracycline, a RR as high as 50% was achieved [38, 39]. In comparative studies, docetaxel alone clearly demonstrated an increase in OS, over other anthracycline-free combinations [40, 41]. A trial compared 3-weekly paclitaxel 175 mg/m² to 3-weekly docetaxel 100 mg/m², in anthracycline-resistant disease, and demonstrated superiority of docetaxel in terms of RR, TTP and OS [42]. However, and as previously mentioned, 3-weekly paclitaxel may not be the optimal schedule of administration. Another option in pretreated patients may be represented by paclitaxel nanoparticles bound to albumin, nab-paclitaxel, an innovative formulation of paclitaxel. In a phase III trial, nab-paclitaxel 260 mg/m² every 3 weeks demonstrated significantly higher RR, significantly longer TTP compared with patients who received conventional 3-weekly paclitaxel. In addition, a retrospective analysis revealed a significantly greater OS in MBC patients treated with second-line or greater therapy [43]. Nab-paclitaxel toxicities included grade 3 neuropathy but no allergic reaction and lower grade 4 neutropenia than paclitaxel. Most recently, nab-paclitaxel 300 mg/m² 3-weekly, 100 mg/m² weekly, 150 mg/m² weekly and docetaxel 100 mg/m² every 3 weeks were compared in untreated MBC patients. Weekly nab-paclitaxel 150 mg/m²/weekly resulted in better RR and PFS than docetaxel (12.9 vs. 7.5 months; p = 0.0065) with less fatigue, neutropenia and febrile neutropenia. Neuropathy was similar among the treatment arms [44].

In MBC patients pretreated with anthracyclines, combinations of taxanes plus antimetabolites have been compared to taxanes alone. A phase III randomized study compared docetaxel associated to capecitabine with docetaxel alone. The combination was proved to be more effective in terms of RR (42% vs. 30%; p = 0.006), TTP (6.1 vs. 4.2 months; HR 0.65; p = 0.00019) and OS (14.5 vs. 11.5 months; HR 0.77; p = 0.01) [45]. While musculoskeletal disorders and febrile neutropenia were more frequent in the docetaxel arm, gastrointestinal side effects and hand–foot syndrome were more common in combination arm, limiting the routine use of this regimen, which almost always requires significant dose reduction. Another study with similar design compared the efficacy and tolerability of the association of paclitaxel and gemcitabine, vs. paclitaxel 175 mg/m^2 every 3 weeks. In this trial, the combination provided a benefit in RR (41.4% vs. 26.2%; p = 0.0002), TTP (6.1 vs. 3.9 months; p = 0.0002) and OS (18.6 vs. 15.8 months; HR 0.78; p = 0.018). Moreover, an improvement in symptoms and in quality of life was observed [46]. However, in this study the single-agent arm was probably suboptimal, since weekly paclitaxel has been proven to be superior to 3-weekly paclitaxel. Another trial was recently reported and evaluated docetaxel-capecitabine vs. docetaxel-gemcitabine in MBC patients. This study failed to identify any significant differences between both arms in term of efficacy but treatment interruption for toxicity was higher in patients receiving docetaxel-capecitabine [47]. For all of these studies, the cross-over to the experimental drug for patients in control arm was not planned and therefore these studies do not allow concluding about the relative merits of both combinations vs. the sequential use of taxanes single agent, followed by an antimetabolite mono-therapy on progression. This issue was addressed by two additional studies. In a first trial, 100 MBC patients were randomized between docetaxel-capecitabine vs. doc-etaxel alone followed with capecitabine on progression: response rate, progression-free survival and overall survival were higher in the combination arm, but 26% of the docetaxel single-agent arm did not actually receive capecitabine [48]. A second trial included 368 patients with MBC and compared the three following options : Capecitabine 1,000 mg/m^2 bid days 1–14 followed after progression by taxane single agent (paclitaxel 175 mg/m^2 or docetaxel 100 mg/m^2 every 3 weeks) vs. doc-etaxel-capecitabine (C 825 mg/m^2 bid days 1–14 + D 75 mg/m^2 day 1 P 175 mg/m^2 day 1) or paclitaxel-capecitabine (C 825 mg/m^2 bid days 1–14 + P 175 mg/m^2 day 1). Response rate was higher with XP and XT, but PFS and OS were similar. The authors concluded that because there was no clear superiority of sequential vs. combined therapy, and patient characteristics are likely to be used to decide which regimen is the most appropriate [49].

In patients with previous exposure to anthracyclines in the adjuvant/neoadju-vant setting, an option to consider may be the reintroduction of anthracyclines, if disease-free interval following last administration is more than 12 months and if cumulative dose-threshold (450–550 mg/m^2 for doxorubicin and 800–1,000 mg/m^2 for epirubicin) are not reached. However, the benefits of this strategy remain dis-cussable. On one hand, two retrospectives studies suggested that response and survival rate in MBC patients first-line anthracycline-based regimens were not different according to the previous use of anthracyclines in the adjuvant setting. Of note, drug cumulative doses were moderate in these studies [50, 51]. On another hand, a small-sized prospective randomized trial compared epirubicin plus doc-etaxel to docetaxel alone in first-line, adjuvant anthracycline-pretreated, MBC patients and revealed no significant differences in efficacy, but tolerance was worse in the combination arm [52]. In addition, another comparative trial in a similar population of first-line, adjuvant anthracycline-pretreated MBC patients, evaluated epirubicin-docetaxel vs. capecitabine-docetaxel. Less than 100 patients were included and no significant differences in progression-free (although a trend was observed in favor of the anthracycline-free group, 12 vs. 9 months, p = 0.08) and overall survival were observed [53].

10.2.3 Chemotherapy and Patients with Previous Exposure to Taxanes and Anthracyclines

As previously mentioned, this is an increasingly frequent situation in MBC patients, and notably in IBC, since taxane/anthracycline-based primary systemic chemotherapy is currently the standard of care in this disease. In this setting, there is no consensual strategy and several options are to be considered. A first pragmatic possibility, although with only limited evidences in the literature, may be the reintroduction of taxanes and/or anthracyclines, if compatible with disease-free interval (in general >12 months) and with anthracycline cumulative dose.

Other options include the use of non-taxane, non anthracycline-based regimen. A large number of molecules have been commonly used in this setting, including alkylators (such as cyclophosphamide, melphalan, thiotepa), platinum derivatives, methotrexate or 5FU. Capecitabine single-agent was extensively studied in anthracyclines and taxane pretreated patients. At least five studies, enrolling 547 anthracyclines- and taxanes pretreated MBC, examined capecitabine single-agent [54–58]. Response rates varied from 15% to 29% and median overall survival ranged from 9.4 to 15.2 months. Tolerance profile was excellent, with hand-foot syndrome being the most relevant toxicity. Of note, most of patients in these trials were receiving capecitabine as second- or third-line treatment. Vinorelbine, a tubulin-binding agent, provides similar response rate as capecitabine in patient previously treated with anthracyclines and taxanes (10–20%), with minimal extra-hematologic toxicity [59]. Gemcitabine alone was also examined in this setting and has minimal but detectable activity [60, 61].

Epothilones are naturally occurring macrolides that share a similar mechanism of action with taxanes. These agents induce microtubule polymerization at submicromolar concentrations In the preclinical setting, epothilones possess potent antiproliferative activity in various tumor cell lines, particularly in the setting of taxane resistance. Epothilones and paclitaxel compete for the same binding pocket on β-tubulin; however, epothilones and the taxanes bind to different sites on β-tubulin. Significantly, epothilones have low susceptibility to multiple mechanisms of tumor resistance, including overexpression of MDR-1, p-glycoprotein,and tubulin mutations [62]. Ixabepilone, the most advanced member of this family in clinical development, was recently evaluated in taxane- and anthracycline-pretreated or -resistant MBC. This compound showed detectable antitumor activity in a phase II study including 126 triple-resistant (anthracyclines, taxanes and capecitabine) MBC patients, providing an objective response rate of 11.5% in this setting. Resistance to each agent was defined as progressive disease within 8 weeks of last dose of drug in the metastatic setting or recurrence within 6 months of adjuvant or neoadjuvant anthracycline or taxane therapy. In addition, 13% experienced stable disease for ≥6 months. Neutropenia (grade 3, 31%; grade 4, 23%), sensory neuropathy (grade 3, 13%; grade 4, 1%), and fatigue (grade 3, 13%; grade 4, 1%) were prominent in the toxicity profile [63]. In a randomized phase III trial enrolling anthracycline-pretreated or resistant- and taxane-resistant MBC patients, ixabepilone was associated to capecitabine and compared to capecitabine alone [64]. Seven hundred fifty-two patients were randomized 1:1 to receive either 40 mg/m² of ixabepilone as a 3-h infusion every 3 weeks and 2,000 mg/m²/day of oral capecitabine in divided doses days 1–14 every 3 weeks or oral capecitabine alone 2,500 mg/m²/day in divided doses on days 1–14 every 3 weeks. Anthracycline and taxane resistance was defined as tumor progression while on treatment or within 3 months of the last dose in the metastatic setting, or recurrence within 6 months of the last adjuvant or neo-adjuvant dose. Patients who were not resistant to anthracyclines but had received a minimum dose of 240 mg/m² doxorubicin or 360 mg/m² epirubicin were eligible. After 377 patients were enrolled, the definition of taxane resistance was broadened to progression within 4 months of the last dose in the metastatic setting or within 12 months of the last adjuvant or neoadjuvant dose. Approximately, 40% of patients had received two prior chemotherapy regimens before enrollment on both arms. The combination achieved a higher response rate (35% vs. 14%; p < 0.0001) and increased median progression-free survival (5.7 vs. 4.1 months; hazard ratio, 0.69; 95% CI 0.58–0.83; p < 0.0001), which was the primary endpoint. No overall survival difference was observed. Peripheral sensory neuropathy and myelosuppression were more common with the combination. There were 12 treatment-related deaths on the combination arm attributed to neutropenia in patients with abnormal liver function tests. These two studies provided the basis fro FDA-approval of ixabepilone either as single-agent in triple-resistant MBC or in combination with capecitabine in anthracycline pretreated or resistant- and taxane-resistant MBC. However, based on the same data, EMEA did not register this compound considering the benefit/risk ratio not favorable to ixabepilone.

Eribulin, a synthetic analog of halichondrin B, a natural product extracted from a marine sponge (*Halichondria okadai*), is another recently developed antimicrotubule. It binds on tubulin on a distinct site of taxane-binding site, induces tubulin sequestration in non functional aggregates and inhibits microtubule dynamics in a specific way [65]. Eribulin provided evidences of antitumor activity at the pre-clinical and clinical levels in taxane-resistant disease. In a phase III randomized study enrolling 762 MBC patients, pretreated with at least two and no more than five chemotherapy regimen (at least two of them in the metastatic setting), including taxanes and anthracyclines, eribulin 1.4 mg/m² D1, D8 every 3 weeks was compared to treatment of physician's choice (defined as any single-agent chemotherapy or hormonal or biological treatment approved for the treatment of cancer and to be administered according to local practice; radiotherapy; or symptomatic treatment alone)[66]. In this heavily pretreated patient population (a median four previous lines of treatment, capecitabine pre-treatment in more than 70% of cases), eribulin increased overall survival (the primary endpoint) from 10.6 to 13.1 months

(HR=0.81, 95 %CI 0.66–0.99; p=0.041). It also increased the response rate (from 5% to 12%, p=0.002), whereas a non-significant trend for progression-free survival improvement was observed (from 2.2 to 3.7 months, HR 0.87, 95%CI 0.71–1.05; p=0.137). Thus, erubulin was recently FDA-approved for treatment of MBC, after at least two regimen of chemotherapy for advanced disease. Similarly, eribulin has received a favorable advice from EMEA.

10.2.4 Mono- or Polychemotherapy

In the most recent meta-analysis assessing this issue in MBC, 43 trials were examined, comparing single agent vs. more than one drug and including 9,742 women, 55% of whom were receiving their first treatment with chemotherapy for metastatic disease. A benefit was found for the combination chemotherapy for survival (HR 0.88, 95% CI 0.83–0.93, p<0.00001), which was also associated with significantly better time to progression (HR 0.78, 95% CI 0.74–0.82, p<0.00001) and response (RR 1.29, 95% CI 1.14–1.45, p<0.0001). However, patients receiving combination had more adverse effects of treatment. It should be noted that this review was not able to address the issue of whether combination regimens are more effective than sequential treatment with different single agents [67]. The only study conducted to compare the concomitant administration of anthracyclines and taxanes to their sequential use, was reported in 2003 and presented above [24]: 739 patients were randomized to receive doxorubicin, paclitaxel, or both (A, P, AP) in a first-line setting. When progression occurred, the patients in the monotherapy arms were treated with the substance they had not received so far. The combination gave rise to higher remission rates (A 34%, P 36%, AP 47%) and a longer progression-free interval (A 6 months, P 6 months, AP 8 months), though toxicity was also higher. However, there were no significant differences in total survival in the three arms (A 19 months, P 22 months, AP 22 months). Thus, polychemotherapy may be preferred when a rapid response is needed, because potentially life-threatening or symptomatic disease; otherwise, single-agent chemotherapy may be sequentially used, with less toxicity and without evidences for less long-term efficacy. This applies to metastatic IBC, with the restriction of patients with synchronous metastatic disease, as previously mentioned, where the sequential or concomitant combination of anthracyclines and taxanes are usually preferred.

10.2.5 High-Dose Chemotherapy

High-dose chemotherapy (HDC) consists of major dose-escalation of alkylators and other chemotherapeutic agents, the main dose-limiting toxicity of which being hematologic, therefore supported by autologous haematopoietic stem cell transplant (ASCT), with the aim of increasing efficacy using the dose–response effect. This concept was extensively developed in high-risk and metastatic breast cancers during the 1990s, including inflammatory breast cancer. Accordingly, a specific chapter is dedicated to this strategy elsewhere.

On a general point of view, eight randomized studies have evaluated HDC plus ASCT in MBC patients. If six of them have shown a significant increase in event-free survival, only one was positive for overall survival. A meta-analysis including all these trials (except two small randomized studies where HDC was administered in both arms, either early or later on progression), confirmed an event-free survival benefit from HDC at 1 year (hazard ratio 1.8, p<0.00001) and at 5 years (hazard ratio 2.8, p=0.04). Although there was no OS difference at 1 year (hazard ratio 1, p=0.9), it approached statistical significance at 5 years (hazard ratio 1.5, p=0.08) [68]. Of note, the procedure-related mortality rates in the HDC and conventional chemotherapy groups were 3.4% and 0.4%, respectively (p=0.01). Accordingly, although potentially effective to delay progression of the disease, its lack of proven impact on overall survival makes HDC not being considered as a standard procedure in MBC patients.

10.2.6 Duration of Chemotherapy

It is not clearly defined what is the optimal duration of chemotherapy in MBC patients. The most recent meta-analysis (on published data) addressing this issue involved 11 randomized trials comparing different durations of chemotherapy and a total of 2,269 patients. Longer first-line chemotherapy duration resulted into a significantly improved PFS (HR, 0.64; 95% CI 0.55–0.76; P<0.001). Impact on OS was also significant but marginal (HR 0.91; 95% CI 0.84–0.99; p=0.046). A general attitude is to consider that when chemotherapy is indicated, it should be continued so long as the therapeutic index is favorable, i.e., so long as the benefit is greater than the side effects. However, the decision to maintain chemotherapy must be taken after a thorough discussion with patient, about symptoms of the disease, side effects of treatment, and quality of life evaluation. When chemotherapy is stopped, maintenance with hormonal therapy may be proposed in hormone receptor positive disease, even though this attitude is not clearly evidence-based.

10.2.7 Combination of Chemotherapy with Bevacizumab

As described in a specific chapter of this book, there is a strong rationale to target angiogenesis in IBC. During the last 10 years, bevacizumab has been extensively evaluated in MBC patients, yet its actual place in the therapeutic armamentarium is not clearly defined.

A first trial (AVF2119g) compared the association of bevacizumab 15 mg/kg/3 weeks with capecitabine 2,500 mg/m² D1 to D14 every 3 weeks vs. capecitabine alone in 462 MBC patients previously treated by anthracyclines and taxanes. The objective response rate was significantly increased in the bevacizumab arm

(19.8% vs. 9.1%, p=0.001), but no significant differences were observed in terms of progression-free and overall survivals. Tolerance was as expected, without drastic alteration of the capecitabine tolerance profile [69]. In 2007, was reported the results of the E2100 trial, comparing in first-line treated HER2-negative MBC patients, bevacizumab 10 mg/mkg on days 1 and 15 plus weekly paclitaxel 90 mg/m² on days 1, 8 and 15 every 28 days vs. paclitaxel alone. Progression-free survival was twice higher in the bevacizumab arm (from 5.9 to 11.8 months, HR 0.6; p<0.001), similarly to the objective response rate which was also significantly increased (36.9% vs. 21.2%, p<0.001). However, the overall survival was not different between the two groups (median, 26.7 vs. 25.2 months; hazard ratio, 0.88; p=0.16), although no cross-over was allowed for patients in control arm. In addition, HTA, proteinuria, headaches, ischemic cerebro-vascular accidents, peripheral neuropathies, as well as infectious episodes were more frequent in the combination arm [70]. At this time, FDA and subsequently EMEA registered bevacizumab in combination with weekly paclitaxel as first-line treatment of HER2-negative MBC patients. For FDA, the authorization was conditional, providing that additional data studies would confirm the amplitude of the benefit and detect an advantage in OS.

A third study (AVADO) randomized docetaxel 100 mg/m² plus bevacizumab 7.5 or 15 mg/kg every 3 weeks vs. docetaxel plus placebo, in 736 HER2-negative first-line treated MBC patients. Objective response rate was 44% in the docetaxel plus placebo arm vs. 55% in docetaxel plus bevacizumab 7.5 mg/kg arm (p=0.07) vs. 64% in docetaxel plus bevacizumab 15 mg/kg arm (p<0.001). Progression-free survival was significantly increased in the 15 mg/kg bevacizumab arm (median PFS from of 8.2 to 10.1 months, HR, 0.77; p=0.006). With a limited follow-up, no difference in survival was observed; of note the design of this study made it possible to have access to bevacizumab at time of progression for both arms. The toxicity profile of docetaxel was not affected drastically but the frequency of grade 3 or more events, including infection and febrile neutropenia, were significantly increased [71]. Based on these results, demonstrating an impact of bevacizumab on docetaxel efficacy, similar to that obtained with paclitaxel but with a much lesser magnitude, EMEA registered this combination as first-line treatment in HER2-negative MBC patients.

Most recently, a fourth study (RIBBON-1) was reported and compared various cytotoxic regimen plus bevacizumab or placebo in 1,237 HER2-negative, first-line treated MBC patients [72]. Before random assignment, investigators chose cohort 1: capecitabine (2,000 mg/m² for 14 days) or cohort 2: taxane-based (nab-paclitaxel 260 mg/m², docetaxel 75 or 100 mg/m²), or anthracycline-based (doxorubicin or epirubicin) combinations (AC, EC, FEC, FAC) chemotherapy administered every 3 weeks. Bevacizumab or placebo was administered at 15 mg/kg every 3 weeks. Response rates were significantly increased in bevacizumab combinations. Median progression-free survival (the primary endpoint) was longer for each bevacizumab combination (Capecitabine cohort: increased from 5.7 to 8.6 months; HR, 0.69; 95% CI 0.56–0.84; log-rank p<0.001; and Tax/Anthra cohort: increased from 8.0 to 9.2 months; HR, 0.64; 95% CI 0.52–0.80; log-rank p<0.001). No statistically significant differences in overall survival between the placebo- and bevacizumab-containing arms were observed. In docetaxel/bevacizumab-treated patients, the hazard ratio for death was non-significantly increased. Toxicities were higher in bevacizumab arms, notably in taxane-treated patients (neutropenia and febrile neutropenia). Based on AVADO and RIBBON-1 data, FDA considered that results of E2100 trials were not confirmed and, in the absence of impact on overall survival together with a significant increase in side effects, recommended to remove the breast cancer indication for bevacizumab. In the EU, EMEA decided to confirm that the benefits of bevacizumab in combination with paclitaxel outweigh its risks and that this combination remains a valuable treatment option for patients suffering from metastatic breast cancer. However, it also concluded that the balance of benefits and risks of bevacizumab in combination with docetaxel was negative and that this combination should no longer be used in the treatment of breast cancer. Finally, based on RIBBON-1 results, EMEA has recently given a favorable advice for registration of bevacizumab in combination with capecitabine, in first-line treated HER2-negative MBC patients in whom treatment with other chemotherapy options, including taxanes or anthracyclines, is not considered appropriate.

10.3 Chemotherapy for HER2-positive Inflammatory MBC

As already mentioned, HER2 is frequently overexpressed in IBC, with a greater frequency than in non-IBC [5, 16]. Trastuzumab, a recombinant humanized monoclonal antibody that binds with high affinity to the extracellular domain of HER2 and inhibits proliferation in human tumor cells that overexpress HER2, has become a major component of treatment of MBC with HER2 overexpression or amplification, as defined by immunohistochemistry and/or FISH (Table 10.3). Trastuzumab, as single agent in previously treated MBC, provided a low but consistent antitumor activity with objective response rates from 10% to 20% [73, 74]. In 2001, Slamon et al. reported a landmark study enrolling 469 first-line treated HER2-overexpressing MBC patients, and randomized to receive chemotherapy alone (3-weekly doxorubicin plus cyclophosphamide, AC or paclitaxel according to previous exposure to anthracyclines) or the same regimen plus weekly trastuzumab [75]. Trastuzumab significantly improved the objective response rate (from 32% to 50%, p<0.001 in the whole population, from 17% to 41% in the paclitaxel cohort and from 42% to 56% in the AC cohort), the median duration of response (from 6.1 to 9.1 months, p<0.001 in the whole population, from 4.5 to 10.5 months in the paclitaxel cohort and from 6.7 to 9.1 months in the AC cohort), the median time to progression (from 4.6 to 7.4 months, p<0.001 in the whole population, from 3 to 6.9 months in the paclitaxel cohort and from 6.1 to 7.8 months in the AC cohort). Overall survival was also significantly increased (from 20.3 to 25.1 months, p<0.046), which was highly relevant, since the design of the study allowed nearly 2/3 of patients in the control arm to receive trastuzumab on progression. In this trial, trastuzumab was also associated with an increased risk of cardiac dysfunction, notably in the anthracyclines arm (27% of cardiac events, including 16% of congestive heart failure), but also in the paclitaxel arm, although to a lesser extent (13% of cardiac events, in a population

Table 10.3 Chemotherapy options for HER2-positive inflammatory MBC

Pre-treatment history	Options
Previously untreated (synchronous metastases)	Sequential Anthracyclines-taxanes + trastuzumab
	Taxanes-trastuzumab
	Vinorelbine-trastuzumab
After trastuzumab-failure	Capecitabine-lapatinib
	Capecitabine-trastuzumab
	Vinorelbine-trastuzumab
	Eribulin

largely exposed to anthracyclines in the adjuvant setting). Based on these results, concomitant association of trastuzumab and anthracyclines are not to be used. A second study from Marty et al., confirmed the dramatic impact of trastuzumab on the efficacy of chemotherapy [76]. In a randomized phase II study comparing docetaxel 100 mg/m² every 3 weeks with or without weekly trastuzumab in a total of 186 HER2-positive MBC patients, the combination significantly increased response rate, (61% vs. 34%; p = .0002), overall survival (median, 31.2 vs. 22.7 months; p = 0.0325), time to disease progression (median, 11.7 vs. 6.1 months; p = 0.0001), time to treatment failure (median, 9.8 vs. 5.3 months; p = 0.0001), and duration of response (median, 11.7 vs. 5.7 months; p = 0.009), with little difference in the number and severity of adverse events between the arms. A third trial was performed comparing weekly paclitaxel plus trastuzumab vs. weekly paclitaxel alone and also revealed significant improvements of efficacy parameters [77]. Thus, trastuzumab-taxane combinations have become the standard of care in first-line treated HER2-positive MBC patients.

Other taxane-based combinations have been evaluated in this setting. Robert et al., compared the triplet 3-weekly carboplatin-paclitaxel plus weekly trastuzumab vs. 3-weekly paclitaxel-weekly trastuzumab and demonstrated an increase in response rate (52% vs. 36%, p = 0.04) and progression-free survival (10.7 vs. 7.1 months, HR = 0.66, p = 0.03), but without detectable impact on overall survival [78]. Of note, a similar study testing the addition of carboplatin to 3-weekly docetaxel-trastuzumab did not show any significant impact [79]. A phase II randomized study also evaluated the addition of capecitabine to 3-weekly docetaxel-trastuzumab and showed similar response rate and overall survival in both regimen, while progression-free survival was significantly lengthened from 12.8 in the control arm to 17.9 months in the docetaxel-capecitabine-trastuzumab arm, probably due to a maintenance effect of capecitabine [80]. Numerous taxane-free regimen have also been investigated in combination with trastuzumab with promising results including vinorelbine, capecitabine, or gemcitabine [81–87]. However, only vinorelbine was evaluated in a phase III randomized study, vs. a taxane-based regimen. In this trial, Andesson et al. compared 3-weekly trastuzumab plus vinorelbine 30–35 mg/m² days 1 and 8 vs. 3-weekly docetaxel-trastuzumab in HER2-positive first-line treated MBC patients. Response rate and survival were similar, but patients treated in the vinorelbine-trastuzumab arm experienced fewer adverse effect [88], making this combination an acceptable alternative as first-line treatment in HER2-positive MBC patients. From a recent retrospective study performed at the MD Anderson Cancer Center, it is clear that the incorporation of trastuzumab in this population has significantly modified the natural history of the disease. In this survey, it was estimated that trastuzumab reduced the risk of death by 44% and it was suggested that the prognosis could be better in HER2-positive than in HER2-negative MBC patients, if trastuzumab-based treatment is administered [15].

After failure of trastuzumab-based regimen for MBC, two randomized studies support the strategy of simultaneous continuation of anti-HER2 targeted therapies with modification of the cytotoxic component. In a phase III trial enrolling 324 s- or third-line treated HER2-positive MBC patients, after previous failure of trastuzumab regimen, capecitabine alone was compared to capecitabine associated with lapatinib, an orally administered dual HER1/HER2 inhibitor. A significant reduction in risk of progression (HR 0.49; p<0.001) and a significant increase in TTP (8.4 vs. 4.4 months) were observed in the lapatinib plus capecitabine arm. The final analysis after a longer follow-up, confirmed preliminary results (TTP 6.2 vs. 4.3 months; HR 0.57; p=0.0001) [89]. Overall survival was not affected, and tolerance was acceptable with cutaneous and digestive toxicity, likely attributable to HER1 modulation induced by lapatinib, and no major cardiotoxicity. Thus, lapatinib was registered in combination with capecitabine, in HER2-positive MBC patients after failure of first-line trastuzumab. Another trial addressed the same question by comparing in a similar population of HER2-positive MBC patients failing trastuzumab, capecitabine alone vs. capecitabine plus trastuzumab [90]. Interestingly, results were very similar in terms of progression-free survival, which was significantly increased without detectable increase in overall survival, making capecitabine-trastuzumab combination an alternative option for HER2-positive MBC patient with previous exposure to trastuzumab-taxane.

Of note, there are no clear data for management of metastatic disease occurring in IBC pretreated with trastuzumab in a neoadjuvant setting for non-metastatic disease. In this case, either a novel trastuzumab-chemotherapy combination or lapatinib-capecitabine may be considered, depending on the disease-free interval.

10.4   Conclusion

Unfortunately, metastases occur frequently in IBC, either on diagnosis or in the outcome, and MBC is considered as an incurable disease, the therapeutic management of which has almost always a palliative intent. Treatment of synchronous metastatic is usually similar to that of non metastatic disease, and frequently includes anthracyclines and taxanes in concomitant or sequential combination, with or without trastuzumab according HER2 status, with the additional issue of the nature of local treatment in responding patients. In metachronous metastatic IBC, current recommendations for cytotoxic treatment are not different from those for non inflammatory MBC and are based on HER2 status. In HER2-negative taxanes, anthracyclines, antimetabolites and novel antimicrotubules may be used alone or in combination depending on disease symptoms, previously administered chemotherapeutic agents, comorbidities, patients choices. Future improvements are expected to come from combining chemotherapy to novel targeted molecular therapies. The actual role of bevacizumab-based cytotoxic combinations is not clear. In HER2-positive disease, chemotherapy must be associated to anti-HER2 targeted therapies. Since IBC is increasingly recognized as a distinct molecular, pathological and clinical entity, specific clinical trials are warranted to better define the optimal use of cytotoxics and their combination to targeted therapies in this disease.

References

1. Cristofanilli M, Valero V, Buzdar AU et al (2007) Inflammatory breast cancer (IBC) and patterns of recurrence. Cancer 110:1436–1444
2. Hance KW, Anderson WF, Devesa SS et al (2005) Trends in inflammatory breast carcinoma incidence and survival: the Surveillance, Epidemiology, and End Results program at the National Cancer Institute. J Natl Cancer Inst 97:966–975
3. Dawood S, Ueno NT, Valero V et al (2011) Differences in survival among women with stage III inflammatory and noninflammatory locally advanced breast cancer appear early: a large population-based study. Cancer 117(9):1819–1826
4. Sutherland S, Ashley S, Walsh G et al (2010) Inflammatory breast cancer – the Royal Marsden Hospital experience: a review of 155 patients treated from 1990 to 2007. Cancer 116:2815–2820
5. Robertson FM, Bondy M, Yang W et al (2010) Inflammatory breast cancer: the disease, the biology, the treatment. CA Cancer J Clin 60:351–375
6. Chia SK, Speers CH, D'Yachkova Y et al (2007) The impact of new chemotherapeutic and hormone agents on survival in a population-based cohort of women with metastatic breast cancer. Cancer 110:973–979
7. Mauri D, Polyzos NP, Salanti G et al (2008) Multiple-treatments meta-analysis of chemotherapy and targeted therapies in advanced breast cancer. J Natl Cancer Inst 100:1780–1791
8. Gennari A, Conte P, Nanni O et al (2005) Multicenter randomised trial of paclitaxel (P) maintenance chemotherapy (CT) vs. control in metastatic breast cancer (MBC) patients achieving a response or stable disease to first-line CT including anthracyclines and paclitaxel: final results from the Italian MANTA study. J Clin Oncol (Meeting Abstracts) 23:522
9. Dawood S, Broglio K, Buzdar AU et al (2010) Prognosis of women with metastatic breast cancer by HER2 status and trastuzumab treatment: an institutional-based review. J Clin Oncol 28:92–98
10. Orlando L, Colleoni M, Fedele P et al (2007) Management of advanced breast cancer. Ann Oncol 18(Suppl 6):vi74–vi76
11. Guarneri V, Giovannelli S, Ficarra G et al (2008) Comparison of HER-2 and hormone receptor expression in primary breast cancers and asynchronous paired metastases: impact on patient management. Oncologist 13:838–844
12. Curigliano G, Bagnardi V, Viale G et al (2011) Should liver metastases of breast cancer be biopsied to improve treatment choice? Ann Oncol. doi:10.1093/annonc/mdq751
13. Simmons C, Miller N, Geddie W et al (2009) Does confirmatory tumor biopsy alter the management of breast cancer patients with distant metastases? Ann Oncol 20:1499–1504
14. Cristofanilli M, Budd GT, Ellis MJ et al (2004) Circulating tumor cells, disease progression, and survival in metastatic breast cancer. N Eng J Med 351:781–791
15. Dawood S, Broglio K, Buzdar AU et al (2009) Prognosis of women with metastatic breast cancer by HER2 status and trastuzumab treatment: an institutional-based review. J Clin Oncol 28:92–98

16. Parton M, Dowsett M, Ashley S et al (2004) High incidence of HER-2 positivity in inflammatory breast cancer. Breast 13:97–103
17. Sawaki M, Ito Y, Akiyama F et al (2006) High prevalence of HER-2/neu and p53 overexpression in inflammatory breast cancer. Breast Cancer 13:172–178
18. Kleer C, van Golen K, Merajver S (2000) Molecular biology of breast metastasis: inflammatory breast cancer - clinical syndrome and molecular determinants. Breast Cancer Res 2:423–429
19. Gilabert M, Bertucci F, Esterni B et al (2011) Capecitabine after anthracycline and taxane exposure in HER2-negative metastatic breast cancer patients: response, survival and prognostic factors. Anticancer Res 31:1079–1086
20. Goncalves A, Deblock M, Esterni B et al (2009) Docetaxel first-line therapy in HER2-negative advanced breast cancer: a cohort study in patients with prospectively determined HER2 status. Anticancer Drugs 20:946–952
21. Johnston S, Pippen J Jr, Pivot X et al (2009) Lapatinib combined with letrozole vs. letrozole and placebo as first-line therapy for postmenopausal hormone receptor-positive metastatic breast cancer. J Clin Oncol 27:5538–5546
22. Kaufman B, Mackey JR, Clemens MR et al (2009) Trastuzumab plus anastrozole vs. anastrozole alone for the treatment of postmenopausal women with human epidermal growth factor receptor 2-positive, hormone receptor-positive metastatic breast cancer: results from the randomized phase III TAnDEM study. J Clin Oncol 27:5529–5537
23. Chan S, Friedrichs K, Noel D et al (1999) Prospective randomized trial of docetaxel vs. doxorubicin in patients with metastatic breast cancer. J Clin Oncol 17:2341–2354
24. Sledge GW, Neuberg D, Bernardo P et al (2003) Phase III trial of doxorubicin, paclitaxel, and the combination of doxorubicin and paclitaxel as front-line chemotherapy for metastatic breast cancer: an intergroup trial (E1193). J Clin Oncol 21:588–592
25. Paridaens R, Biganzoli L, Bruning P et al (2000) Paclitaxel vs. doxorubicin as first-line single-agent chemotherapy for metastatic breast cancer: a European organization for research and treatment of cancer randomized study with cross-over. J Clin Oncol 18:724–733
26. Verrill MW, Lee J, Cameron DA et al (2007) Anglo-Celtic IV: first results of a UK National Cancer Research Network randomized phase III pharmacogenetic trial of weekly compared to 3 weekly paclitaxel in patients with locally advanced or metastatic breast cancer (ABC). J Clin Oncol (Meeting Abstracts) 25:LBA1005
27. Seidman AD, Berry D, Cirrincione C et al (2008) Randomized phase III trial of weekly compared with every-3-weeks paclitaxel for metastatic breast cancer, with trastuzumab for all HER-2 overexpressors and random assignment to trastuzumab or not in HER-2 nonoverexpressors: final results of cancer and leukemia group B protocol 9840. J Clin Oncol 26:1642–1649
28. Mauri D, Kamposioras K, Tsali L et al (2010) Overall survival benefit for weekly vs. three-weekly taxanes regimens in advanced breast cancer: a meta-analysis. Cancer Treat Rev 36:69–74
29. Jassem J, Pienkowski T, Pluzanska A et al (2001) Doxorubicin and paclitaxel vs. fluorouracil, doxorubicin, and cyclophosphamide as first-line therapy for women with metastatic breast cancer: final results of a randomized phase III multicenter trial. J Clin Oncol 19:1707–1715
30. Langley RE, Carmichael J, Jones AL et al (2005) Phase III trial of epirubicin plus paclitaxel compared with epirubicin plus cyclophosphamide as first-line chemotherapy for metastatic breast cancer: United Kingdom National Cancer Research Institute trial AB01. J Clin Oncol 23:8322–8330
31. Biganzoli L, Cufer T, Bruning P et al (2002) Doxorubicin and paclitaxel vs. doxorubicin and cyclophosphamide as first-line chemotherapy in metastatic breast cancer: the European organization for research and treatment of cancer 10961 multicenter phase III trial. J Clin Oncol 20:3114–3121
32. Nabholtz JM, Falkson C, Campos D et al (2003) Docetaxel and doxorubicin compared with doxorubicin and cyclophosphamide as first-line chemotherapy for metastatic breast cancer: results of a randomized, multicenter, phase III trial. J Clin Oncol 21:968–975
33. Bontenbal M, Creemers GJ, Braun HJ et al (2005) Phase II to III study comparing doxorubicin and docetaxel with fluorouracil, doxorubicin, and cyclophosphamide as first-line chemotherapy in patients with metastatic breast cancer: results of a Dutch community setting trial for the clinical trial group of the comprehensive Cancer centre. J Clin Oncol 23:7081–7088

34. Bonneterre J, Dieras V, Tubiana-Hulin M et al (2004) Phase II multicentre randomised study of docetaxel plus epirubicin vs 5-fluorouracil plus epirubicin and cyclophosphamide in metastatic breast cancer. Br J Cancer 91:1466–1471
35. Piccart-Gebhart MJ, Burzykowski T, Buyse M et al (2008) Taxanes alone or in combination with anthracyclines as first-line therapy of patients with metastatic breast cancer. J Clin Oncol 26:1980–1986
36. O'Brien ME, Wigler N, Inbar M et al (2004) Reduced cardiotoxicity and comparable efficacy in a phase III trial of pegylated liposomal doxorubicin HCl (CAELYX/Doxil) vs. conventional doxorubicin for first-line treatment of metastatic breast cancer. Ann Oncol 15:440–449
37. Batist G, Ramakrishnan G, Rao CS et al (2001) Reduced cardiotoxicity and preserved antitumor efficacy of liposome-encapsulated doxorubicin and cyclophosphamide compared with conventional doxorubicin and cyclophosphamide in a randomized, multicenter trial of metastatic breast cancer. J Clin Oncol 19:1444–1454
38. Ravdin PM, Burris HA 3rd, Cook G et al (1995) Phase II trial of docetaxel in advanced anthracycline-resistant or anthracenedione-resistant breast cancer. J Clin Oncol 13:2879–2885
39. Valero V, Holmes FA, Walters RS et al (1995) Phase II trial of docetaxel: a new, highly effective antineoplastic agent in the management of patients with anthracycline-resistant metastatic breast cancer. J Clin Oncol 13:2886–2894
40. Sjostrom J, Blomqvist C, Mouridsen H et al (1999) Docetaxel compared with sequential methotrexate and 5-fluorouracil in patients with advanced breast cancer after anthracycline failure: a randomised phase III study with crossover on progression by the Scandinavian Breast Group. Eur J Cancer 35:1194–1201
41. Nabholtz JM, Senn HJ, Bezwoda WR et al (1999) Prospective randomized trial of docetaxel vs. mitomycin plus vinblastine in patients with metastatic breast cancer progressing despite previous anthracycline-containing chemotherapy. 304 study group. J Clin Oncol 17:1413–1424
42. Jones SE, Erban J, Overmoyer B et al (2005) Randomized phase III study of docetaxel compared with paclitaxel in metastatic breast cancer. J Clin Oncol 23:5542–5551
43. Gradishar WJ, Tjulandin S, Davidson N et al (2005) Phase III trial of nanoparticle albumin-bound paclitaxel compared with polyethylated castor oil-based paclitaxel in women with breast cancer. J Clin Oncol 23:7794–7803
44. Gradishar WJ, Krasnojon D, Cheporov S et al (2009) Significantly longer progression-free survival with nab-paclitaxel compared with docetaxel as first-line therapy for metastatic breast cancer. J Clin Oncol 27:3611–3619
45. O'Shaughnessy J, Miles D, Vukelja S et al (2002) Superior survival with capecitabine plus docetaxel combination therapy in anthracycline-pretreated patients with advanced breast cancer: phase III trial results. J Clin Oncol 20:2812–2823
46. Albain KS, Nag SM, Calderillo-Ruiz G et al (2008) Gemcitabine plus paclitaxel vs. paclitaxel monotherapy in patients with metastatic breast cancer and prior anthracycline treatment. J Clin Oncol 26:3950–3957
47. Chan S, Romieu G, Huober J et al (2009) Phase III study of gemcitabine plus docetaxel compared with capecitabine plus docetaxel for anthracycline-pretreated patients with metastatic breast cancer. J Clin Oncol 27:1753–1760
48. Beslija S, Obralic N, Basic H et al (2006) Randomized trial of sequence vs. combination of capecitabine (X) and docetaxel (T): XT vs. T followed by X after progression as first-line therapy for patients (pts) with metastatic breast cancer (MBC). J Clin Oncol (Meeting Abstracts) 24:571
49. Soto C, Torrecillas L, Reyes S et al (2006) Capecitabine (X) and taxanes in patients (pts) with anthracycline-pretreated metastatic breast cancer (MBC): sequential vs. combined therapy results from a MOSG randomized phase III trial. J Clin Oncol (Meeting Abstracts) 24:570
50. Gennari A, Bruzzi P, Orlandini C et al (2004) Activity of first-line epirubicin and paclitaxel in metastatic breast cancer is independent of type of adjuvant therapy. Br J Cancer 90:962–967
51. Venturini M, Bruzzi P, Del Mastro L et al (1996) Effect of adjuvant chemotherapy with or without anthracyclines on the activity and efficacy of first-line cyclophosphamide, epidoxorubicin, and fluorouracil in patients with metastatic breast cancer. J Clin Oncol 14:764–773

52. Pacilio C, Morabito A, Nuzzo F et al (2006) Is epirubicin effective in first-line chemotherapy of metastatic breast cancer (MBC) after an epirubicin-containing adjuvant treatment? A single centre phase III trial. Br J Cancer 94:1233–1236

53. Bachelot T, Luporsi E, Bajard A et al (2008) Randomized trial of first-line docetaxel + capecitabine (XT) vs. docetaxel + epirubicin (ET) for metastatic breast cancer (MBC): efficacy results of ERASME-4/CAPEDOC-EPIDOC. J Clin Oncol (Meeting Abstracts) 26:1049

54. Blum JL, Jones SE, Buzdar AU et al (1999) Multicenter phase II study of capecitabine in paclitaxel-refractory metastatic breast cancer. J Clin Oncol 17:485–493

55. Blum JL, Dieras V, Lo Russo PM et al (2001) Multicenter, phase II study of capecitabine in taxane-pretreated metastatic breast carcinoma patients. Cancer 92:1759–1768

56. Reichardt P, Von Minckwitz G, Thuss-Patience PC et al (2003) Multicenter phase II study of oral capecitabine (Xeloda(")) in patients with metastatic breast cancer relapsing after treatment with a taxane-containing therapy. Ann Oncol 14:1227–1233

57. Fumoleau P, Largillier R, Clippe C et al (2004) Multicentre, phase II study evaluating capecitabine monotherapy in patients with anthracycline- and taxane-pretreated metastatic breast cancer. Eur J Cancer 40:536–542

58. Wist EA, Sommer HH, Ostenstad B et al (2004) Oral capecitabine in anthracycline- and taxane-pretreated advanced/metastatic breast cancer. Acta Oncol 43:186–189

59. Degardin M, Bonneterre J, Hecquet B et al (1994) Vinorelbine (navelbine) as a salvage treatment for advanced breast cancer. Ann Oncol 5:423–426

60. Heinemann V (2003) Role of gemcitabine in the treatment of advanced and metastatic breast cancer. Oncology 64:191–206

61. Rha SY, Moon YH, Jeung HC et al (2005) Gemcitabine monotherapy as salvage chemotherapy in heavily pretreated metastatic breast cancer. Breast Cancer Res Treat 90:215–221

62. Cortes J, Baselga J (2007) Targeting the microtubules in breast cancer beyond taxanes: the epothilones. Oncologist 12:271–280

63. Perez EA, Lerzo G, Pivot X et al (2007) Efficacy and safety of ixabepilone (BMS-247550) in a phase II study of patients with advanced breast cancer resistant to an anthracycline, a taxane, and capecitabine. J Clin Oncol 25:3407–3414

64. Thomas ES, Gomez HL, Li RK et al (2007) Ixabepilone plus capecitabine for metastatic breast cancer progressing after anthracycline and taxane treatment. J Clin Oncol 25:5210–5217

65. Jordan MA, Kamath K, Manna T et al (2005) The primary antimitotic mechanism of action of the synthetic halichondrin E7389 is suppression of microtubule growth. Mol Cancer Ther 4:1086–1095

66. Cortes J, O'Shaughnessy J, Loesch D et al (2011) Eribulin monotherapy vs. treatment of physician's choice in patients with metastatic breast cancer (EMBRACE): a phase 3 open-label randomised study. Lancet 377:914–923

67. Carrick S, Parker S, Thornton CE et al (2009) Single agent vs. combination chemotherapy for metastatic breast cancer. Cochrane Database Syst Rev 2009:CD003372. doi:003310.00 1002/14651858.CD14003372.pub14651853

68. Nieto Y, Shpall EJ (2009) High-dose chemotherapy for high-risk primary and metastatic breast cancer: is another look warranted? Curr Opin Oncol 21:150–157

69. Miller KD, Chap LI, Holmes FA et al (2005) Randomized phase III trial of capecitabine compared with bevacizumab plus capecitabine in patients with previously treated metastatic breast cancer. J Clin Oncol 23:792–799

70. Miller K, Wang M, Gralow J et al (2007) Paclitaxel plus bevacizumab vs. paclitaxel alone for metastatic breast cancer. N Engl J Med 357:2666–2676

71. Miles DW, Chan A, Dirix LY et al (2010) Phase III study of bevacizumab plus docetaxel compared with placebo plus docetaxel for the first-line treatment of human epidermal growth factor receptor 2-negative metastatic breast cancer. J Clin Oncol. doi:10.1200/JCO.2008.21.6457

72. Robert NJ, Dieras V, Glaspy J et al (2011) RIBBON-1: randomized, double-blind, placebo-controlled, phase III trial of chemotherapy with or without bevacizumab for first-line treatment of human epidermal growth factor receptor 2-negative, locally recurrent or metastatic breast cancer. J Clin Oncol 29:1252–1260

73. Baselga J, Tripathy D, Mendelsohn J et al (1996) Phase II study of weekly intravenous recombinant humanized anti-p185HER2 monoclonal antibody in patients with HER2/neu-overexpressing metastatic breast cancer. J Clin Oncol 14:737–744

74. Cobleigh MA, Vogel CL, Tripathy D et al (1999) Multinational study of the efficacy and safety of humanized anti-HER2 monoclonal antibody in women who have HER2-overexpressing metastatic breast cancer that has progressed after chemotherapy for metastatic disease. J Clin Oncol 17:2639–2648

75. Slamon DJ, Leyland-Jones B, Shak S et al (2001) Use of chemotherapy plus a monoclonal antibody against HER2 for metastatic breast cancer that overexpresses HER2. N Engl J Med 344:783–792

76. Marty M, Cognetti F, Maraninchi D et al (2005) Randomized phase II trial of the efficacy and safety of trastuzumab combined with docetaxel in patients with human epidermal growth factor receptor 2-positive metastatic breast cancer administered as first-line treatment: the M77001 study group. J Clin Oncol 23:4265–4274

77. Gasparini G, Gion M, Mariani L et al (2007) Randomized phase II trial of weekly paclitaxel alone vs. trastuzumab plus weekly paclitaxel as first-line therapy of patients with Her-2 positive advanced breast cancer. Breast Cancer Res Treat 101:355–365

78. Robert N, Leyland-Jones B, Asmar L et al (2006) Randomized phase III study of trastuzumab, paclitaxel, and carboplatin compared with trastuzumab and paclitaxel in women with HER-2-overexpressing metastatic breast cancer. J Clin Oncol 24:2786–2792

79. Valero V, Forbes J, Pegram MD et al (2011) Multicenter phase III randomized trial comparing docetaxel and trastuzumab with docetaxel, carboplatin, and trastuzumab as first-line chemotherapy for patients with HER2-gene-amplified metastatic breast cancer (BCIRG 007 study): two highly active therapeutic regimens. J Clin Oncol 29:149–156

80. Wardley AM, Pivot X, Morales-Vasquez F et al (2010) Randomized phase II trial of first-line trastuzumab plus docetaxel and capecitabine compared with trastuzumab plus docetaxel in HER2-positive metastatic breast cancer. J Clin Oncol 28:976–983

81. Jahanzeb M, Mortimer JE, Yunus F et al (2002) Phase II trial of weekly vinorelbine and trastuzumab as first-line therapy in patients with HER2(+) metastatic breast cancer. Oncologist 7:410–417

82. Burstein HJ, Harris LN, Marcom PK et al (2003) Trastuzumab and vinorelbine as first-line therapy for HER2-overexpressing metastatic breast cancer: multicenter phase II trial with clinical outcomes, analysis of serum tumor markers as predictive factors, and cardiac surveillance algorithm. J Clin Oncol 21:2889–2895

83. Chan A, Martin M, Untch M et al (2006) Vinorelbine plus trastuzumab combination as first-line therapy for HER 2-positive metastatic breast cancer patients: an international phase II trial. Br J Cancer 95:788–793

84. O'Shaughnessy JA, Vukelja S, Marsland T et al (2004) Phase II study of trastuzumab plus gemcitabine in chemotherapy-pretreated patients with metastatic breast cancer. Clin Breast Cancer 5:142–147

85. O'Shaughnessy J (2003) Gemcitabine and trastuzumab in metastatic breast cancer. Semin Oncol 30:22–26

86. Bartsch R, Wenzel C, Altorjai G et al (2007) Capecitabine and trastuzumab in heavily pretreated metastatic breast cancer. J Clin Oncol 25:3853–3858

87. Schaller G, Fuchs I, Gonsch T et al (2007) Phase II study of capecitabine plus trastuzumab in human epidermal growth factor receptor 2 overexpressing metastatic breast cancer pretreated with anthracyclines or taxanes. J Clin Oncol 25:3246–3250

88. Andersson M, Lidbrink E, Bjerre K et al (2011) Phase III randomized study comparing docetaxel plus trastuzumab with vinorelbine plus trastuzumab as first-line therapy of metastatic or locally advanced human epidermal growth factor receptor 2-positive breast cancer: the HERNATA study. J Clin Oncol 29:264–271

89. Geyer CE, Forster J, Lindquist D et al (2006) Lapatinib plus capecitabine for HER2-positive advanced breast cancer. N Engl J Med 355:2733–2743

90. von Minckwitz G, du Bois A, Schmidt M et al (2009) Trastuzumab beyond progression in human epidermal growth factor receptor 2-positive advanced breast cancer: a German breast group 26/breast international group 03–05 study. J Clin Oncol 27:1999–2006

Chapter 11
The Role of the Multidisciplinary Team in Inflammatory Breast Cancer

Nabila Chowdhury and Sandra M. Swain

Abstract During the past three decades multidisciplinary teams have played an increasingly prominent role in the care of patients with inflammatory breast cancer (IBC). A multidisciplinary approach provides a rational and coordinated mechanism for evaluation and treatment of patients with IBC by bringing providers in the surgical, medical, radiation oncology, pathology, and radiology disciplines together. The approach is enhanced with the involvement of a dedicated care coordinator who manages the care process. This figure plays an important role in communication of the care plan to the patient as well as seeing that the care needed is arranged and delivered. The psychosocial and palliative care services are also closely involved in the care of the patient. This care process enables the patient to make informed treatment decisions and be reassured that all her physicians are working in close conjunction for better management of her case. This in turn leads to more patient satisfaction and ultimately to more favorable outcomes for the patient. In this article we discuss the benefits of multidisciplinary team and its role in the management of a patient diagnosed with IBC.

Keywords IBC: inflammatory breast cancer • MOCS: multidisciplinary oncology consultation services

N. Chowdhury
National Cancer Institute/National Institutes of Health, Bethesda, MD, USA
e-mail: chowdhuryn@mail.nih.gov

S.M. Swain (⊠)
Washington Cancer Institute, Washington Hospital Center, Washington, DC, USA
e-mail: Sandra.m.swain@medstar.net

N.T. Ueno and M. Cristofanilli (eds.), *Inflammatory Breast Cancer: An Update*,
DOI 10.1007/978-94-007-3907-9_11, © Springer Science+Business Media B.V. 2012

11.1 Introduction

Multidisciplinary meetings are commonplace in the management of breast cancer. These meetings represent a gathering of medical professionals, known as the multidisciplinary team, to form comprehensive management plans for the patient. The multidisciplinary management of inflammatory breast cancer (IBC) includes neoadjuvant chemotherapy, surgery, radiotherapy, hormonal therapy in hormone receptor positive disease, and trastuzumab in Her2 positive disease. It not only requires the active participation of different medical and surgical entities but also the involvement of a dedicated care coordinator who helps in the development and communication of the care plan and ensures that all the care needed is arranged and delivered. The team also includes psychosocial and palliative care services. The multidisciplinary team is therefore meant to streamline care and improve efficacy of health service delivery in the management of IBC.

11.2 Role of Multidisciplinary Team in Inflammatory Breast Cancer

Inflammatory breast cancer (IBC) is the most aggressive manifestation of primary breast carcinoma, with the clinical and biological characteristics of a rapidly proliferating disease. Often patients present with skin involvement and diffuse erythema as well as edema involving more than two thirds of the breast [1]. Presently the standard of care requires having a team of dedicated and experienced specialists involved in the complex management of this entity. After the initial clinical diagnosis of IBC a multidisciplinary assessment and initial evaluation of the case is conducted. Neoadjuvant or preoperative chemotherapy is recommended for patients with Stage III disease which is the mainstay of treatment in IBC. Locoregional treatment also continues to play a major role. After initial chemotherapy a response is assessed by the multidisciplinary team. The majority of the cases are expected to have an optimal response with resolution of the characteristic skin changes and are considered surgical candidates for a modified radical mastectomy and axillary lymphnode dissection followed by radiotherapy [2]. During this time the patient care coordinator is responsible for coordinating care, educating the patient and providing access to community resources and other support services.

 In the case of IBC where the diagnosis and treatment is quite complicated a conventional tumor board falls short as it typically focuses on a wide range of tumors and the sessions are not ideal for the subspecialty expertise needed to optimize tumor specific management, like IBC. Moreover most of the cases discussed in a tumor board are retrospective which is different from the prospective treatment planning that happens at a multidisciplinary meeting. In the case of IBC a multidisciplinary team is involved every step of the way in the management of the disease and also dealing with the psychosocial and emotional needs of the patient.

11.3 Benefits of a Multidisciplinary Team in Inflammatory Breast Cancer

A multidisciplinary team can lead to a more accurate evaluation of a patient diagnosed with IBC. After a clinical diagnosis has been made and confirmed by pathology a multidisciplinary team is formed for the initial evaluation of the patient. This involves the pathologist, medical oncologists, radiation oncologists, surgical oncologists, reconstructive surgeon, radiologists and also psychologist and social workers. The involvement of these different entities has been shown to result in greater adherence to evidence based care [3]. The patients are referred to the MOCS (multidisciplinary oncology consultation services) after diagnosis and the same day consultation allows for efficient evaluation by the specialists who formulate a care plan as a multidisciplinary team. After the initial assessment the patient is followed closely by the multidisciplinary team all throughout her course of chemotherapy, surgery, radiation and beyond. The care coordinator is responsible for delegating the different appointments and educating the patient. This care process enables the patient to make informed treatment decision and be reassured that all her physicians are working in close conjunction for better management of her case. This in turn leads to more patient satisfaction and less fragmentation of care. It also provides prompt medical management of this complex disease. The referral to the MOCS (multidisciplinary oncology consultation services) in turn provides optimal intercommunication among the specialists and ensures higher level of provider satisfaction. All these measures together lead to overall improved patient outcomes.

11.4 Components of Multidisciplinary Team in IBC

Presently the standard of care requires having a team of dedicated and experienced specialists, e.g. pathologist, surgical oncologist, radiation oncologist, radiologist, reconstructive surgeon, and medical oncologist who are all involved in the complex management of this disease.

The initial diagnosis of IBC is made clinically with a positive histopathologic diagnosis. The diagnostic criteria for IBC include pathological confirmation of invasive carcinoma in the core biopsy. It is also strongly recommended that every patient who meets the diagnostic criteria for IBC undergo adequate skin biopsy to possibly document dermal lymphvascular tumor emboli [4]. Thus the pathologist plays a vital role in the initial diagnosis of the disease. After the diagnosis has been confirmed the patient with IBC also undergoes a series of imaging studies which includes a diagnostic mammogram and an accompanying ultrasound of the breast and regional lymphnodes. Systemic staging studies with a CT and a bone scan is also recommended [4, 7]. The radiologist helps to define the extent of the disease and its initial clinical stage.

Chemotherapy as the initial treatment is the recommendation because if surgery is attempted upfront the probability of residual disease being left behind is high. Therefore it is strongly recommended that all women with a diagnosis of IBC be referred to a medical oncologist [4] Primary systemic chemotherapy is usually recommended by the medical oncologist as the first line of treatment with the goal to allow for definitive surgery as per the National Comprehensive Cancer Network (NCCN) guidelines [7]. Prior to start of the chemotherapy the patient is also seen by the surgical oncologist, radiation oncologist, and reconstructive surgeon before the case is presented at the multidisciplinary clinic. After the initiation of the chemotherapy the close involvement of the medical oncologist continues with regular clinic visits for assessing the response to chemotherapy and physical exams are conducted every 6–8 weeks [5]. The radiologist is also closely involved as radiological assessments are carried out at the end of the primary treatment and compared to the baseline results. Sometimes mid treatment assessments are done to confirm or refute results of the clinical assessment.

After the initial systemic therapy is completed the multidisciplinary team again evaluates the patient and assesses the response. The patient is then recommended for locoregional therapy which includes involvement of the breast surgeon, radiation oncologist and reconstructive surgeon. Because of the high likelihood of residual disease and also the fact that despite a clinical response residual disease may still be present in the affected skin women with IBC are only offered definitive surgery with a modified radical mastectomy [4, 7]. The primary concern in surgical planning is that the operative field needs to be wide enough to encompass all secondary skin changes. While as much skin as necessary should be removed, tension should be avoided in closing the skin flaps, as this would make the site unsuitable for radiotherapy. Sometimes reconstructive surgery is needed for immediate flap reconstruction if extensive skin needs to be excised during mastectomy [6]. Immediate reconstruction is not recommended. After the surgery a thorough pathological evaluation of the mastectomy specimen is done by the pathologist. The patient is then referred to a radiation oncologist as all patients with IBC are recommended to receive postmastectomy radiation [7]. Additionally IBC patients who have hormone receptor positive disease receive 5 year of hormonal therapy and a year of adjuvant trastuzumab if the tumor is Her2 positive [7] (Fig. 11.1).

During their treatment an appointed care coordinator for the patient helps them navigate the health system, making appointments, explaining procedures and reinforcing information from all health care providers and ensuring comprehensive recording of patient information in health records. They help in providing advocacy, support, education and monitoring the progress of the patient.

During the multidisciplinary conference, patients and their support groups can also attend a separate educational session outlining the important aspects of their diagnosis and treatment. The recommendations of the multidisciplinary clinic are disclosed here and the side effects of the therapy, the survival, local and distant recurrences and the cosmetic outcome of IBC is discussed in detail.

It is to be taken into consideration that all these treatment options appear to be overwhelming to a patient with newly diagnosed IBC as they are faced with the

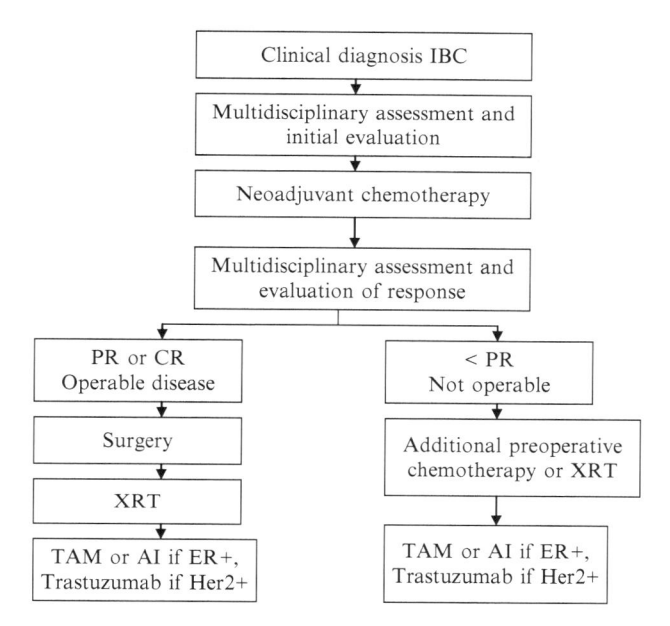

Fig. 11.1 Schematic representation of the proposed optimal sequence of treatment of newly diagnosed IBC. Abbreviations: *XRT* radiotherapy, *TAM* tamoxifen, *AI* aromatase inhibitor

formidable task of making timely wise decisions during this very stressful period of their lives. This is why psychosocial care is also needed to help patients manage the physical, mental and emotional effects of the diagnosis of IBC that can impact their response to treatment. In advanced cases of IBC the focus of care for the patients is considerably different. Treatment is given with a palliative intent and so psychosocial and spiritual needs of the patients needs to be addressed. Palliative care services, i.e. pain management also take a higher priority at this time.

11.5   Conclusion

A multidisciplinary approach targeting both the local and systemic disease of IBC has resulted in improved survival outcomes compared to those reported historically for this aggressive disease. During the past three decades multidisciplinary teams have played an increasingly prominent role in the care of a patient with IBC. Of paramount importance is employing a highly dedicated and sincere care coordinator who provides personal attention to the patient from diagnosis to treatment and follows up. Thus a multidisciplinary approach provides a rational and coordinated mechanism for evaluation and treatment of patients with this complex disease by bringing health care providers of different disciplines together.

References

1. Haagensen C (1971) Diseases of the breast. Philadelphia, Saunders
2. Fleming RY, Asmar L, Budzar AU et al (1997) Effectiveness of mastectomy by response to induction chemotherapy for control of inflammatory breast carcinoma. Ann Surg Oncol 4:452–461
3. Vinod S, Sidhom M, Delaney G et al (2010) Do multidisciplinary meetings follow guideline based care? J Oncol Prac 6:276–281
4. Dawood S, Merajver SD, Viens P et al (2011) International expert panel on inflammatory breast cancer: consensus statement and standardized diagnosis and treatment. Ann Oncol 22:515–523
5. Kaufmann M, von Minckwitz G, Bear HD et al (2007) Recommendations from an international expert panel on the use of neoadjuvant (primary) systemic treatment of operable breast cancer. Ann Oncol 18:1927–1934
6. Singletary SE et al (2008) Surgical management of inflammatory breast cancer. Semin Oncol 35:72–77
7. NCCN (2011) Clinical practice guidelines in oncology. Vol. 2 Inflammatory Breast Cancer. Available at http://www.nccn.org

Chapter 12
High-Dose Chemotherapy with Autologous Hematopoietic Stem Cell Transplantation in Inflammatory Breast Cancer

Yee Chung Cheng and Naoto T. Ueno

Keywords Dose intensity • High-dose chemotherapy • Hematopoietic stem cell transplantation (HSCT) • Autologous HSCT • West German Study Group • PEGASE 01 • PEGASE 04 • Cancer registry data • Autologous Blood and Marrow Transplant Registry (ABMTR) • European Group for Blood and Marrow Transplantation (EBMT) • PEGASE 05 • PEGASE 02 • PEGASE 07 • Center for International Blood and Marrow Transplant Research (CIBMTR) • Meta-analysis

Inflammatory breast cancer (IBC) is a rare type of invasive breast cancer with only about 5% of all breast cancer cases. However, it is one of the most aggressive forms of invasive breast cancer. It frequently presents with regional lymph node involvement at presentation and is followed by rapid disease progression to distant involvement from micrometastasis in the natural course of disease. With locoregional treatment only, long-term survival is less than 5% [1]. With the addition of systemic cytotoxic chemotherapy together with locoregional treatment, the long term survival has improved significantly but still at the range of 30–50% [2]. Inflammatory breast cancer being a systemic disease and also a chemo-sensitive disease, it makes sense that systemic cytotoxic therapy is the main force of treatment. The main issue is how to improve the systemic treatment to achieve a better survival outcome. One way to improve the systemic treatment is through the concept of dose intensity of cytotoxic chemotherapy.

Y.C. Cheng, M.D. (✉)
Division of Hematology and Oncology, Department of Medicine,
Medical College of Wisconsin, Milwaukee, WI, USA
e-mail: ycheng@mcw.edu

N.T. Ueno, M.D., Ph.D., F.A.C.P.
Morgan Welch Inflammatory Breast Cancer Program and Clinic, Department of Breast
Medical Oncology, The University of Texas, MD Anderson Cancer Center,
Unit 1354, Holcombe Blvd. 1515, Houston, TX, USA
e-mail: nueno@mdanderson.org

N.T. Ueno and M. Cristofanilli (eds.), *Inflammatory Breast Cancer: An Update*,
DOI 10.1007/978-94-007-3907-9_12, © Springer Science+Business Media B.V. 2012

In the mid-1980s, Hryniuk and colleagues suggested a linear dose–response relationship in cases of primary and metastatic breast cancer treated with cytotoxic agents particularly the alkylating agents [3–5]. Increasing the dose of the cytotoxic alkylating chemotherapy might be expected to result in more tumor cells being killed. However, normal cells, such as bone marrow cells, in the body are also susceptible to the cytotoxic effect of high-dose chemotherapy (HDC). To address this dilemma, hematopoietic stem cell transplantation (HSCT) was developed as a rescue process for HDC treatment. In this process, hematopoietic stem cells of the patient is collected and stored before given HDC to the patient. After the HDC treatment, the hematopoietic stem cells collected previously will be re-infused back to the patient to restore normal hematopoietic system. This concept led to the use of HDC with autologous HSCT in the treatment of breast cancer.

In the late 1980s and early 1990s, multiple phase II studies of the use of HDC with autologous HSCT in either high-risk primary breast cancer or metastatic breast cancer demonstrated significant favorable outcomes compared with historical data. These positive results prompted significantly increased use of HDC with autologous HSCT in breast cancer as a routine treatment. However, the true benefit of this treatment in breast cancer needed to be proven in randomized phase III trials. Since the late 1990s, a total of 15 randomized phase III trials of HDC with autologous HSCT in high-risk primary breast cancer and 8 randomized phase III trials in metastatic breast cancer have been described.

Of the 15 trials in high-risk primary breast cancer [6–20], 13 were already published, with 4 of them updated after longer follow-up. Two were still in preliminary form; one of these has been updated. Together, these 15 trials enrolled a total of more than 6,000 patients. One study, that of the West German Study Group reported by Nitz et al. [16], showed significant benefit in both relapse-free survival and overall survival. A second study, the PEGASE 01 study reported by Roché et al. [8], showed significant benefit in relapse-free survival but not in overall survival. However, the PEGASE 01 study was only presented in preliminary form in 2001, and it has not been updated. In 2011, Berry et al. [21] reported the first meta-analysis using individual data from all 15 trials; this analysis showed a significant benefit of HDC with autologous HSCT in relapse-free survival with a hazard ratio of 0.87 ($p < 0.001$) but not in overall survival (hazard ratio of 0.94, $p = 0.13$). Subgroup analysis failed to show a benefit in any particular subpopulation.

Of the 8 trials in metastatic breast cancer [22–30], 7 were already published, with 1 of them updated after longer follow-up. One was still in preliminary form. Together, these 8 trials enrolled a total of more than 1,000 patients. Six trials showed significant benefit in progression-free survival but not in overall survival. One of them (the PEGASE 04 study) showed significant benefit in both progression-free survival and overall survival [26]. In 2011, Berry et al. [31] reported the first meta-analysis using individual data from 6 of the 8 trials; this analysis showed a significant benefit in progression-free survival with a hazard ratio of 0.76 ($p < 0.001$) but not in overall survival (hazard ratio of 0.89, $p = 0.13$). Subgroup analysis failed to show a benefit in any particular subpopulation.

However, with the rarity of IBC, not many cases were included in the above randomized phase III trials. Some of the IBC cases were included in the locally advanced breast cancer group including non-inflammatory stage III breast cancer during the survival analysis. Therefore those randomized phase III trials did not particularly address the role of HDC with autologous HSCT in IBC. We hereby review the available clinical data including cancer registry data, phase II studies, randomized phase III trial and current study of the use of HDC with autologous HSCT in IBC.

12.1   Cancer Registry Data

In 1997, Antman et al. [32] published the first report of HDC with autologous HSCT for breast cancer in North America using data in the Autologous Blood and Marrow Transplant Registry (ABMTR). Between January 1, 1989 and June 30, 1995, a total of 5,886 patients received HDC with autologous HSCT for breast cancer were reported to ABMTR. Of these, 260 patients were cases of non-metastatic IBC. The most commonly used high-dose conditioning regimen was cyclophosphamide and thiotepa; or cyclophosphamide, thiotepa and carboplatin; or cyclophosphamide, carmustine or cisplatin. The 3-year Kaplan-Meier estimates of progression-free survival were 42% (95% confidence interval of 31–53%) and the 3-year Kaplan-Meier estimates of overall survival were 52% (95% confidence interval of 40–64%).

In 2003, Pedrazzoli et al. [33] published their report of HDC with autologous HSCT for breast cancer in Europe using data in the European Group for Blood and Marrow Transplantation (EBMT) Registry. Between 1990 and 1999, a total of 7,471 patients received HDC with autologous HSCT for breast cancer were reported to the EBMT Registry but only 5,895 were eligible for data analysis. Of these, 921 patients were cases of non-metastatic IBC. This 10-year number of IBC cases is much more than the ABMTR data of 260 cases in 6.5 years. One possible reason for this discrepancy is the more likely used of HDC with autologous HSCT approach for IBC in Europe. The most commonly used high-dose conditioning regimen was STAMP V regimen, which composed of cyclophosphamide, thiotepa and carboplatin; or its variant. The 5-year Kaplan-Meier estimates of progression-free survival were 42% and the 5-year Kaplan-Meier estimates of overall survival were 53% (Table 12.1).

12.2   Phase II Studies

Since 1997, there were 10 phase II studies of HDC with autologous HSCT for IBC exclusively and 3 other phase II studies for high-risk primary breast cancer including IBC but had separated survival analysis for IBC subgroup. With these 13 studies, 12 were already published and one (PEGASE 05 trial) was still in the preliminary form.

Among the three phase II studies for high risk primary breast cancer but had separated survival analysis for IBC subgroup, Ayash et al. [34] in 1998 included the

Table 12.1 Cancer Registry Data

Author, year and study	Number of patients	Number of IBC cases	Disease-free survival (95% CI)	Overall survival (95% CI)
Antman et al. 1997 [32] ABMTR	5,886	260	42% (31–53%) at 3 years	52% (40–64%) at 3 years
Pedrazzoli et al. 2003 [33] EBMT	5,895	921	42% at 5 years	53% at 5 years

IBC inflammatory breast cancer, *CI* confidence interval

most number of IBC cases, a total of 42 among 47 evaluable high risk primary breast cancer patients. After standard induction chemotherapy, high-dose conditioning chemotherapy of cyclophosphamide, thiotepa and carboplatin with autologous HSCT was given as neoadjuvant consolidation treatment before the primary surgery. Thirty months relapse-free survival and overall survival were 64% and 89% respectively. Somlo et al. [35] in 1997 had 22 among 114 high risk breast cancer patients. After the primary surgery, high-dose conditioning chemotherapy of either cyclophosphamide, etoposide and doxorubicin, or cyclophosphamide, etoposide and cisplatin was given as adjuvant consolidation treatment. Three and a half-year relapse-free survival and overall survival were 50% and 72% respectively. We reported our study in 2004 with 18 cases among 117 high-risk breast cancer patients [36]. After the primary surgery, patients received the cyclophosphamide, etoposide and cisplatin for stem cell mobilization, followed by high-dose conditioning regimen of cyclophosphamide, carmustine and thiotepa with autologous HSCT as adjuvant consolidation treatment. Five-year relapse-free survival and overall survival rate were 28% and 36% respectively (Table 12.2). Although our study had the lower survival rate, it was comparable with historical data.

Among the ten phase II studies for IBC exclusively; PEGASE 02 trial reported by Viens et al. [37] in 1999 had the most number of patients, which were 95 cases. After two cycles of high-dose cyclophosphamide and doxorubicin followed by hematopoietic stem cells collection each, patient received two more cycles of high-dose cyclophosphamide, doxorubicin and 5-fluorouracil with stem cells infusion each as a neoadjuvant consolidation treatment before the primary surgery. One patient died from septic shock after becoming aplasia. After the primary surgery, pathologic complete response rate was 32%. Three-year relapse-free survival and overall survival were 44% and 70% respectively. The other nine phase II studies enrolled patients from 17 to 56 cases. Like PEGASE 2 trial, 3 of them used the HDC and autologous HSCT as neoadjuvant consolidation treatment before the primary surgery (Table 12.3). PEGASE 05 trial reported by Palangie et al. [40] in 2006 as a preliminary form had 54 cases. The extreme intense high-dose conditioning chemotherapy regimens used included two cycles of high-dose cyclophosphamide and doxorubicin with hematopoietic stem cells collection each, followed by docetaxel for three cycles, followed by another two cycles of high-dose cyclophosphamide and doxorubicin with hematopoietic stem cells infusion each. Pathologic complete response rate was 35%. Five-year relapse-free survival and overall survival were 42%

Table 12.2 Phase II studies for high risk breast cancer including inflammatory breast cancer

Author and year	Number of patients	Number of IBC cases	HDC	Treatment-related death	Disease-free survival (95% CI)	Overall survival (95% CI)
Somlo et al. 1997 [35]	114	22	CEA or CEP	1	50% (29–71%) at 3.5 years	72% (53–91%) at 3.5 years
Ayash et al. 1998 [34]	47	42	CTCb	0	64% (49–84%) at 30 months	89% (79–100%) at 30 months
Cheng et al. 2004 [36]	117	18	CBT	0	28% at 5 years	36% at 5 years

C cyclophosphamide, *E* etoposide, *A* doxorubicin, *P* cisplatin, *T* Thiotepa, *Cb* carboplatin, *B* carmustine

and 62% respectively. However, the trial was prematurely stopped due to increased toxicity and two treatment-related deaths. Viens et al. [38] initially report a small single institution phase II study of 17 patients in 1998. High-dose conditioning chemotherapy regimen of cyclophosphamide, mitoxantrone and melphalan was given before the primary surgery. No treatment-related death. Pathologic complete response rate was 39%. Three-year relapse-free survival and overall survival were 66% and 68% respectively. Dazzi et al. [39] reported another small phase II study of 20 patients. High-dose conditioning chemotherapy regimen of cyclophosphamide, mitoxantrone and thiotepa was given before the primary surgery. One patient died from treatment-related cardiac toxicity. Pathologic complete response rate was reported as 55%. Four-year relapse-free survival and overall survival were 58% and 74% respectively. These three studies reported the pathologic complete response rate from 35% to 55% after neoadjuvant HDC with autologous HSCT, which is higher than that from standard neoadjuvant chemotherapy regimen. Whether higher pathologic complete response rate will translate into better survival outcome remains to be determined. The other six phase II studies used the HDC with autologous HSCT as adjuvant treatment after the primary surgery [41–46] (Table 12.4). The high-dose conditioning regimens varied but mostly composed of high-dose cyclophosphamide-based regimen. Survival rates also varied among the different studies but were comparable to historical data.

12.3   Randomized Phase III Trial

The result of the two phase II studies – PEGASE 02 and 05 trials suggested that increased intensity of the HDC given before the primary surgery might increase pathologic complete response rate which in turn might improve the ultimate survival

Table 12.3 Phase II studies for inflammatory breast cancer (neoadjuvant approach)

Author, year and study	Number of patients	Median age (range)	Median follow up (range)	HDC	pCR	Treatment-related death	Disease-free survival (95% CI)	Overall survival (95% CI)
Viens et al. 1998 [38]	17	46 years (24–54)	36 months (17–52)	CMMe	39%	0	66% (44–88) 3 years	68% (40–89) 3 years
Viens et al. 1999 [37] PEGASE 02	95	46 years (26–59)	36 months	FAC×2	32%	1	44% (33–54) 3 years	70% (60–79) 3 years
Dazzi et al. 2001 [39]	20	46 years (29–56)	48 months	CMT	55%	1	58% 4 years	74% 4 years
Palangie et al. 2006 [40] PEGASE 05	54	NR	NR	AC×2/D×3/ AC×2	35%	2	42% 5 years	62% 5 years

NR not reported, *M* mitoxantrone, *Me* melphalan, *F* 5-fluorouracil, *D* docetaxel, *pCR* pathologic complete response

Table 12.4 Phase II studies for inflammatory breast cancer (adjuvant approach)

Author and year	Number of patients	Median age (range)	Median follow up (range)	HDC	Treatment-related death	Disease-free survival (95% CI)	Overall survival (95% CI)
Cagnoni et al. 1998 [41]	30	12.5 years (26–45)	19 months (4–44)	CBT	1	70% (51–86%) at 19 months	NR
Schwartzberg et al. 1999 [42]	56	46 years (26–63)	44 months (15–76)	CTCb	2	53% at 3 years	72% at 3 years
Adkins et al. 1999 [43]	47	44 years (25–61)	22 months (0.5–82)	MeECb or CT±Cb or CBP or BuMeT	2	56.4% at 4 years	54.4% at 4 years
Arun et al. 1999 [44]	24	45 years (32–58)	18 months (8–68)	CCb	0	71% (55–87%) at 2 years	73% (53–93%) at 2 years
Yalamanchili et al. 2008 [45]	28	45 years (29–58)	141 months (mean)	CMT	0	40 months (median)	49.5 months (median)
Sportes et al. 2009 [46]	20	50 years (35–67)	8.3 years	MeE	1	60% at 3 years	75% at 3 years

Bu busulfan

outcome. However, increased cycles of HDC regimen given before the primary surgery also increase the treatment-related morbidity and mortality. Another unsolved issue is the role of adjuvant or maintenance chemotherapy in patients received intense neoadjuvant treatment including HDC with autologous HSCT. Based on this question, PEGASE group launched another trial PEGASE 07 in 2000 [47]. PEGASE 07 trial was the only randomized phase III study of the use of HDC with autologous HSCT for patients with IBC. In this trial, all patients received four cycles of high-dose cyclophosphamide and epirubicin with the hematopoietic stem cells collected after the cycle 1 and re-infused after cycle 2, 3 and 4 upon enrollment. Then patients proceeded to locoregional therapy of primary surgery and radiation therapy. After the locoregional therapy, patients were randomized to either observation with no chemotherapy or another 4 cycles of adjuvant chemotherapy of docetaxel and 5-fluorouracil. The primary endpoint was 3-year disease-free survival. Secondary endpoints were pathologic complete response rate, overall survival and quality of life. The trial was closed on June 2005 after the expected accrual of 175 patients. Result was not yet reported at this moment [48].

12.4 Current Study

In 2004, a new organization named Center for International Blood and Marrow Transplant Research (CIBMTR) joined together the research programs of the National Marrow Donor Program® (NMDP) and the International Bone Marrow Transplant Registry (IBMTR) at the Medical College of Wisconsin. Center for International Blood and Marrow Transplant Research collaborates with the global scientific community to advance hematopoietic cell transplantation and cellular therapy research worldwide. It also facilitates critical research that has led to increased survival and an enriched quality of life for thousands of patients.

Currently we are conducting a study – CIBMTR ST10-01 that is a retrospective study to determine the value of HDC and autologous HSCT in patients with high risk or metastatic IBC. The three aims of the study are (1) to determine the overall outcome of patients with IBC who underwent HDC and autologous HSCT in high-risk setting or metastatic setting, (2) to determine the prognostic factors that select patients with IBC who benefit from HDC and autologous HSCT and, (3) to compare the overall outcome of patients with IBC who underwent HDC and autologous HSCT in high risk setting or metastatic setting and that of patients with non-IBC who underwent HDC and autologous HSCT in high risk setting or metastatic setting.

12.5 Conclusion

Since the introduction of multidisciplinary approach especially the use of systemic cytotoxic chemotherapy as early as possible in the course of IBC management, there has not been any other major breakthrough in the treatment of IBC. Inflammatory breast cancer remains as one of the invasive breast cancers with poor prognosis. Pre-clinical research is needed in understanding the biology of this unique type of invasive breast cancer. Well-design clinical trial is needed in testing the efficacy of new treatment modalities in IBC based on the biology information. Clinical trial is also needed in refining existing treatment modalities such as HDC and autologous HSCT. From the current data we have reviewed, we cannot completely deny the role of HDC and autologous HSCT in IBC. High-dose chemotherapy and autologous HSCT is not for every patient with IBC, but certain subgroup of patient definitely benefit from this treatment modality. Therefore, instead of simply giving up on a potential treatment modality, it is more logical and practical to refine and improve this existing modality in addition to developing new modalities in the clinical trial setting [49].

References

1. Ueno NT, Buzdar AU, Singletary SE et al (1997) Combined-modality treatment of inflammatory breast carcinoma: twenty years of experience at M. D. Anderson Cancer Center. Cancer Chemother Pharmacol 40:321–329
2. Jaiyesimi IA, Buzdar AU, Hortobagyi G (1992) Inflammatory breast cancer: a review. J Clin Oncol 10:1014–1024
3. Hryniuk W, Bush H (1984) The importance of dose intensity in chemotherapy of metastatic breast cancer. J Clin Oncol 2:1281–1288
4. Hryniuk W, Levine MN (1986) Analysis of dose intensity for adjuvant chemotherapy trials in stage II breast cancer. J Clin Oncol 4:1162–1170
5. Hryniuk WM, Levine MN, Levin L (1986) Analysis of dose intensity for chemotherapy in early (stage II) and advanced breast cancer. NCI Monogr 1986 (1):87–94
6. Wilking N, Lidbrink E, Wiklund T et al (2007) Long-term follow-up of the SBG 9401 study comparing tailored FEC-based therapy versus marrow-supported high-dose therapy. Ann Oncol 18:694–700
7. Hanrahan EO, Broglio K, Frye D et al (2006) Randomized trial of high-dose chemotherapy and autologous hematopoietic stem cell support for high-risk primary breast carcinoma: follow-up at 12 years. Cancer 106:2327–2336
8. Roché HH, Pouillart P, Meyer N et al (2001) Adjuvant high-dose chemotherapy (HDC) improves early outcome for high risk (N > 7) breast cancer patients: the PEGASE 01 trial. Proc Am Soc Clin Oncol 20 :abstr 102
9. Gianni A, Bonadonna G (2007) Updated 12-year results of a randomized clinical trial comparing standard-dose versus high-dose myeloablative chemotherapy in the adjuvant treatment of breast cancer with more than 3 positive nodes (LN+). Proc Am Soc Clin Oncol 25 :abstr 549
10. Schrama JG, Faneyte IF, Schornagel JH et al (2002) Randomized trial of high-dose chemotherapy and hematopoietic progenitor-cell support in operable breast cancer with extensive lymph node involvement: final analysis with 7 years of follow-up. Ann Oncol 13:689–698
11. Rodenhuis S, Bontenbal M, Beex LV et al (2003) High-dose chemotherapy with hematopoietic stem-cell rescue for high-risk breast cancer. N Engl J Med 349:7–16
12. Tallman MS, Gray R, Robert NJ et al (2003) Conventional adjuvant chemotherapy with or without high-dose chemotherapy and autologous stem-cell transplantation in high-risk breast cancer. N Engl J Med 349:17–26
13. Leonard RC, Lind M, Twelves C et al (2004) Conventional adjuvant chemotherapy versus single-cycle, autograft-supported, high-dose, late-intensification chemotherapy in high-risk breast cancer patients: a randomized trial. J Natl Cancer Inst 96:1076–1083

14. Zander AR, Schmoor C, Kroger N et al (2008) Randomized trial of high-dose adjuvant chemotherapy with autologous hematopoietic stem-cell support versus standard-dose chemotherapy in breast cancer patients with 10 or more positive lymph nodes: overall survival after 6 years of follow-up. Ann Oncol 19:1082–1089
15. Coombes RC, Howell A, Emson M et al (2005) High dose chemotherapy and autologous stem cell transplantation as adjuvant therapy for primary breast cancer patients with four or more lymph nodes involved: long-term results of an international randomised trial. Ann Oncol 16:726–734
16. Nitz UA, Mohrmann S, Fischer J et al (2005) Comparison of rapidly cycled tandem high-dose chemotherapy plus peripheral-blood stem-cell support versus dose-dense conventional chemotherapy for adjuvant treatment of high-risk breast cancer: results of a multicentre phase III trial. Lancet 366:1935–1944
17. Peters WP, Rosner GL, Vredenburgh JJ et al (2005) Prospective, randomized comparison of high-dose chemotherapy with stem-cell support versus intermediate-dose chemotherapy after surgery and adjuvant chemotherapy in women with high-risk primary breast cancer: a report of CALGB 9082, SWOG 9114, and NCIC MA-13. J Clin Oncol 23:2191–2200
18. Basser RL, O'Neill A, Martinelli G et al (2006) Multicycle dose-intensive chemotherapy for women with high-risk primary breast cancer: results of International Breast Cancer Study Group Trial 15–95. J Clin Oncol 24:370–378
19. Moore HC, Green SJ, Gralow JR et al (2007) Intensive dose-dense compared with high-dose adjuvant chemotherapy for high-risk operable breast cancer: Southwest Oncology Group/Intergroup study 9623. J Clin Oncol 25:1677–1682
20. Tokuda Y, Tajima T, Narabayashi M et al (2008) Phase III study to evaluate the use of high-dose chemotherapy as consolidation of treatment for high-risk postoperative breast cancer: Japan Clinical Oncology Group study, JCOG 9208. Cancer Sci 99:145–151
21. Berry D, Ueno N, Johnson MM et al (2011) High-dose chemotherapy with autologous stem-cell support as adjuvant therapy in breast cancer: overview of 15 randomized trials. J Clin Oncol 29:3214–3223
22. Stadtmauer EA, O'Neill A, Goldstein LJ et al (2000) Conventional-dose chemotherapy compared with high-dose chemotherapy plus autologous hematopoietic stem-cell transplantation for metastatic breast cancer. Philadelphia Bone Marrow Transplant Group. N Engl J Med 342:1069–1076
23. Stadtmauer EA, O'Neill A, Goldstein LJ et al (2002) Conventional-dose chemotherapy compared with high-dose chemotherapy (HDC) plus autologous stem cell transplantation (SCT) for metastatic breast cancer: 5-year update of the 'Philadelphia Trial' (PBT-01). Proc Am Soc Clin Oncol 21 :abstr 169
24. Crown J, Perey L, Lind M et al (2003) Superiority of tandem high-dose chemotherapy (HDC) versus optimized conventionally-dosed chemotherapy (CDC) in patients (pts) with metastatic breast cancer (MBC): the International Breast Cancer Dose Intensity Study (IBDIS 1). Proc Am Soc Clin Oncol 22 :abstr 88
25. Schmid P, Schippinger W, Nitsch T et al (2005) Up-front tandem high-dose chemotherapy compared with standard chemotherapy with doxorubicin and paclitaxel in metastatic breast cancer: results of a randomized trial. J Clin Oncol 23:432–440
26. Lotz JP, Cure H, Janvier M et al (2005) High-dose chemotherapy with haematopoietic stem cell transplantation for metastatic breast cancer patients: final results of the French multicentric randomised CMA/PEGASE 04 protocol. Eur J Cancer 41:71–80
27. Vredenburgh JJ, Coniglio D, Broadwater G et al (2006) Consolidation with high-dose combination alkylating agents with bone marrow transplantation significantly improves disease-free survival in hormone-insensitive metastatic breast cancer in complete remission compared with intensive standard-dose chemotherapy alone. Biol Blood Marrow Transplant 12:195–203
28. Vredenburgh JJ, Madan B, Coniglio D et al (2006) A randomized phase III comparative trial of immediate consolidation with high-dose chemotherapy and autologous peripheral blood

progenitor cell support compared to observation with delayed consolidation in women with metastatic breast cancer and only bone metastases following intensive induction chemotherapy. Bone Marrow Transplant 37:1009–1015

29. Biron P, Durand M, Roche H et al (2008) Pegase 03: a prospective randomized phase III trial of FEC with or without high-dose thiotepa, cyclophosphamide and autologous stem cell transplantation in first-line treatment of metastatic breast cancer. Bone Marrow Transplant 41:555–562

30. Crump M, Gluck S, Tu D et al (2008) Randomized trial of high-dose chemotherapy with autologous peripheral-blood stem-cell support compared with standard-dose chemotherapy in women with metastatic breast cancer: NCIC MA.16. J Clin Oncol 26:37–43

31. Berry D, Ueno N, Johnson MM et al (2011) High-dose chemotherapy with autologous hematopoietic stem-cell transplantation in metastatic breast cancer: overview of 6 randomized trials. J Clin Oncol 29:3224–3231

32. Antman KH, Rowlings PA, Vaughan WP et al (1997) High-dose chemotherapy with autologous hematopoietic stem-cell support for breast cancer in North America. J Clin Oncol 15:1870–1879

33. Pedrazzoli P, Ferrante P, Kulekci A et al (2003) Autologous hematopoietic stem cell transplantation for breast cancer in Europe: critical evaluation of data from the European Group for Blood and Marrow Transplantation (EBMT) registry 1990–1999. Bone Marrow Transplant 32:489–494

34. Ayash LJ, Elias A, Ibrahim J et al (1998) High-dose multimodality therapy with autologous stem-cell support for stage IIIB breast carcinoma. J Clin Oncol 16:1000–1007

35. Somlo G, Doroshow JH, Forman SJ et al (1997) High-dose chemotherapy and stem-cell rescue in the treatment of high-risk breast cancer: prognostic indicators of progression-free and overall survival. J Clin Oncol 15:2882–2893

36. Cheng YC, Rondon G, Yang Y et al (2004) The use of high-dose cyclophosphamide, carmustine, and thiotepa plus autologous hematopoietic stem cell transplantation as consolidation therapy for high-risk primary breast cancer after primary surgery or neoadjuvant chemotherapy. Biol Blood Marrow Transplant 10:794–804

37. Viens P, Palangie T, Janvier M et al (1999) First-line high-dose sequential chemotherapy with rG-CSF and repeated blood stem cell transplantation in untreated inflammatory breast cancer: toxicity and response (PEGASE 02 trial). Br J Cancer 81:449–456

38. Viens P, Penault-Llorca F, Jacquemier J et al (1998) High-dose chemotherapy and haematopoietic stem cell transplantation for inflammatory breast cancer: pathologic response and outcome. Bone Marrow Transplant 21:249–254

39. Dazzi C, Cariello A, Rosti G et al (2001) Neoadjuvant high dose chemotherapy plus peripheral blood progenitor cells in inflammatory breast cancer: a multicenter phase II pilot study. Haematologica 86:523–529

40. Palangie T, Pouillart P, Roche H et al (2006) Five year update of sequential high dose doxorubicin, cyclophosphamide and docetaxel in inflammatory breast cancer; PEGASE05 trial on behalf of FNLCC. Proc Am Soc Clin Oncol 24 :abstr 10773

41. Cagnoni PJ, Nieto Y, Shpall EJ et al (1998) High-dose chemotherapy with autologous hematopoietic progenitor-cell support as part of combined modality therapy in patients with inflammatory breast cancer. J Clin Oncol 16:1661–1668

42. Schwartzberg L, Weaver C, Lewkow L et al (1999) High-dose chemotherapy with peripheral blood stem cell support for stage IIIB inflammatory carcinoma of the breast. Bone Marrow Transplant 24:981–987

43. Adkins D, Brown R, Trinkaus K et al (1999) Outcomes of high-dose chemotherapy and autologous stem-cell transplantation in stage IIIB inflammatory breast cancer. J Clin Oncol 17:2006–2014

44. Arun B, Slack R, Gehan E et al (1999) Survival after autologous hematopoietic stem cell transplantation for patients with inflammatory breast carcinoma. Cancer 85:93–99

45. Yalamanchili K, Lalmuanpuii J, Waheed F et al (2008) High-dose chemotherapy with autologous stem cell rescue in stage IIIB inflammatory breast cancer. Anticancer Res 28:3139–3142

46. Sportes C, Steinberg SM, Liewehr DJ et al (2009) Strategies to improve long-term outcome in stage IIIB inflammatory breast cancer: multimodality treatment including dose-intensive induction and high-dose chemotherapy. Biol Blood Marrow Transplant 15:963–970
47. Roche H, Viens P, Biron P et al (2003) High-dose chemotherapy for breast cancer: the French PEGASE experience. Cancer Control 10:42–47
48. Viens P, Tarpin C, Roche H et al (2010) Systemic therapy of inflammatory breast cancer from high-dose chemotherapy to targeted therapies: the French experience. Cancer 116:2829–2836
49. Cheng YC, Ueno NT (2010) Is high-dose chemotherapy with autologous hematopoietic stem cell transplantation in breast cancer patients a done deal? Womens Health (Lond Engl) 6:481–485

Chapter 13
Models of Inflammatory Breast Cancer

Lara Lacerda and Wendy A. Woodward

Abstract Inflammatory Breast Cancer (IBC) is a rare and difficult to characterize subtype of breast cancer for which few in vitro and in vivo models are currently available. In this chapter we describe the characteristics and limitations of the models that have been published to further study the pathology of IBC and to develop therapeutic approaches for IBC. Published information regarding receptor status, E-cadherin expression, 2D and 3D culture, xenografts, ability to form metastases and identified tumor-initiation cell sub-populations are reviewed.

Keywords Xenografts • Inflammatory breast cancer • Animal models • Mary-X • SUM149 • SUM190 • KLP4 • WIBC-9 • MDA-IBC-3

13.1 Introduction

An ideal animal model for any disease should faithfully recapitulate the clinical and pathologic findings associated with that disease. Currently, the most widely referenced definition of inflammatory breast cancer (IBC) is that of the American Joint Committee on Cancer [1], which states in part that "*inflammatory carcinoma is a clinicopathologic entity characterized by diffuse erythema and edema (peau d'orange) of the breast, often without an underlying mass... It is important to remember that inflammatory carcinoma is primarily a clinical diagnosis. Involvement of the dermal lymphatics alone does not indicate inflammatory carcinoma in the absence of clinical findings.*" Unfortunately, most of the models for IBC while derived from human IBC tumors, fail to recapitulate the clinicopathologic findings

L. Lacerda • W.A. Woodward (✉)
Department of Radiation Oncology, Unit 1202, The University of Texas MD Anderson Cancer Center, 1515 Holcombe Blvd., Houston, TX 77030, USA
e-mail: wwoodward@mdanderson.org

N.T. Ueno and M. Cristofanilli (eds.), *Inflammatory Breast Cancer: An Update*,
DOI 10.1007/978-94-007-3907-9_13, © Springer Science+Business Media B.V. 2012

of skin erythema and invasion of the dermal lymphatics. Efforts have been made to identify molecular signatures that define IBC to better identify true IBC pathology, however most of the available signatures are heavily influenced by the relative paucity of the luminal A and B subtypes among IBC patients compared with non-IBC patients [2–4]. Both the rarity of this disease and the limited availability of IBC models contribute to the difficulty in defining IBC at the molecular level and understanding the pathobiology sufficiently to lead to novel therapies.

While significant progress has been made in identifying individual genes and proteins differentially regulated in IBC compared to non-IBC, including RhoC [5–8], WISP3 [9–11], E-cadherin [12, 13], and EIF4GI [14], the lack of abundant and ideal IBC models inherently limits the investigation of these and other potential IBC regulators. Although dermal lymphatic invasion is not identified in the majority of IBC patients, when associated with the clinical signs of IBC it remains the sine qua non of the diagnosis; however, to date, only one IBC model recapitulates this phenotype in the mouse [15]. Studies in this model and others have suggested that IBC tumors have properties of tumor stem cell biology [16, 17], and indeed, microarray studies in IBC have demonstrated increased expression of genes associated with breast cancer stem cells [18]. Furthermore, an independent study has confirmed the expression of the stem cell marker aldehyde dehydrogenase 1 (ALDH1) as prognostic in IBC patient samples [16]. Ideally, to facilitate and accelerate the study of this disease, this chapter would describe a broad array of IBC cell lines and animal models that fully recapitulate the clinical and pathobiologic IBC phenomena described and span the spectrum of intrinsic breast cancer subtypes seen in IBC. Not surprisingly given the rarity of the disease, however, while progress has been made, the available IBC models remain somewhat limited. Herein we describe the development and characteristics of each (Table 13.1).

13.2 IBC Models Established *In Vitro*

13.2.1 *KPL-4*

The KPL-4 cell line was established at Kawasaki Medical School in Okayama (Japan) with cells obtained from a pleural effusion collected from a woman diagnosed in 1995 with recurrent breast cancer and inflammatory skin metastasis [19]. Following centrifugation, cells from the pleural effusion were directly plated into plastic cell culture flasks, maintained in 2D culture, and passaged more than 70 times over a year. *In vitro*, KPL-4 cells have a polygonal shape and a large nucleus and grow in a monolayer fashion like cobblestones with a doubling time of about 2 days [19, 26]. In addition, this cell line can also grow in anchorage-independent soft agar cultures [19, 27].

In vivo, the KPL-4 cell line develops fast-growing tumors (detectable 1–2 weeks after injections) at an efficiency of 100% in both nude and severe combined immunodeficient (SCID) mice (1×10^7 cells) [19, 26, 27]. The tumors have massive

Table 13.1 Established IBC models

Model	Origin	ER/PgR/HER2 status	E-cadherin Status	Mutation status	IBC characteristics	Reference
KPL-4	Malignant pleural effusion of a breast cancer patient with an inflammatory skin metastasis	−/−/+	n.a.	Chromosomal abnormalities	Very aggressive phenotype	[19]
MARY-X	Biopsy of patient with IBC	−/−/−	Positive	p53 positive	Erythema in the overlying mouse skin and development of tumor emboli	[13, 15]
SUM149	Primary tumor from IBC patient	−/−/−	Positive	p53 positive	Aggressive local disease, tumor mass grows in nodes/clusters with small necrotic areas, local and distant metastases, and invasion of skin (ulcerative tumors)	[20–23]
SUM190	Primary tumor from IBC patient	−/−/+	Positive[a]	p53 positive	n.a.	[20, 21]
WIBC-9	Surgically resected tumor from patient with IBC	−/−/+	Positive	Chromosomal abnormalities	Exhibited erythema of the overlying skin, marked lymphatic permeation, and high rate of metastasis	[24]
MDA-IBC-3	Pleural effusion from IBC patient	−/−/+[a]	Positive	p53 positive	Erythema and loss of fur on the overlying skin, local metastasis, and invasion of skin[a]	[25]

n.a. – not available

[a]Unpublished data from Dr. Woodward's lab

central necrosis and occasionally can invade surrounding tissues (skin and muscles). This cell line has also been described as spontaneously forming micrometastases in the lymph nodes and lungs; mice became cachexic and die 3–4 weeks after cell injections [19]. Both *in vitro* and *in vivo*, KPL-4 cells express cytokeratin, carcino-embryonic antigen, CA15-3, and HER2; do not express vimentin, estrogen receptor (ER), or progesterone receptor (PgR); and secrete high levels of interleukin (IL)-6 [19]. The cell line KPL-4 has been used as a model to study the connection between IL-6 secretion and cancer-induced cachexia [26] and as a model of trastuzumab resistance because it expresses p95HER2, the NH_2-terminal truncated HER2 fragment that is associated with clinical resistance to trastuzumab and poor clinical outcome [27].

13.2.2   SUM149

Cell line SUM149 was established at the University of Michigan Medical School in Ann Arbor (USA) from a primary tumor of a patient with invasive ductal carcinoma [20, 28, 29]. This karyotypically abnormal cell line was isolated and grown in optimized 2D culture conditions (Table 13.2) and expresses luminal cytokeratins 8, 18, and 19 [21]. Nevertheless, SUM149 can also be cultured and remain viable in several 3D conditions (Table 13.2), such as soft agar, methylcellulose, and liquid suspension [20, 32]. It has been shown that the expression of E-cadherin by SUM149 is key in its invasion and motility ability *in vitro* [22, 35].

SUM149 cells have highly tumorigenic behavior *in vivo*. Primary tumor frequency for xenografts of SUM149 is 100%, with tumors of 1 cm in diameter 6–8 weeks after injection of 1×10^6 cells (in diluted Matrigel) into the mammary glands of nonobese diabetic (NOD)/SCID mice [33] or subcutaneously in nude mice [34]. Tumors also develop when 2×10^6 SUM149 cells, diluted in Matrigel or not, are injected orthotopically in athymic nude mice [23]. Tumors are described to grow in multiple nodes/clusters with small necrotic cores and invade the skin very aggressively [23]. Furthermore, SUM149 can produce spontaneous micrometastases in the lungs upon tail-vein injection of 2×10^6 cells [33] and in the lungs and legs following implantation in the mammary fat pad [23].

Recently, studies regarding the identification of chemo- and radiotherapy-resistant subpopulations of cells that may mediate metastasis (cancer stem cells or tumor-initiating cells) have described such subpopulations in the cell line SUM149 as $CD44^+/CD24^{-/low}/ESA^+$ [32] and $ALDH1^+$ [16] cells.

13.2.3   SUM190

The cell line SUM190 is another karyotypically abnormal cell line established at the University of Michigan Medical School in Ann Arbor (USA) from a primary tumor of a patient with invasive ductal breast carcinoma [20, 28, 29]. SUM190 cells were

Table 13.2 Conditions for *in vitro* and *in vivo* maintenance of IBC models

Model	2D culture	3D culture	Xenografts	Spontaneous metastasis	TICs	Reference
KPL-4	Dulbecco's modified Eagle's medium supplemented with 5% FBS	Soft agar	Injected into mammary fat pads of female athymic nude and SCID mice; subcutaneously in nude mice	Lungs and lymph nodes	n.a.	[19, 27]
MARY-X	n.a.	Keratinocyte serum-free medium or MEM medium with 10% FCS	Implanted subcutaneously in female athymic nude and SCID mice	Lungs, confined to within vessels	CD44$^+$/CD24$^{-/low}$, ALDH1$^+$, and CD133$^+$	[13, 15, 16, 30, 31]
SUM149	Ham's F-12 medium supplemented with 5 µg/ml insulin, 1 mg/ml hydrocortisone and 5% FBS	Soft agar; methylcellulose; serum-free MEM supplemented with 20 ng/ml bFGF, 20 ng/ml EGF, B27, 1% pen-strep and 4 µg/ml gentamycin	Injected into mammary fat pads of female athymic nude and NOD/SCID mice; injected by tail vein in NOD/SCID mice	Lungs and legs	CD44$^+$/CD24$^{-/low}$, ESA$^+$, ALDH1$^+$	[16, 20, 21, 23, 25, 32–34]
SUM190	Ham's F-12 medium supplemented with 5 µg/ml insulin and 1 mg/ml hydrocortisone	Soft agar; serum-free MEM supplemented with 20 ng/ml bFGF, 20 ng/ml EGF, B27, 1% penstrep and 1% gentamycin[a]	Implanted subcutaneously in female nude mice and into mammary fat pads of female NOD/SCID mice; injected by tail vein into NOD/SCID mice	No	n.a.	[20, 21, 33, 34]
WIBC-9	n.a.	n.a.	Implanted subcutaneously in female BALB/c nude and SCID mice	Lungs	n.a.	[24]
MDA-IBC-3	Ham's F-12 medium supplemented with 5 µg/ml insulin, 10% FBS, 1 mg/ml hydrocortisone, and 1% antibiotic/ antimycotic	Serum-free MEM supplemented with 20 ng/ml bFGF, 20 ng/ml EGF, B27, 1% penstrep and 1% gentamycin	Injected into mammary fat pads of female SCID/Beige mice and subcutaneously in NOD/SCID mice	Locally	CD44$^+$/CD24$^-$	[25]

FBS fetal bovine serum, *SCID* severe combined-immunodeficient, *MEM* minimal essential medium, *bFGF* basic fibroblast growth factor, *EGF* epidermal growth factor, *NOD* nonobese diabetic, *TICs* tumor-initiating cells
[a]Unpublished data from Dr. Woodward's lab

initially isolated in a complex medium supplemented with epidermal growth factor (EGF) and lysophosphatidic acid and later cultured in a serum-free medium (Table 13.2). This cell line also expresses luminal cytokeratins 8, 18, and 19 [21]. Anchorage-independent cultures can be prepared with soft agar [20] and liquid medium (Table 13.2).

In vivo, SUM190 cells form primary tumors of 1 cm in diameter with an efficacy of 100% within 6–8 weeks after implantation of 1×10^6 cells (in diluted Matrigel) into the mammary glands of NOD/SCID mice [33] or subcutaneously in nude mice [34]. Unfortunately, this cell line is unable to metastasize spontaneously, whether it is injected orthotopically, intraperitoneally, or by tail vein [33].

13.3   IBC Models Established *In Vivo*

13.3.1   *MARY-X*

The first human transplantable IBC xenograft was established with pieces of a biopsy from a woman diagnosed with IBC; the specimens were directly implanted subcutaneously in SCID and athymic nude mice at the School of Medicine of the University of California, Los Angeles (USA) [15]. *In vivo*, MARY-X grows exclusively nestled within murine lymphatic and blood vessel channels (tumor emboli) and shows erythema of the overlying skin, recapitulating the human IBC phenotype of extensive lymphovascular invasion *in situ*. This xenograft is 100% tumorigenic, has a latency time of one week and grows rapidly once established. Moreover, spontaneous metastases can develop within vessels in the lungs [15].

MARY-X can also be cultured *in vitro* as spheroids in suspension for up to 3 months (Table 13.2) or attached to monolayers of normal human mammary epithelial cells and human umbilical-vein endothelial cells. In order to obtain MARY-X spheroids, tumors collected from mice need to be minced and agitated in culture medium at 4°C for 2 min. Then, released sheets of cells and single cells from the tumor are pelleted and finally plated. These cells form tight, compact clumps designated as "MARY-X spheroids." Interestingly, while MARY-X tumors have a 30% murine component (surrounding stroma and lymphatic and blood vessels) and 70% human IBC cell component (tumor cell emboli), their spheroids are 99% human tumor cells [15, 30].

The unique IBC phenotype displayed by MARY-X *in vivo* and *in vitro* has allowed researchers to study in detail the molecular mechanisms of lymphovascular invasion and lymphovascular emboli formation in this experimental model, making it a reference in studies regarding IBC, micrometastasis, and E-cadherin [13, 30, 36, 37]. MARY-X is positive for p53 and EGFR; is negative for ER, PgR, and HER2; and overexpresses E-cadherin (a property maintained through the metastatic progression) and MUC1 [13, 15, 30]. Furthermore, MARY-X cells express the cancer stem cell markers CD44$^+$/CD24$^{-/low}$, CD133, and ALHD1, and these subpopulations are tumorigenic and able to proliferate and self-renew [16, 17, 31].

13.3.2 WIBC-9

The WIBC-9 xenograft was established at the National Cancer Center Research Institute in Tokyo (Japan) with pieces of a resected tumor from a patient with IBC; the specimens were directly implanted into BALB/c nude and SCID mice. Tumors were re-transplanted successfully over 3 years with subcutaneous inoculations of tumor pieces into the mammary pads of both strains of mice [24]. WIBC-9 is 100% tumorigenic, has a latency of 2 weeks, and grows rapidly. Macroscopically, this xenograft exhibits skin erythema. Histologic analysis of WIBC-9 tumors shows hypervascularity, blood pooling without a lining of endothelia and absence of central necrosis or fibrosis. Moreover, metastatic foci and tumor cell leakage from pre-existing vessels can be found in the lungs [24]. Cells resulting from the digestion of WIBC-9 xenografts can be cultured *in vitro* in a collagen-coated dish, and they form tube-like structures and loops in the basement membrane matrix; however, the maintenance of WIBC-9 cultures *in vitro* has not been established. WIBC-9 tumor cells express IL-1, IL-8, basic fibroblast growth factor (bFGF), and vascular endothelial growth factor (VEGF) [24].

Two distinctive features of WIBC-9, the blood pooling without a lining of endothelial cells and the tube-like structures and loops in the central tumor, make WIBC-9 a unique IBC model for studying the hemodynamics of vasculogenic mimicry and angiogenesis of IBC [38–42] and the tumor-infiltrating endothelial cells [41].

13.3.3 MDA-IBC-3

The MDA-IBC-3 model was generated in 2008 at The University of Texas MD Anderson Cancer Center in Houston (USA) in collaboration with Baylor College of Medicine, also in Houston, with cells isolated from a pleural effusion obtained from a patient with IBC [25]. Tumor cells were selected by serial transplant of xenograft pieces into the cleared mammary fat pad of SCID/Beige immunocompromised mice over nine transplants, and the resulting tumor tissue was later digested and passaged *in vitro* in monolayer and 3D cultures, generating as well a new IBC cell line (Table 13.2).

In vivo, MDA-IBC-3 tumors can develop within 4 weeks following subcutaneous injections of 1×10^6 cells [25]. Xenografts of MDA-IBC-3 form solid and expansive tumors and exhibit skin erythema and loss of fur on the overlying skin. Histologically, tumor cells grossly invade the skin and adjacent muscle; however, gross metastatic disease has not been observed, and specific dermal lymphatic invasion has not been identified (Fig. 13.1). *In vitro*, MDA-IBC-3 grows in clusters of large and round attaching cells in 2D cultures; these clusters are able to form well-defined spheres when plated in serum-free conditions in ultra-low-attachment culture plates at a concentration of 20,000 cells/ml (Fig. 13.2). MDA-IBC-3 2D cultures grow slowly, and cells need be subcultured only once or twice a week. Cells from xenografts and *in vitro* cultures are ER and PgR negative, HER2 positive, and p53

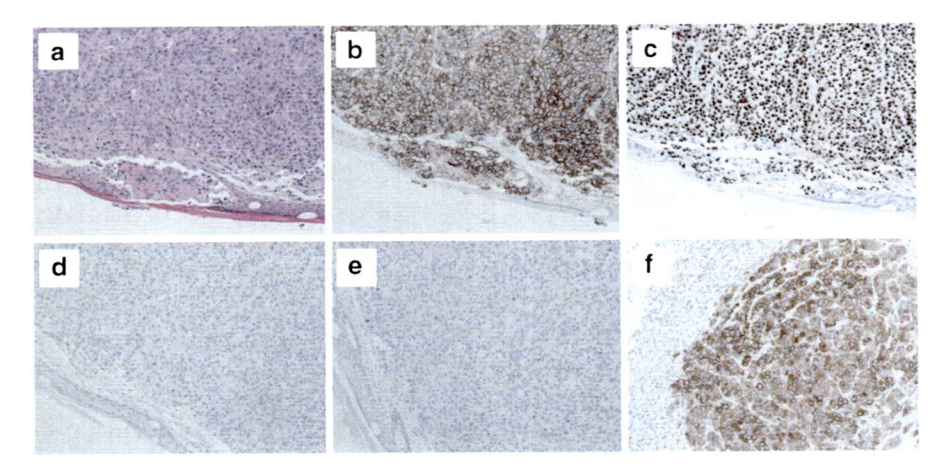

Fig. 13.1 MDA-IBC-3 tumor xenograft. Invasive carcinoma in subcutaneous tissue, poorly differentiated with sheets of large cells with prominent nucleolus, moderate nuclear pleomorphism and significant mitotic activity (**a**). The invasive carcinoma is strongly and diffusely positive for E-cadherin (**b**), note the prominent membranous staining of the cells for E-cadherin; and strongly and diffusely positive for p53 (**c**), note the strongly nuclear positivity of the tumor cells for p53. The invasive carcinoma is also entirely negative for estrogen (**d**) and progesterone (**e**) receptors; and diffusely positive for HER2/neu protein overexpression (**f**), note that the majority of the tumor cells show strong membranous positivity for HER2/neu

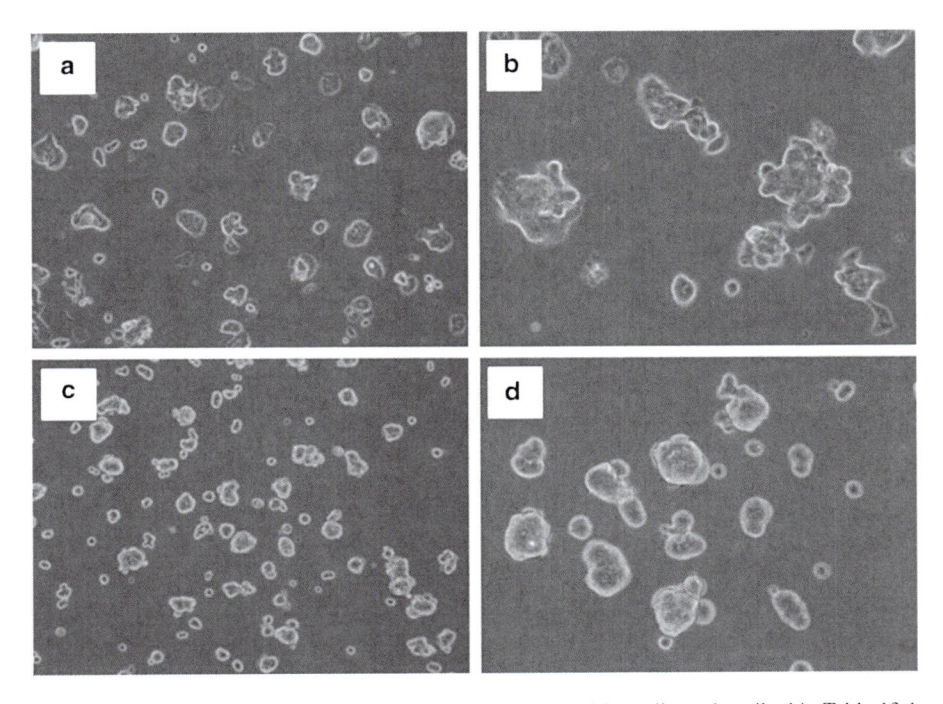

Fig. 13.2 MDA-IBC-3 cell line grown in vitro. 2D culture with media as described in Table 13.1 at 10× amplification (**a**) and 20× amplification (**b**). 3D culture with media as described in Table 13.1 at 10× amplification (**c**) and 20× amplification (**d**)

and E-cadherin positive (Fig. 13.1). Based on short tandem repeat analysis, MDA-IBC-3 represents a new, unique cell line, and it is the most recent IBC model described [25].

13.4 Conclusion

The available IBC models have been critical to establishing the IBC pathobiology known so far, but more work is needed. IBC is a biologically heterogeneous disease not likely fully represented by the limited number of available models and cell lines. Clinically, the disease progresses heterogeneously as well, with some patients developing strong local disease features with uncontrollable disease spread beyond the breast and other patients developing predominantly distant disease features. The biology of secondary IBC, IBC presenting as a recurrence after a non-IBC primary breast cancer, is even less well understood and modeled. Without question, additional work is needed to model and understand this aggressive disease.

Acknowledgments We would like to thank Dr. Savitri Krisnamurthy for helping to describe MDA-IBC-3 xenografts.

Funding

This work has been supported by the National Institutes of Health grants R01CA138239-01 and CA016672 (MD Anderson's Cancer Center Support Grant); the State of Texas Grant for Rare and Aggressive Cancers; and American Airlines Komen Foundation Promise Grant KGO81287.

References

1. Greene FL, Page DL, Fleming ID, Fritz AG, Balch CM, Haller DG, Morrow M (2002) Breast cancer. In: AJCC cancer staging handbook, 6th edn, TNM classification of malignant tumors. Springer, New York, pp 255–281
2. Nguyen DM, Sam K, Tsimelzon A, Li X, Wong H, Mohsin S, Clark GM, Hilsenbeck SG, Elledge RM, Allred DC, O'Connell P, Chang JC (2006) Molecular heterogeneity of inflammatory breast cancer: a hyperproliferative phenotype. Clin Cancer Res 12(17):5047–5054. doi:12/17/5047 [pii]10.1158/1078-0432.CCR-05-2248
3. Van der Auwera I, Van Laere SJ, Van den Eynden GG, Benoy I, van Dam P, Colpaert CG, Fox SB, Turley H, Harris AL, Van Marck EA, Vermeulen PB, Dirix LY (2004) Increased angiogenesis and lymphangiogenesis in inflammatory versus noninflammatory breast cancer by real-time reverse transcriptase-PCR gene expression quantification. Clin Cancer Res 10(23):7965–7971. doi:10/23/7965 [pii]10.1158/1078-0432.CCR-04-0063
4. Van den Eynden GG, Van der Auwera I, Van Laere S, Colpaert CG, van Dam P, Merajver S, Kleer CG, Harris AL, Van Marck EA, Dirix LY, Vermeulen PB (2004) Validation of a tissue microarray to study differential protein expression in inflammatory and non-inflammatory breast cancer. Breast Cancer Res Treat 85(1):13–22. doi:10.1023/B:BREA.0000021028.33926. a85256693 [pii]

5. van Golen KL, Davies S, Wu ZF, Wang Y, Bucana CD, Root H, Chandrasekharappa S, Strawderman M, Ethier SP, Merajver SD (1999) A novel putative low-affinity insulin-like growth factor-binding protein, LIBC (lost in inflammatory breast cancer), and RhoC GTPase correlate with the inflammatory breast cancer phenotype. Clin Cancer Res 5(9):2511–2519
6. van Golen KL, Wu ZF, Qiao XT, Bao LW, Merajver SD (2000) RhoC GTPase, a novel transforming oncogene for human mammary epithelial cells that partially recapitulates the inflammatory breast cancer phenotype. Cancer Res 60(20):5832–5838
7. Kleer CG, van Golen KL, Zhang Y, Wu ZF, Rubin MA, Merajver SD (2002) Characterization of RhoC expression in benign and malignant breast disease: a potential new marker for small breast carcinomas with metastatic ability. Am J Pathol 160(2):579–584. doi:S0002-9440(10)64877-8 [pii]10.1016/S0002-9440(10)64877-8
8. Kleer CG, Griffith KA, Sabel MS, Gallagher G, van Golen KL, Wu ZF, Merajver SD (2005) RhoC-GTPase is a novel tissue biomarker associated with biologically aggressive carcinomas of the breast. Breast Cancer Res Treat 93(2):101–110. doi:10.1007/s10549-005-4170-6
9. Kleer CG, Zhang Y, Pan Q, Gallagher G, Wu M, Wu ZF, Merajver SD (2004) WISP3 and RhoC guanosine triphosphatase cooperate in the development of inflammatory breast cancer. Breast Cancer Res 6(2):R110–R115
10. Kleer CG, Zhang Y, Merajver SD (2007) CCN6 (WISP3) as a new regulator of the epithelial phenotype in breast cancer. Cells Tissues Organs 185(1–3):95–99. doi:000101308 [pii]10.1159/000101308
11. Kleer CG, Zhang Y, Pan Q, Merajver SD (2004) WISP3 (CCN6) is a secreted tumor-suppressor protein that modulates IGF signaling in inflammatory breast cancer. Neoplasia 6(2):179–185. doi:10.1593/neo.03316
12. Kleer CG, van Golen KL, Braun T, Merajver SD (2001) Persistent E-cadherin expression in inflammatory breast cancer. Mod Pathol 14(5):458–464. doi:10.1038/modpathol.3880334
13. Tomlinson JS, Alpaugh ML, Barsky SH (2001) An intact overexpressed E-cadherin/alpha, beta-catenin axis characterizes the lymphovascular emboli of inflammatory breast carcinoma. Cancer Res 61(13):5231–5241
14. Silvera D, Arju R, Darvishian F, Levine PH, Zolfaghari L, Goldberg J, Hochman T, Formenti SC, Schneider RJ (2009) Essential role for eIF4GI overexpression in the pathogenesis of inflammatory breast cancer. Nat Cell Biol 11(7):903–908. doi:ncb1900 [pii]10.1038/ncb1900
15. Alpaugh ML, Tomlinson JS, Shao ZM, Barsky SH (1999) A novel human xenograft model of inflammatory breast cancer. Cancer Res 59(20):5079–5084
16. Charafe-Jauffret E, Ginestier C, Iovino F, Tarpin C, Diebel M, Esterni B, Houvenaeghel G, Extra JM, Bertucci F, Jacquemier J, Xerri L, Dontu G, Stassi G, Xiao Y, Barsky SH, Birnbaum D, Viens P, Wicha MS (2010) Aldehyde dehydrogenase 1-positive cancer stem cells mediate metastasis and poor clinical outcome in inflammatory breast cancer. Clin Cancer Res 16(1):45–55. doi:1078-0432.CCR-09-1630 [pii]10.1158/1078-0432.CCR-09-1630
17. Xiao Y, Ye Y, Zou X, Jones S, Yearsley K, Shetuni B, Tellez J, Barsky SH (2011) The lymphovascular embolus of inflammatory breast cancer exhibits a Notch 3 addiction. Oncogene 30(3):287–300. doi:onc2010405 [pii]10.1038/onc.2010.405
18. Van Laere S, Van der Auwera I, Van den Eynden GG, Fox SB, Bianchi F, Harris AL, van Dam P, Van Marck EA, Vermeulen PB, Dirix LY (2005) Distinct molecular signature of inflammatory breast cancer by cDNA microarray analysis. Breast Cancer Res Treat 93(3):237–246. doi:10.1007/s10549-005-5157-z
19. Kurebayashi J, Otsuki T, Tang CK, Kurosumi M, Yamamoto S, Tanaka K, Mochizuki M, Nakamura H, Sonoo H (1999) Isolation and characterization of a new human breast cancer cell line, KPL-4, expressing the Erb B family receptors and interleukin-6. Br J Cancer 79(5–6):707–717. doi:10.1038/sj.bjc.6690114
20. Ignatoski KM, Ethier SP (1999) Constitutive activation of pp125fak in newly isolated human breast cancer cell lines. Breast Cancer Res Treat 54(2):173–182
21. Forozan F, Veldman R, Ammerman CA, Parsa NZ, Kallioniemi A, Kallioniemi OP, Ethier SP (1999) Molecular cytogenetic analysis of 11 new breast cancer cell lines. Br J Cancer 81(8):1328–1334. doi:10.1038/sj.bjc.6695007

22. Dong HM, Liu G, Hou YF, Wu J, Lu JS, Luo JM, Shen ZZ, Shao ZM (2007) Dominant-negative E-cadherin inhibits the invasiveness of inflammatory breast cancer cells in vitro. J Cancer Res Clin Oncol 133(2):83–92. doi:10.1007/s00432-006-0140-6

23. Singh B, Cook KR, Martin C, Huang EH, Mosalpuria K, Krishnamurthy S, Cristofanilli M, Lucci A (2010) Evaluation of a CXCR4 antagonist in a xenograft mouse model of inflammatory breast cancer. Clin Exp Metastasis 27(4):233–240. doi:10.1007/s10585-010-9321-4

24. Shirakawa K, Tsuda H, Heike Y, Kato K, Asada R, Inomata M, Sasaki H, Kasumi F, Yoshimoto M, Iwanaga T, Konishi F, Terada M, Wakasugi H (2001) Absence of endothelial cells, central necrosis, and fibrosis are associated with aggressive inflammatory breast cancer. Cancer Res 61(2):445–451

25. Klopp AH, Lacerda L, Gupta A, Debeb BG, Solley T, Li L, Spaeth E, Xu W, Zhang X, Lewis MT, Reuben JM, Krishnamurthy S, Ferrari M, Gaspar R, Buchholz TA, Cristofanilli M, Marini F, Andreeff M, Woodward WA (2010) Mesenchymal stem cells promote mammosphere formation and decrease E-cadherin in normal and malignant breast cells. PLoS One 5(8):e12180. doi:10.1371/journal.pone.0012180

26. Kurebayashi J, Yamamoto S, Otsuki T, Sonoo H (1999) Medroxyprogesterone acetate inhibits interleukin 6 secretion from KPL-4 human breast cancer cells both in vitro and in vivo: a possible mechanism of the anticachectic effect. Br J Cancer 79(3–4):631–636. doi:10.1038/sj.bjc.6690099

27. Damiano V, Garofalo S, Rosa R, Bianco R, Caputo R, Gelardi T, Merola G, Racioppi L, Garbi C, Kandimalla ER, Agrawal S, Tortora G (2009) A novel toll-like receptor 9 agonist cooperates with trastuzumab in trastuzumab-resistant breast tumors through multiple mechanisms of action. Clin Cancer Res 15(22):6921–6930. doi:1078-0432.CCR-09-1599 [pii]10.1158/1078-0432.CCR-09-1599

28. Garcia R, Yu CL, Hudnall A, Catlett R, Nelson KL, Smithgall T, Fujita DJ, Ethier SP, Jove R (1997) Constitutive activation of Stat3 in fibroblasts transformed by diverse oncoproteins and in breast carcinoma cells. Cell Growth Differ 8(12):1267–1276

29. Flanagan L, Van Weelden K, Ammerman C, Ethier SP, Welsh J (1999) SUM-159PT cells: a novel estrogen independent human breast cancer model system. Breast Cancer Res Treat 58(3):193–204

30. Morales J, Alpaugh ML (2009) Gain in cellular organization of inflammatory breast cancer: a 3D in vitro model that mimics the in vivo metastasis. BMC Cancer 9:462. doi:1471-2407-9-462 [pii]10.1186/1471-2407-9-462

31. Xiao Y, Ye Y, Yearsley K, Jones S, Barsky SH (2008) The lymphovascular embolus of inflammatory breast cancer expresses a stem cell-like phenotype. Am J Pathol 173(2):561–574. doi:S0002-9440(10)61631-8 [pii]10.2353/ajpath.2008.071214

32. Fillmore CM, Kuperwasser C (2008) Human breast cancer cell lines contain stem-like cells that self-renew, give rise to phenotypically diverse progeny and survive chemotherapy. Breast Cancer Res 10(2):R25. doi:bcr1982 [pii]10.1186/bcr1982

33. Kuperwasser C, Dessain S, Bierbaum BE, Garnet D, Sperandio K, Gauvin GP, Naber SP, Weinberg RA, Rosenblatt M (2005) A mouse model of human breast cancer metastasis to human bone. Cancer Res 65(14):6130–6138. doi:65/14/6130 [pii]10.1158/0008-5472.CAN-04-1408

34. Wang Y, Liu X, Chen L, Cheng D, Rusckowski M, Hnatowich DJ (2009) Tumor delivery of antisense oligomer using trastuzumab within a streptavidin nanoparticle. Eur J Nucl Med Mol Imaging 36(12):1977–1986. doi:10.1007/s00259-009-1201-2

35. Hoffmeyer MR, Wall KM, Dharmawardhane SF (2005) In vitro analysis of the invasive phenotype of SUM 149, an inflammatory breast cancer cell line. Cancer Cell Int 5(1):11. doi:1475-2867-5-11 [pii]10.1186/1475-2867-5-11

36. Alpaugh ML, Tomlinson JS, Kasraeian S, Barsky SH (2002) Cooperative role of E-cadherin and sialyl-Lewis X/a-deficient MUC1 in the passive dissemination of tumor emboli in inflammatory breast carcinoma. Oncogene 21(22):3631–3643. doi:10.1038/sj.onc.1205389

37. Alpaugh ML, Barsky SH (2002) Reversible model of spheroid formation allows for high efficiency of gene delivery ex vivo and accurate gene assessment in vivo. Hum Gene Ther 13(10):1245–1258. doi:10.1089/104303402320139023

38. Kobayashi H, Shirakawa K, Kawamoto S, Saga T, Sato N, Hiraga A, Watanabe I, Heike Y, Togashi K, Konishi J, Brechbiel MW, Wakasugi H (2002) Rapid accumulation and internalization of radiolabeled herceptin in an inflammatory breast cancer xenograft with vasculogenic mimicry predicted by the contrast-enhanced dynamic MRI with the macromolecular contrast agent G6-(1B4M-Gd)(256). Cancer Res 62(3):860–866

39. Shirakawa K, Furuhata S, Watanabe I, Hayase H, Shimizu A, Ikarashi Y, Yoshida T, Terada M, Hashimoto D, Wakasugi H (2002) Induction of vasculogenesis in breast cancer models. Br J Cancer 87(12):1454–1461. doi:10.1038/sj.bjc.66006106600610 [pii]

40. Shirakawa K, Kobayashi H, Heike Y, Kawamoto S, Brechbiel MW, Kasumi F, Iwanaga T, Konishi F, Terada M, Wakasugi H (2002) Hemodynamics in vasculogenic mimicry and angiogenesis of inflammatory breast cancer xenograft. Cancer Res 62(2):560–566

41. Shirakawa K, Shibuya M, Heike Y, Takashima S, Watanabe I, Konishi F, Kasumi F, Goldman CK, Thomas KA, Bett A, Terada M, Wakasugi H (2002) Tumor-infiltrating endothelial cells and endothelial precursor cells in inflammatory breast cancer. Int J Cancer 99(3):344–351. doi:10.1002/ijc.10336

42. Shirakawa K, Wakasugi H, Heike Y, Watanabe I, Yamada S, Saito K, Konishi F (2002) Vasculogenic mimicry and pseudo-comedo formation in breast cancer. Int J Cancer 99(6):821–828. doi:10.1002/ijc.10423

Chapter 14
Signaling Pathways in Inflammatory Breast Cancer

Dongwei Zhang and Naoto T. Ueno

Abstract The biology of inflammatory breast cancer (IBC) has some important differences from the biology of other types of breast cancer. Gene expression profiling, real-time reverse-transcription polymerase chain reaction, immunohistochemistry, and in situ hybridization have been used to detect unique characteristics that are found in the majority of IBC tumors but not in non-IBC tumors. Recent research has revealed some differences between IBC and non-IBC, including overexpression of RhoC GTPase and loss of expression of WISP3 in IBC. In this chapter, we summarize the current understanding of the biological signaling pathways of IBC, mainly cell proliferation pathways. At present, therapies that target cell proliferation pathways are the most promising targeted therapies for IBC. Identification of molecular findings unique to IBC will provide a rationale for developing novel treatment strategies targeting IBC.

Keywords EGFR • HER2 • MAPK • p27 • WISP3 • RhoC • GTPase • IGF • p53

The biology of inflammatory breast cancer (IBC) has some important differences from the biology of other types of breast cancer. Gene expression profiling, real-time reverse-transcription polymerase chain reaction, immunohistochemistry, and in situ hybridization have been used to detect unique characteristics that are found in the majority of IBC tumors but not in non-IBC tumors. Recent research has revealed some differences between IBC and non-IBC, including overexpression of

D. Zhang, M.D., Ph.D. (✉) • N.T. Ueno, M.D., Ph.D., F.A.C.P.
Morgan Welch Inflammatory Breast Cancer Program and Clinic, Department of Breast Medical Oncology, The University of Texas, MD Anderson Cancer Center, Unit 1354, Holcombe Blvd. 1515, Houston, TX, USA
e-mail: dwzhang@mdanderson.org; nueno@mdanderson.org

N.T. Ueno and M. Cristofanilli (eds.), *Inflammatory Breast Cancer: An Update*, DOI 10.1007/978-94-007-3907-9_14, © Springer Science+Business Media B.V. 2012

RhoC GTPase and loss of expression of WISP3 in IBC. In this chapter, we summarize the current understanding of the biological signaling pathways of IBC, mainly cell proliferation pathways. At present, therapies that target cell proliferation pathways are the most promising targeted therapies for IBC. Identification of molecular findings unique to IBC will provide a rationale for developing novel treatment strategies targeting IBC.

14.1 EGFR

The ErbB receptor family consists of typical cell membrane receptor tyrosine kinases that are activated following ligand binding and receptor dimerization and regulate diverse biologic responses, including proliferation, differentiation, cell motility, and survival. The ErbB receptor tyrosine kinase family consists of four cell surface receptors: ErbB1 (also called epidermal growth factor receptor [EGFR] or HER1), ErbB2 (also called HER2/neu or simply HER2), ErbB3 (HER3), and ErbB4 (HER4).

EGFR is frequently overexpressed in human malignant tumors and is known to drive tumor growth, progression, and metastasis [1–4]. EGFR overexpression is associated with poor prognosis and reduced overall survival in cancer patients [5, 6]. Therefore, the EGFR signaling pathway has emerged as a promising target for cancer therapy. A number of tyrosine kinase inhibitors (TKIs) that target EGFR, such as erlotinib and gefitinib, have been developed and used successfully to treat cancer, especially non–small cell lung cancer [7, 8]. Recent studies have shown that EGFR may play an important role in the progression of IBC. EGFR overexpression was detected in 30% of IBC patients by immunohistochemical staining. Patients with EGFR-expressing IBC have a significantly worse 5-year overall survival rate than that of patients with EGFR-negative IBC, and EGFR expression was also associated with increased risk of IBC recurrence [9]. The association of EGFR expression with poor prognosis and increased risk of recurrence indicates that EGFR may represent a potential therapeutic target in IBC. One *in vitro* study showed that inhibition of EGFR with gefitinib suppresses the growth of SUM149 IBC cells [10]. Another study reported that erlotinib shows significant antitumor activity against IBC. Erlotinib also has the potential to prevent metastasis of IBC through inhibition of epithelial-mesenchymal transition [11].

14.2 HER2

Another member of the ErbB receptor tyrosine kinase family, HER2, is also known to drive tumor growth and progression. HER2 is amplified and/or overexpressed in 20–30% of all types of breast cancers [12, 13]. The incidence of HER2 protein overexpression in IBC is even higher (52%) [14]. In a study of the prognostic impact of HER2 status on survival outcomes of 179 patients with IBC, no statistically significant difference was observed for either recurrence-free or overall survival between patients who had HER2-positive disease and those who had HER2-negative disease. Even though HER2 status does not appear to significantly affect recurrence-free survival of patients with IBC, the addition of trastuzumab, a monoclonal antibody that targets the HER2 receptor, in the metastatic setting significantly improved the overall survival in the HER2-positive group compared with the HER2-negative group [15]. Another drug that can be used to target HER2 is the TKI lapatinib, an oral reversible inhibitor of both HER2 and EGFR. In a phase II trial of lapatinib monotherapy in heavily treated patients with IBC, the response rate was 50% among the 30 patients with HER2-positive IBC, compared with only 7% among the 15 patients with HER2-negative, EGFR-positive tumors [16]. These findings illustrate that HER2 is a promising target for IBC.

14.3 Mitogen-Activated Protein Kinase (MAPK) – Extracellular Signal-Regulated Kinase (ERK)

The MAPK-ERK pathway is known to promote cell proliferation, differentiation, survival, and metastasis [17, 18]. It has been reported that blockade of the MAPK pathway suppresses growth of colon tumors and melanoma metastasis *in vivo* [19, 20], supporting the therapeutic value of blocking ERK signaling in cancer. High levels of activated ERK have been shown in IBC cell lines SUM149 and KPL-4 [11]. When ERK was knocked down using short interfering RNA (siRNA) in these cells, erlotinib exhibited significantly more antiproliferative activity, suggesting that combining erlotinib therapy with inhibition of the ERK pathway may improve the therapeutic outcome in IBC [11]. The combination of an inhibitor of MAPK signaling, U0126, and an EGFR TKI, PKI166, decreased MAPK signaling and induced p27^{kip1} expression in SUM149 cells and led to cell apoptosis and G_1 cell-cycle arrest [21] (see the next section for more details).

14.4 p27^{kip1}

p27^{kip1} is a cyclin-dependent kinase inhibitor that negatively regulates cellular proliferation by inhibiting progression through the cell cycle [22]. It triggers G_1 cell-cycle arrest and might be involved in apoptosis induction, cell adhesion, promotion of cell differentiation, and drug resistance. An increase in p27^{kip1} levels causes proliferating cells to exit the cell cycle [22, 23], in part through direct binding between p27^{kip1} and Cdk2, which inhibits the kinase activity of Cdk2 [24–26]. One study of 38 patients with IBC previously treated with chemotherapy showed that downregulation of p27^{kip1} correlated with poor clinical outcome [27]. As mentioned earlier, upregulation of p27[kip1] can be induced by combining inhibitors of MAPK and EGFR, and therefore blocks the breast cancer cell growth [21]. The phosphorylation status of p27[kip1] is known to affect its nuclear-cytoplasmic localization. Dephosphorylation of p27[kip1] at serine 10 inhibits p27 nuclear export and promotes its assembly into cyclin–CDK complexes, which inhibits cell proliferation [28–31]. A recent study reported that inhibiting serine 10 phosphorylation of p27 by siRNA knockdown of the kinase-interacting stathmin gene enhances erlotinib-induced inhibition of breast tumor growth in IBC [32].

14.5   WNT-1 Inducible Signaling Pathway Protein 3 (WISP3)

The WISP3 gene is located on chromosome 6q22-23. WISP3 (also called LIBC [lost in inflammatory breast cancer]) is a secreted protein and has been identified as a member of the nephroblastoma overexpressed gene (also called CCN) family of proteins, which have important biological functions in normal physiology as well as in carcinogenesis [33]. Among 38 archival stage III IBC tumor specimens, loss of expression of WISP3 was detected in 80% of IBC samples versus only 20% of non-IBC tumors by in situ hybridization [34]. Loss of WISP3 expression contributes to the phenotype of IBC by regulating tumor cell growth, invasion, and angiogenesis. Restoration of WISP3 expression in SUM149 cells resulted in a significant decrease in anchorage-independent growth in soft agar and cellular proliferation, as well as a drastic decrease in the cells' invasive capabilities, and resulted in a biologically relevant decrease in the levels of angiogenic factors (vascular endothelial growth factor, basic fibroblast growth factor, and interleukin-6) in the conditioned media of the cells. *In vivo*, restoration of WISP3 expression in SUM149 cells caused a drastic decrease in tumor volume and rate of tumor growth when injected into nude mice [35]. Furthermore, WISP3 can be secreted into the extracellular medium and into the lumens of normal breast ducts. The secreted WISP3 can decrease the growth rate of IBC cells [36]. These studies suggest that WISP3 is a tumor suppressor gene in IBC.

14.6   RhoC GTPase

The three closely related proteins RhoA, RhoB, and RhoC are members of the Ras superfamily of small GTPases. Activation of Rho proteins by soluble factors, such as serum or growth factors, leads to the assembly of actin–myosin contractile filaments and focal adhesion complexes [37, 38]. In breast cancer, the prognostic and predictive value of RhoC GTPase expression was investigated by analyzing tissue microarrays of 801 breast cancer tissue samples from 280 patients [39]. High RhoC GTPase expression correlated with high histologic grade, positive lymph nodes, and negative hormone receptor status, but not with tumor stage, tumor size, lymphovascular invasion status, or HER2 status. Patients with high RhoC GTPase expression had a significantly worse overall survival and responded poorly to doxorubicin-based chemotherapy. RhoC GTPase was overexpressed in 90% of archival stage III IBC tumor samples, but not in stage-matched, non-IBC tumors [34]. RhoC GTPase has been defined as a transforming oncogene involved in conferring the metastatic phenotype in breast cancer. Overexpression of RhoC GTPase in human mammary epithelial cells results in a highly motile and invasive phenotype that recapitulates IBC [40]. The induction of motility and invasion by RhoC GTPase is mediated through activation of the ERK and p38 arms of the MAPK pathway in IBC [41].

Reversal of RhoC GTPase expression is being investigated as a potential cancer therapy. Farnesyl transferase inhibitors have been shown to be effective in modulating tumor growth in Ras-transformed tumor cells [42, 43]. Treatment of RhoC GTPase-overexpressing SUM149 cells with a farnesyl transferase inhibitor L-744832 resulted in a significant decrease in anchorage-independent growth, motility, and invasion, possibly by increasing the level of geranylgeranylated RhoB [44]. On the basis of these preclinical findings, farnesyl transferase inhibitors (for example, tipifarnib) are currently being investigated in clinical trials in combination with chemotherapy as a potential novel targeted therapy for tumors that overexpress Rho, including IBC.

14.7 Insulin-Like Growth factor (IGF)

The IGF system is critically involved in the development and maintenance of breast cancer. For example, IGF-1 and its major receptor, IGF-1 receptor (IGF-1R), play an important role in normal breast biology and in the development of breast cancer [45, 46]. IGF receptors require ligand binding to trigger the appropriate downstream pathways, including the PI3K survival pathway and MAPK pathway, which link to cell growth and proliferation. Binding of IGF-binding proteins (IGFBPs) to IGFs normally blocks the interaction between IGFs and IGF receptors and blocks IGF-regulated proliferation. WISP3, described above, is a member of the low-affinity IGFBP family, and its loss was highly correlated with IBC [34]. Several molecular events lead to modulation of IGF-1R signaling pathways and cellular growth. For example, RhoC GTPase activity promotes IGF-1-stimulated migration and invasion in prostate cancer [47]. WISP3 decreases the IGF-1-induced activation of IGF-IR and two of its main downstream signaling molecules, IRS1 and ERK-1/2, in SUM149 cells [36]. Because RhoC GTPase and WISP3 are concordantly altered in the majority of IBC tumors but not in non-IBC tumors [34], the IGF pathway might be an effective target for therapeutic intervention for IBC.

14.8   Cooperation of WISP3 and Other Cell
Proliferation Pathways

It seems that WISP3 appears to act as a modulator of other cell proliferation pathways in IBC growth. WISP3 transfection into the IBC cell line SUM149 has been shown to increase levels of $p27^{kip1}$ and $p21^{waf1}$ [35]. As described above, secreted extracellular WISP3 decreased the IGF-1-induced activation of IGF-1R and two of its main downstream signaling cascades, IRS1 and ERK-1/2, therefore decreasing the growth rate of IBC cells [36]. In the study that compared archival stage III breast cancer samples, alterations of both WISP3 and RhoC GTPase were observed in 91% of the IBC specimens but none of the non-IBC specimens. Restoration of WISP3 expression in SUM149 cells decreased the expression of RhoC GTPase protein [34]. Investigators have hypothesized that overexpression of RhoC GTPase and loss of WISP3 act together to promote aggressiveness of IBC, and in support of that hypothesis, an *in vitro* study has shown that RhoC GTPase expression is modulated by WISP3 expression [48]. Although further investigations are required, modulating both genes simultaneously might help control the aggressiveness of IBC.

14.9   p53

Mutation of p53 (also known as TP53 in humans) remains the most common genetic change identified in human neoplasia. In breast cancer, p53 mutation was found to be associated with worse survival in a comprehensive meta-analysis of the effect of somatic p53 mutations on prognosis in breast cancer [49]. p53 mutation or overexpression has been found in 41%–58% of IBC patients [50–52]. The prevalence of the p53 mutation was much higher in IBC than in other types of breast cancer (for example, locally advanced breast cancer), even though histological grade was independent of p53 status in IBC tumors [52]. The prognostic role of p53 in IBC has also been studied. IBC patients with p53-positive tumors were younger and tended to have lower 5-year progression-free survival rates and overall survival rates [51]. Studies examining whether p53 expression in IBC predicts response to neoadjuvant therapy have not been conclusive [53]. In spite of studies suggesting that p53 status is an important characteristic of IBC, additional investigation will be required to determine whether this gene is a relevant target for treatment.

14.10   Conclusion

The unique molecular changes in signaling pathways of IBC have not been well defined. Further extensive work using molecular analysis technology is imperative in order to determine differential gene expression and fully reveal a signature profile of IBC. Thus far, the HER2 and EGFR pathways have been tested in preclinical and

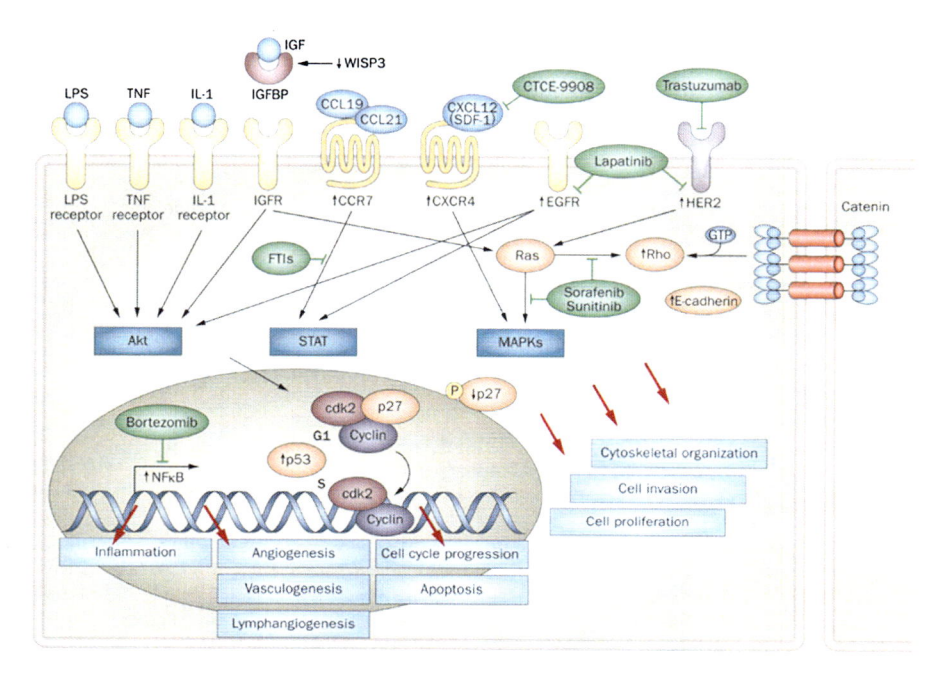

Fig. 14.1 Signaling Pathways in Inflammatory Breast Cancer. Reprinted with permission of Nature Publishing Group from [54] Molecular targets for treatment of inflammatory breast cancer. *Nat Rev Clin Oncol* doi:10.1038/nrclinonc.2009.73. Abbreviations: CCL, chemokine ligand, CCR, chemokine receptor; CXCL, chemokine ligand; CXCR, chemokine receptor; FTIs, farnesyl transferase inhibitors; HER2, human epidermal growth factor receptor 2; IGF, insulin-like growth factor; IGFBP, insulin-like growth factor binding protein; IGFR, insulin-like growth factor receptor; IL-1, interleukin 1; LPS, lipopolysaccharide; MAPK, mitogen-activated protein kinase; NF B, nuclear factor kappaB; SDF-1, stromal-cell-derived factor 1; STAT, signal transducers and activators of transcription protein; TNF, tumor necrosis factor; WISP3, WNT1 inducible signaling pathway protein 3

clinical trials as targets for IBC treatment. Continued research will allow us to understand the molecular basis of the aggressiveness of IBC so that we may accurately identify markers of disease, improve diagnostic tools and predictors of response to treatment, and suggest targeted IBC-specific therapies that afford improved survival.

References

1. Berger MS, Gullick WJ, Greenfield C, Evans S, Addis BJ, Waterfield MD (1987) Epidermal growth factor receptors in lung tumours. J Pathol 152:297–307
2. Olayioye MA, Neve RM, Lane HA, Hynes NE (2000) The ErbB signaling network: receptor heterodimerization in development and cancer. EMBO J 19:3159–3167
3. Seshadri R, McLeay WR, Horsfall DJ, McCaul K (1996) Prospective study of the prognostic significance of epidermal growth factor receptor in primary breast cancer. Int J Cancer 69:23–27
4. Yarden Y, Sliwkowski MX (2001) Untangling the ErbB signalling network. Nat Rev Mol Cell Biol 2:127–137

5. Cox G, Jones JL, O'Byrne KJ (2000) Matrix metalloproteinase 9 and the epidermal growth factor signal pathway in operable non-small cell lung cancer. Clin Cancer Res 6:2349–2355

6. Ohsaki Y, Tanno S, Fujita Y, Toyoshima E, Fujiuchi S, Nishigaki Y, Ishida S, Nagase A, Miyokawa N, Hirata S, Kikuchi K (2000) Epidermal growth factor receptor expression correlates with poor prognosis in non-small cell lung cancer patients with p53 overexpression. Oncol Rep 7:603–607

7. Moore MJ, Goldstein D, Hamm J, Figer A, Hecht JR, Gallinger S, Au HJ, Murawa P, Walde D, Wolff RA, Campos D, Lim R, Ding K, Clark G, Voskoglou-Nomikos T, Ptasynski M, Parulekar W (2007) Erlotinib plus gemcitabine compared with gemcitabine alone in patients with advanced pancreatic cancer: a phase III trial of the National Cancer Institute of Canada Clinical Trials Group. J Clin Oncol 25:1960–1966

8. Shepherd FA, Rodrigues Pereira J, Ciuleanu T, Tan EH, Hirsh V, Thongprasert S, Campos D, Maoleekoonpiroj S, Smylie M, Martins R, van Kooten M, Dediu M, Findlay B, Tu D, Johnston D, Bezjak A, Clark G, Santabarbara P, Seymour L (2005) Erlotinib in previously treated non-small-cell lung cancer. N Engl J Med 353:123–132

9. Cabioglu N, Gong Y, Islam R, Broglio KR, Sneige N, Sahin A, Gonzalez-Angulo AM, Morandi P, Bucana C, Hortobagyi GN, Cristofanilli M (2007) Expression of growth factor and chemokine receptors: new insights in the biology of inflammatory breast cancer. Ann Oncol 18:1021–1029

10. Stratford AL, Habibi G, Astanehe A, Jiang H, Hu K, Park E, Shadeo A, Buys TP, Lam W, Pugh T, Marra M, Nielsen TO, Klinge U, Mertens PR, Aparicio S, Dunn SE (2007) Epidermal growth factor receptor (EGFR) is transcriptionally induced by the Y-box binding protein-1 (YB-1) and can be inhibited with Iressa in basal-like breast cancer, providing a potential target for therapy. Breast Cancer Res 9:R61

11. Zhang D, LaFortune TA, Krishnamurthy S, Esteva FJ, Cristofanilli M, Liu P, Lucci A, Singh B, Hung MC, Hortobagyi GN, Ueno NT (2009) Epidermal growth factor receptor tyrosine kinase inhibitor reverses mesenchymal to epithelial phenotype and inhibits metastasis in inflammatory breast cancer. Clin Cancer Res 15:6639–6648

12. Slamon DJ, Clark GM, Wong SG, Levin WJ, Ullrich A, McGuire WL (1987) Human breast cancer: correlation of relapse and survival with amplification of the HER-2/neu oncogene. Science 235:177–182

13. Slamon DJ, Godolphin W, Jones LA, Holt JA, Wong SG, Keith DE, Levin WJ, Stuart SG, Udove J, Ullrich A et al (1989) Studies of the HER-2/neu proto-oncogene in human breast and ovarian cancer. Science 244:707–712

14. Parton M, Dowsett M, Ashley S, Hills M, Lowe F, Smith IE (2004) High incidence of HER-2 positivity in inflammatory breast cancer. Breast 13:97–103

15. Dawood S, Broglio K, Gong Y, Yang WT, Cristofanilli M, Kau SW, Meric-Bernstam F, Buchholz TA, Hortobagyi GN, Gonzalez-Angulo AM (2008) Prognostic significance of HER-2 status in women with inflammatory breast cancer. Cancer 112:1905–1911

16. Johnston S, Trudeau M, Kaufman B, Boussen H, Blackwell K, LoRusso P, Lombardi DP, Ben Ahmed S, Citrin DL, DeSilvio ML, Harris J, Westlund RE, Salazar V, Zaks TZ, Spector NL (2008) Phase II study of predictive biomarker profiles for response targeting human epidermal growth factor receptor 2 (HER-2) in advanced inflammatory breast cancer with lapatinib monotherapy. J Clin Oncol 26:1066–1072

17. Roberts PJ, Der CJ (2007) Targeting the Raf-MEK-ERK mitogen-activated protein kinase cascade for the treatment of cancer. Oncogene 26:3291–3310

18. Treisman R (1996) Regulation of transcription by MAP kinase cascades. Curr Opin Cell Biol 8:205–215

19. Sebolt-Leopold JS, Dudley DT, Herrera R, Van Becelaere K, Wiland A, Gowan RC, Tecle H, Barrett SD, Bridges A, Przybranowski S, Leopold WR, Saltiel AR (1999) Blockade of the MAP kinase pathway suppresses growth of colon tumors in vivo. Nat Med 5:810–816

20. Collisson EA, De A, Suzuki H, Gambhir SS, Kolodney MS (2003) Treatment of metastatic melanoma with an orally available inhibitor of the Ras-Raf-MAPK cascade. Cancer Res 63:5669–5673

21. Lev DC, Kim LS, Melnikova V, Ruiz M, Ananthaswamy HN, Price JE (2004) Dual blockade of EGFR and ERK1/2 phosphorylation potentiates growth inhibition of breast cancer cells. Br J Cancer 91:795–802

22. Sherr CJ, Roberts JM (1999) CDK inhibitors: positive and negative regulators of G1-phase progression. Genes Dev 13:1501–1512

23. Loda M, Cukor B, Tam SW, Lavin P, Fiorentino M, Draetta GF, Jessup JM, Pagano M (1997) Increased proteasome-dependent degradation of the cyclin-dependent kinase inhibitor p27 in aggressive colorectal carcinomas. Nat Med 3:231–234

24. Polyak K, Lee MH, Erdjument-Bromage H, Koff A, Roberts JM, Tempst P, Massague J (1994) Cloning of p27[Kip1], a cyclin-dependent kinase inhibitor and a potential mediator of extracellular antimitogenic signals. Cell 78:59–66

25. Toyoshima H, Hunter T (1994) p27, a novel inhibitor of G1 cyclin-Cdk protein kinase activity, is related to p21. Cell 78:67–74

26. Sherr CJ (1996) Cancer cell cycles. Science 274:1672–1677

27. Gonzalez-Angulo AM, Guarneri V, Gong Y, Cristofanilli M, Morales-Vasquez F, Sneige N, Hortobagyi GN, Esteva FJ (2006) Downregulation of the cyclin-dependent kinase inhibitor p27kip1 might correlate with poor disease-free and overall survival in inflammatory breast cancer. Clin Breast Cancer 7(4):326–330

28. Boehm M, Yoshimoto T, Crook MF, Nallamshetty S, True A, Nabel GJ, Nabel EG (2002) A growth factor-dependent nuclear kinase phosphorylates p27(Kip1) and regulates cell cycle progression. EMBO J 21:3390–3401

29. Liang J, Zubovitz J, Petrocelli T, Kotchetkov R, Connor MK, Han K, Lee JH, Ciarallo S, Catzavelos C, Beniston R, Franssen E, Slingerland JM (2002) PKB/Akt phosphorylates p27, impairs nuclear import of p27 and opposes p27-mediated G1 arrest. Nat Med 8:1153–1160

30. Shin I, Yakes FM, Rojo F, Shin NY, Bakin AV, Baselga J, Arteaga CL (2002) PKB/Akt mediates cell-cycle progression by phosphorylation of p27(Kip1) at threonine 157 and modulation of its cellular localization. Nat Med 8:1145–1152

31. Viglietto G, Motti ML, Bruni P, Melillo RM, D'Alessio A, Califano D, Vinci F, Chiappetta G, Tsichlis P, Bellacosa A, Fusco A, Santoro M (2002) Cytoplasmic relocalization and inhibition of the cyclin-dependent kinase inhibitor p27(Kip1) by PKB/Akt-mediated phosphorylation in breast cancer. Nat Med 8:1136–1144

32. Zhang D, Tari AM, Akar U, Arun BK, LaFortune TA, Nieves-Alicea R, Hortobagyi GN, Ueno NT (2010) Silencing kinase-interacting stathmin gene enhances erlotinib sensitivity by inhibiting Ser(1) p27 phosphorylation in epidermal growth factor receptor-expressing breast cancer. Mol Cancer Ther 9:3090–3099

33. Perbal B (2001) NOV (nephroblastoma overexpressed) and the CCN family of genes: structural and functional issues. Mol Pathol 54:57–79

34. van Golen KL, Davies S, Wu ZF, Wang Y, Bucana CD, Root H, Chandrasekharappa S, Strawderman M, Ethier SP, Merajver SD (1999) A novel putative low-affinity insulin-like growth factor-binding protein, LIBC (lost in inflammatory breast cancer), and RhoC GTPase correlate with the inflammatory breast cancer phenotype. Clin Cancer Res 5:2511–2519

35. Kleer CG, Zhang Y, Pan Q, van Golen KL, Wu ZF, Livant D, Merajver SD (2002) WISP3 is a novel tumor suppressor gene of inflammatory breast cancer. Oncogene 21:3172–3180

36. Kleer CG, Zhang Y, Pan Q, Merajver SD (2004) WISP3 (CCN6) is a secreted tumor-suppressor protein that modulates IGF signaling in inflammatory breast cancer. Neoplasia 6:179–185

37. Ridley AJ (1997) The GTP-binding protein Rho. Int J Biochem Cell Biol 29:1225–1229

38. Hall A (1998) Rho GTPases and the actin cytoskeleton. Science 279:509–514

39. Kleer CG, Griffith KA, Sabel MS, Gallagher G, van Golen KL, Wu ZF, Merajver SD (2005) RhoC-GTPase is a novel tissue biomarker associated with biologically aggressive carcinomas of the breast. Breast Cancer Res Treat 93:101–110

40. van Golen KL, Wu ZF, Qiao XT, Bao LW, Merajver SD (2000) RhoC GTPase, a novel transforming oncogene for human mammary epithelial cells that partially recapitulates the inflammatory breast cancer phenotype. Cancer Res 60:5832–5838

41. van Golen KL, Bao LW, Pan Q, Miller FR, Wu ZF, Merajver SD (2002) Mitogen activated protein kinase pathway is involved in RhoC GTPase induced motility, invasion and angiogenesis in inflammatory breast cancer. Clin Exp Metastasis 19:301–311
42. Rowinsky EK, Windle JJ, Von Hoff DD (1999) Ras protein farnesyltransferase: a strategic target for anticancer therapeutic development. J Clin Oncol 17:3631–3652
43. Cohen LH, Pieterman E, van Leeuwen RE, Overhand M, Burm BE, van der Marel GA, van Boom JH (2000) Inhibitors of prenylation of Ras and other G-proteins and their application as therapeutics. Biochem Pharmacol 60:1061–1068
44. van Golen KL, Bao L, DiVito MM, Wu Z, Prendergast GC, Merajver SD (2002) Reversion of RhoC GTPase-induced inflammatory breast cancer phenotype by treatment with a farnesyl transferase inhibitor. Mol Cancer Ther 1:575–583
45. Bartucci M, Morelli C, Mauro L, Ando S, Surmacz E (2001) Differential insulin-like growth factor I receptor signaling and function in estrogen receptor (ER)-positive MCF-7 and ER-negative MDA-MB-231 breast cancer cells. Cancer Res 61:6747–6754
46. Furstenberger G, Senn HJ (2002) Insulin-like growth factors and cancer. Lancet Oncol 3:298–302
47. Yao H, Dashner EJ, van Golen CM, van Golen KL (2006) RhoC GTPase is required for PC-3 prostate cancer cell invasion but not motility. Oncogene 25:2285–2296
48. Kleer CG, Zhang Y, Pan Q, Gallagher G, Wu M, Wu ZF, Merajver SD (2004) WISP3 and RhoC guanosine triphosphatase cooperate in the development of inflammatory breast cancer. Breast Cancer Res 6(2):R110–R115
49. Pharoah PD, Day NE, Caldas C (1999) Somatic mutations in the p53 gene and prognosis in breast cancer: a meta-analysis. Br J Cancer 80:1968–1973
50. McCarthy NJ, Yang X, Linnoila IR, Merino MJ, Hewitt SM, Parr AL, Paik S, Steinberg SM, Hartmann DP, Mourali N, Levine PH, Swain SM (2002) Microvessel density, expression of estrogen receptor alpha, MIB-1, p53, and c-erbB-2 in inflammatory breast cancer. Clin Cancer Res 8:3857–3862
51. Gonzalez-Angulo AM, Sneige N, Buzdar AU, Valero V, Kau SW, Broglio K, Yamamura Y, Hortobagyi GN, Cristofanilli M (2004) p53 expression as a prognostic marker in inflammatory breast cancer. Clin Cancer Res 10:6215–6221
52. Turpin E, Bieche I, Bertheau P, Plassa LF, Lerebours F, de Roquancourt A, Olivi M, Espie M, Marty M, Lidereau R, Vidaud M, de The H (2002) Increased incidence of ERBB2 overexpression and TP53 mutation in inflammatory breast cancer. Oncogene 21:7593–7597
53. Kandioler-Eckersberger D, Ludwig C, Rudas M, Kappel S, Janschek E, Wenzel C, Schlagbauer-Wadl H, Mittlbock M, Gnant M, Steger G, Jakesz R (2000) TP53 mutation and p53 overexpression for prediction of response to neoadjuvant treatment in breast cancer patients. Clin Cancer Res 6:50–56
54. Yamauchi H, Cristofanilli M, Nakamura S et al (2009) Molecular targets for treatment of inflammatory breast cancer. Nat Rev Clin Oncol 6:387–394

Chapter 15
Molecules That Drive the Invasion and Metastasis of Inflammatory Breast Cancer

Madhura Joglekar and Kenneth L. van Golen

Abstract Invasion and metastasis represent two of the most critical and rate limiting steps of cancer progression. It is very well known that IBC is lympho-angioinvasive and appears to be metastatic upon inception. Therefore, identifying and targeting molecules that regulate these critical steps formulate a logical treatment approach for IBC. This chapter focuses on the advancements that have taken place so far in terms of identifying unique molecular determinants that potentially drive IBC invasion and metastasis. Studies before 2000 established SUM149 and SUM190 IBC cell lines, identified hormonal status, differential expression of RhoC GTPase, LIBC (now known as WISP3) and E-cadherin, as potential metastatic markers along with creation of the MARY-X xenograft model. These findings developed a strong foundation for studies post 2001 that investigated various pre- and posttranslational signaling events, pro-angiogenic factors and potential targeted therapy approaches for IBC. We conclude this chapter with a comprehensive model summarizing all the breakthrough findings and their potential interdependence that could ultimately produce a unique response of preventing IBC invasion and metastasis.

Keywords Metastatic spread • RhoC GTPase • WISP3 • Inflammatory breast cancer cell lines • Differential display • Tissue microarray • IBC xenograft • E-cadherin • MUC1 • Caveolin-1 • eIF4G1 • p120 catenin • HDACs • Lymphangiogenesis • Farnesyl transferase inhibitors • Akt

M. Joglekar
The Department of Biological Sciences, The Center for Translational Cancer Research,
The University of Delaware, Newark, DE, USA

K.L. van Golen (✉)
The Helen F. Graham Cancer Center, Newark, DE, USA

The University of Delaware, 320 Wolf Hall, Newark, DE 19350, USA
e-mail: klvg@udel.edu

N.T. Ueno and M. Cristofanilli (eds.), *Inflammatory Breast Cancer: An Update*,
DOI 10.1007/978-94-007-3907-9_15, © Springer Science+Business Media B.V. 2012

Abbreviations

Abl	Abelson proto-oncogene
Ang-1	Angiopoietin 1
bFGF	basic Fibroblast Growth Factor
BRCA	Breast Cancer Susceptibility Protein
CCR-7	C-C motif chemokine receptor type 7
Cox-2	cyclooxygenase-2
CXCR-4	C-X-C motif chemokine receptor type 4
EGF(R)	Epidermal Growth Factor Receptor
eIF4G1	Eukaryotic Translation Initiation factor 4 Gamma 1
ER	Estrogen Receptor
ERK(1/2)	Extracellular-signal-Regulated Kinases
EST	Expressed Sequence Tag
FTI	Farnesyl Transferase Inhibitor
GAP	GTPase Activating Protein
GDI	Guanosine Dissociation Inhibitor
GEF	Guanosine Exchange Factor
GIST	Gastro Intestinal Stromal Tumors
H19	Imprinted maternally expressed transcript (non-protein coding)
HDAC	Histone Deacetylase
HMEC	Human Mammary Epithelial Cells
HMG-CoA	3-hydroxy-3-methylglutaryl-coenzyme A
IGFBP	Insulin Growth Factor Binding Protein
IGFBP-rp9	Insulin Growth Factor Binding Protein Related Protein 9
IGF(R) (I/II)	Insulin Growth Factor Receptor (I/II)
IL	Interleukin
IRES	Internal Ribosomal Entry Site
IRS-1	Insulin Receptor Substrate-1
KDR	Kinase Insert Domain Receptor
LIBC	Lost in Inflammatory Breast Cancer
MAPK	Mitogen Activated Protein Kinase
MMP-2	Matrix Metalloprotease-2
mTOR	Mammalian Target of Rapamycin
NFκB	nuclear factor kappa-light-chain-enhancer of activated B cells
PDGF(R)	Platelet Derived Growth Factor Receptor
PGE-2	Prostaglandin E2
pHER-2/neu	phospho - Human Epidermal Growth Factor Receptor- 2
PR	Progesteron Receptor
Prox-1	Prospero homeobox 1
Rex-1	RNA exonuclease 1 homolog
SCID	Severe Combined Immunodeficiency
SEER	Surveillance epidemiology and end results
sLex/a	sialyl-Lewis(x/a)

TGF (α/β)   Transforming Growth Factor
Tie (1/2)   Tyrosine kinase with Immunoglobulin-like and EGF-like domains
VEGF   Vascular Endothelial Growth Factor
WISP 3   WNT1 Inducible Signaling pathway Protein 3

15.1 Introduction

The term 'Inflammatory Breast Cancer' (IBC) was first introduced in 1924, when Drs. Lee and Tannenbaum used it to describe a phenotypically distinct and aggressive presentation of locally advanced breast cancer (LABC). Based on clinical and pathological findings IBC unified what was thought to be several distinct entities of LABC as a single disease [1]. Clinically, Lee and Tannenbaum recognized what appeared to be a classical immune inflammatory response with erythema, edema, swelling, intense pain and peau d'orange appearance of the breast; thus the use of the phrase "inflammatory" in the description of the disease [2–9]. This term has proven to be a misnomer as the involvement of a true immunologically driven inflammatory response is rarely seen. Instead, pathological findings indicate the presence of tumor emboli invading the dermal lymphatic vessels of the skin overlying the breast [3, 10, 11]. It is thought that the poor prognosis of this disease is due to its ability to rapidly disseminated via the dermal lymphatic system.

Diagnostic criteria that are being followed today include assessment of the peculiar clinical symptoms described above, a rapid progression of disease and a lympho-angioinvasive nature of the tumor apparently from its inception. The lympho-angiogenic nature and tendency to invade dermal lymphatic vessels contribute significantly to the metastatic nature of this disease [12–14]. IBC typically does not involve a palpable lump in the breast and hence, its development usually goes unnoticed until occurrence of marked changes in the physical appearance of the breast [5, 15]. By definition IBC is a T4d tumor and patients are diagnosed with stage IIIB or IV disease. Most patients show axillary lymph node involvement and almost 30% patients show gross distant metastasis in organs such as lungs, liver and bone at their first clinical presentation [16].

Clearly, IBC is distinct and unique as compared to other forms of breast cancer. By virtue of its ability to invade the dermal lymphatic vessels, a property that defines IBC, it is highly invasive and metastatic. Thus, IBC is a paradigm for lymphovascular invasion. An understanding of the severity and urge to fight this disease has opened a several avenues for the worldwide research community to study this disease at molecular level particularly as it pertains to the invasive properties of the disease. Efforts that have been undertaken in this particular direction for last decade or so have contributed significantly to know this disease in depth and we now have reached a stage where we are aware of the fact that IBC, not only phenotypically but also genetically, is entirely a distinct entity compared to conventional breast cancer cases. This chapter focuses on the advancements that have taken place so far in terms of identifying molecular determinants that potentially drive IBC invasion and metastasis, important rate limiting steps in the progression of this deadly disease. A "new era" in IBC research appeared to begin over the past decade. Therefore, this chapter will focus on IBC research prior to and then after the year 2000.

15.2   IBC Research Prior to 2000

Since its identification and classification, IBC has remained a misunderstood and underrepresented form of breast cancer in terms of research focus. In addition, its inclusion as a distinct entity has been argued for the better part of a half-century. A detailed review of the literature over the span of 80 years starting from 1924 suggests that the rarity of IBC coupled with its frequent misdiagnosis, as 'mastitis' could be the main contributing factors of IBC being an understudied entity for such a long period of time [17–20]. Moreover, it also appears from the literature that due to the rare occurrence of this particular condition as compared to conventional breast cancer, it was initially difficult to understand the urgent need to study the molecular aspects of IBC exclusively. Most early investigations included individual or a small number of IBC samples incidentally, along with conventional breast cancers. These studies attempted to relate IBC to conventional breast cancers and most molecular studies focused on expression of genes and proteins associated with breast cancer. Few investigators had the insight to focus on IBC as distinct entity, however some of these types of studies were performed.

15.2.1   *Early Assessment of Treatment on Metastatic Spread and Clinical Outcome*

Initial retrospective studies of IBC prior to 2000 were mainly focused on understanding the clinical and histopathology of tumor that could improve diagnostic criteria and establish the disease as a distinct form of breast cancer. However, many of these studies helped us in understanding the metastatic profile of IBC. In 1978, Lucas and his group carried out a study involving 58 IBC patients showing clinical signs and symptoms and 15 patients with occult IBC to review if the diagnosis of IBC is clinical or pathological. Lesions of clinically apparent and occult inflammatory carcinoma demonstrated similar gross and microscopic growth patterns, histologic types, axillary involvement and early widespread metastases. Regardless of pathologic evidence of dermal lymphatic tumor, patients with clinical inflammation had rapid deterioration. Cases with only a pathological diagnosis were slightly less fulminant in progression. Thus, either clinical or pathologic criteria were able to justify the use of the term "inflammatory breast carcinoma" [2].

Until the late 1990s, treatment options for IBC cases were same as those were for treating LABC in general. However, later on it became clear that surgery and irradiation alone have little effect on the natural history or course of IBC since lymphatic invasion and distinct metastasis are often present at initial presentation. Therefore, it was proposed that IBC should be considered as a systemic disease as opposed to a locally advanced disease and should be treated with aggressive combined multi-modality therapy including multidrug chemotherapy along with surgery and irradiation [21–24]. There are various retrospective studies listed in the literature that demonstrate initial treatment strategies to treat IBC. Several of these studies included chemotherapy with three cycles of 5-Fluorouracil, Doxorubicin and cyclophosphamide along with radiation and/or radical mastectomy [24–31].

Nonetheless, IBC was still a dreadful disease in terms of overall and disease free survival rate due to its propensity to invade distant organs. Review of data from the National Cancer Institute's SEER program for the period 1975–1992, showed that IBC patients were significantly younger at diagnosis than non-IBC patients. Overall survival was significantly worse for IBC patients than for non-IBC patients and for African Americans than for whites [32]. Throughout each of these studies, florid lymphovascular invasion was noted and attributed to the poor prognosis of the disease.

15.2.2 Steroid and Growth Factor Receptor Status of IBC

Treating IBC as a conventional LABC or as systemic disease was not enough to improve the prognosis and survival rate. This is when a thought to study IBC at molecular level was taken into consideration. The first step towards this goal was to determine whether the estrogen receptor (ER) and progesterone receptor (PR) status in IBC patient tumors was similar to conventional breast cancer [33, 34]. One initial study performed by Paradiso et al. showed that the percentage of ER+ and PR+ cases were lower in IBC compared to stage matched LABC (ER+, 44% versus 64%; PR+, 30% versus 51%, respectively), pertaining to both premenopausal and postmenopausal women. They also put forth an idea that IBC is a heterogeneous biological entity for which hormone receptors and cell kinetics could be useful in identifying patients with different prognoses and therefore candidates for personalized therapy [35]. Charpin and his group carried out similar study using immunocytochemical analysis on frozen sections of IBC samples using antibodies against pHER-2/neu, ER and PR. They found that all tumors were strongly pHER-2/neu positive and less than 40% were slightly ER, PR immunoreactive [36]. Thus, these results correlated with the high degree of malignancy and shorter disease-free survival time due to metastasis and overall poor clinical outcome of IBC patients [3].

In order to investigate the relationship between ER expression and the expression of the proto-oncogene c-myb in breast cancer, Guerin et al. conducted an analysis of 112 non-IBC specimens and 57 IBC specimens. The proto-oncogene c-myb is a transcriptional regulator associated with differentiation and proliferation. However, recent studies suggest it has a role in hepatocellular invasion and homing of several cancer types to the bone marrow [37, 38]. Expression of the ER and PR genes, c-myb, HER-2 (pHER-2/neu), c-myc, c-fos, the epidermal growth factor receptor

(EGFR) gene, and pS2 (a small secreted protein isolated from MCF7 cells after induction by 17β-estradiol) were analyzed in that study. The IBC specimens were found to be positive for the EGFR gene (58%) and HER-2 (60%). Expression of c-myb was found to correlate inversely with c-erb2 expression, and was higher in non-IBC samples (63% versus 38%). Expression of the other genes was approximately the same for non-IBC and IBC specimens, and no statistically significant differences were found [39, 40]. These results are consistent with studies demonstrating that c-myb expression is post-translationally regulated in ER+ breast cancers suggesting it is linked to ER status and not tumor progression [41, 42]. These experiments helped establish the ER, PR, EGFR and HER-2 status in IBC. These factors have all been found to be important in the metastatic phenotype of a number of cancers including IBC.

15.2.3   Status of p53 in IBC

The next milestone in the discovery of prognostic factors was identification of p53 status in IBC samples. The role of p53 in controlling tumor growth as well as metastasis is known for breast cancer [43]. Mutations at the p53 locus have been thought of as the most common mechanism to inactivate the negative regulatory effects of p53 upon cell proliferation in almost all types of cancer. Cells that over express wild type p53 are blocked near the G1/S phase of the cell cycle, suggesting a specific role for controlling cell replication [44–46]. Many different human cancers bear mutant forms of p53 proteins and hence can no longer suppress cell division [47]. A study done by Moll et al. screened 27 cases of IBC for the presence of p53 protein. Among the 27 cases, three groups were detected. Eight cases had higher levels of p53 in the nucleus, nine cases had a complete lack of staining and ten cases showed cytoplasmic staining with no nuclear staining at all. Further, sequencing analysis showed that nuclear staining was associated with mutated p53 expression and overall weak signal for wild type p53 as shown in nine cases. The last 37% of specimens had accumulated p53 in the cytoplasm and almost all of these cases revealed wild-type p53 sequences. Therefore, the study concluded with the finding that IBC cases show two distinct mechanisms for p53 function; direct mutation and cytoplasmic sequestration of the wild type p53 protein [48].

   The same study was extended to look at the relation between p53 status and prognosis. Patients with p53 nuclear expression were found to have poor clinical outcome. In relation to ER status, the group of patients who were ER negative and had nuclear over expression of p53 had 17.9-fold higher risk of death, compared with 2.8-fold for those women who had p53 nuclear over expression alone. Thus, it was evident from this study that p53, ER, PR status strongly influence IBC overall survival [49]. Studies of conventional breast cancer patient samples suggest that p53 status and ER expression may be different in a patients' primary tumor compared to metastases [50]. Since IBC is inherently metastatic the studies highlighted above provide a relevant insight into the relationship of p53 and ER expression, which may affect patterns of IBC metastasis [51–54].

Table 15.1 Updated table of genes identified using modified differential display comparing immortalized human mammary epithelial cells, lymphocytes and the SUM149 IBC cell line

Transcript	Identification	Transcript	Identification
N1	H-NUC/cdc27	T1	*SPIRE1*
N2	*GDP-O-fucosyltransferase*	T2	Deoxyhypusine synthase
N3	28s rRNA variable Region	T3	*CGGBP1*
N4	Olfactory-R Family	T5	Overexpressed breast tumor protein
N5/6	*ARPP19*	T6	**RhoC GTPase**
N7	HMG-CoA Reductase	T7	TI277H/mt gDNA
N8	**WISP3 (a.k.a LIBC, CCN9, IGFBP-rP9)**	T9	28s rRNA variable Region

Transcripts beginning with N# were not expressed by the tumor cell line compared with normal cells, while those beginning with T# were expressed by tumor cells but not normal cells. Bold transcripts are found to be specifically altered in IBC versus stage-matched non-IBC patient samples. Italicized transcripts were previously published as unknown genes corresponding to EST, KIA and THC transcripts

15.2.4   Gene Discovery in IBC: RhoC GTPase and WISP3

To this point IBC research was effectively able to study the role of these prognostic factors on overall survival of IBC patients in a manner similar to studying non-IBC. Although these prognostic factors ultimately play a role in and impact metastasis, none of these studies addressed the invasive nature of IBC. In regards to the unique clinical presentation of IBC compared to non-IBC, there was hardly anything known about the contrasting features between these two-breast cancer types with respect to their genetic makeup. Clearly, a study of these genetic determinants was important to understand the biology behind the invasive and metastatic behavior of IBC. Our laboratory was one of the first few labs that started looking at the genetic dissimilarities within these two cancer groups.

In 1999, van Golen and Merajver hypothesized that a limited number of genetic alterations give rise to IBC and that the disease is metastatic almost upon its inception. In this study, using a modified differential display technique, expression of transcripts from a primary IBC cell line (SUM149), immortalized human mammary epithelial cells and lymphocytes from the patient that the SUM149 was derived from, were compared. Seventeen differentially expressed genes were identified; a partial list of the identified genes is given in Table 15.1. Differential expression was confirmed and also compared in another IBC cell line, SUM190, in addition to several non-IBC cell lines by Southern analysis. To determine which genes were unique to IBC, *in* situ hybridization was performed on IBC patient samples and stage-matched non-IBC specimens. Two transcripts were found to be specifically altered in IBC patient samples. A novel gene that was cloned and called Lost in Inflammatory Breast Cancer (LIBC) and RhoC GTPase. Expression of LIBC was lost in 80% of inflammatory tumors and 21% of non-inflammatory tumors. RhoC GTPase was over expressed in 90% of inflammatory tumors, whereas only 38% of non-inflammatory tumors [55]. Results of this study were confirmed by Vermeulen and colleagues 5 years later using tissue microarray analysis [56, 57].

The LIBC gene encodes a protein with 331 amino acids and 36.9 kDa protein. It is a member of IGFBP family and also termed as IGFBP-rP9 [58]. It contains 36 cysteine residues and the IGF binding domain, GCGCCKIC, starting at amino acid 48. LIBC is found to be N-linked glycosylated and has several predicted myristilation sites that may help LIBC to localize at the plasma membrane and aid in its interaction with IGF and insulin receptors [55]. LIBC is considered as a strong candidate for a tumor suppressor gene in IBC. Close to the time LIBC was cloned and found to be lost in IBC, it was also cloned and found to be over expressed in colorectal carcinoma suggesting it to be both a tumor suppressor and an oncogene [59]. Over time LIBC has been known as IGF binding protein-related protein 9 (IGFBP-rP9), CCN9 and Wnt1-inducible secreted protein 3 (WISP3) [60]. The later is its current designation.

The second differentially expressed gene - RhoC GTPase is a member of Rho family of small GTP binding proteins [61]. Rho proteins are involved in actin cytoskeletal rearrangements and thus are found to modulate cell motility, invasion and metastasis in cancer [62–67]. Rho activity is maintained through the cyclic events called (GTPase cycle) in which Rho proteins operate in GTP bound active form and GDP bound inactive form. These cyclic events take place under the control of Rho regulatory proteins Guanosine exchange factor (GEF), Gauanosine dissociation inhibitor (GDI) and GTPase activating protein (GAP) [68–73]. The first Rho gene was identified in 1985 from the sea slug *Aplysia californicus* by virtue of its close homology to Ras [74]. Rho family members RhoA and RhoC share closest homology with 84% similarity at mRNA level and 91% similarity at protein level [75, 76]. Unlike Ras, the transformation ability of Rho proteins is not bestowed upon any sort of gain-of-function mutations but the over expression and increased activity in its GTP bound form [55, 77–79]. So it is the ratio of GTP bound active form of the protein and total protein that decides the functional response elicited by Rho proteins.

The transforming ability of Rho family members in various other tissue culture systems has been documented. Expression of constitutively active RhoA into NIH3T3, Swiss 3T3 and other similar cell types has resulted in the rapid formation of stress fibers and inhibition of cellular motility and invasion [62, 80, 81]. To study the role of RhoC GTPase in contributing towards IBC like phenotype, our lab generated stable transfectants of human mammary epithelial (HME) cells over expressing the RhoC gene. The HME-RhoC transfectants formed colonies under anchorage independent growth conditions. They were found to be more motile, invasive and produced pro-angiogenic factors. Moreover, orthotopic injection into immunocompromised nude mice led to tumor formation. Thus, this was the very first study that showed how RhoC GTPase transfected mammary epithelial cells carry ability to generate cellular effects that strikingly resemble *in vivo* IBC phenotype [82, 83]. Therefore, identification of RhoC GTPase as one of the prognostic markers in IBC that exhibit differential expression with respect to normal cells and its ability to mimic aggressive IBC phenotype in RhoC transfected mammary cells, indeed gave an important direction to the study of IBC biology.

Of additional interest, HMG-CoA reductase was found to have differential expression compared to normal breast epithelial cells but at the same time, it was not specific to the IBC. HMG-CoA reductase gene resides on chromosomal location 5q13-12.14, which is found to be an area of frequent loss of heterozygosity in breast cancer. This can be correlated with increased chances of BRCA1 and BRCA2 germ line mutations [55]. HMG-CoA reductase participates in many functions that are required for cellular proliferation and prenylation of Ras and Rho proteins [84–87]. As a result, HMG-CoA bears the potential to be prognostic marker in IBC and is the subject of current research in at least two different IBC laboratories.

Several genes like HMG-CoA reductase were found to be differentially expressed by IBC compared to normal epithelial cells but when analyzed were found to not be specific for IBC. Many of these genes were novel transcripts and at the time of the study correlated to an expressed sequence tag (EST). In writing this chapter 12 years after publication of the original study, the novel sequences were re-analyzed using BLAST and several genes that may be involved in invasion and metastasis identified (Table 15.1). Of particular note is SPIRE1, an actin nucleation factor that associates directly with Rho GTPases. Like RhoC GTPase, SPIRE1 is over expressed in IBC cells.

15.2.5   *In Vivo Modeling of IBC Growth and Metastasis: The Establishment of MARY-X*

To study lymphovascular invasion associated with IBC, Barsky and his group established a transplantable human inflammatory breast carcinoma xenograft (MARY-X) in SCID/nude mice [88]. MARY-X grows exclusively in murine lymphatics and blood vessels in the form of several tight tumor emboli. Also, similar to the *in vivo* presentation in patients, it shows erythema of the overlying skin. Molecular studies of MARY-X revealed that it is ER, PR, HER-2/neu negative and p53, EGFR positive.

In a comparative study with non-inflammatory xenografts, MARY-X showed 10–20 fold increased over expression of E-cadherin and MUC1 similar to what is typically seen in IBC patients. Kleer et al. also found strong expression of E-cadherin in 100% of 20 human IBC tumors and in only 68% of 22 stage-matched non-IBC tumors [89]. Based on this data, it was proposed that these molecules might contribute to the characteristic IBC homotypic and heterotypic interactions.

15.3   Progress from 2001-Present

Following on the avenues that were opened with the establishment of the SUM149 and SUM190 IBC cell lines, the identification of RhoC GTPase, LIBC and E-cadherin as potential prognostic markers and creation of the MARY-X model, a significant amount of progress has been made in the IBC field since 2000. This has helped generate a great amount of hope and awareness in researchers, doctors and patients. This section of the chapter discusses several of such milestones in the molecular study of IBC from 2001 till today.

15.3.1 Expression of Cell Adhesion Molecules in IBC Cells and Tumor Emboli

Numerous studies have observed that the expression of E-cadherin and related adhesion molecules is lost in malignant progression [90–92]. Hence, over expression of E-cadherin in IBC tumor emboli was perceived as something unusual. Using the IBC xenograft model MRAY-X, Barsky and colleagues discovered an over expressed and functioning E–cadherin/α-catenin/β-catenin axis in IBC compared to non-IBC cell lines/xenografts. This finding was based on immunoreactivity studies that showed increased membrane but not cytoplasmic localization of E–cadherin/ α-catenin/β-catenin. Moreover, spheroids of MARY-X completely disadhered when placed in media without calcium or when treated with anti-E-cadherin antibodies as well as expression of a dominant negative mutant E-cadherin. Altered E-cadherin expression in IBC was later attributed to the presence of E-cadherin fragments that can preserve the interaction between E-cadherin and β-catenin [93].

They also found that in contrast to strong homotypic tumor cell adhesion, heterotypic interaction to endothelial cells was absent. Subsequently, it was determined that lack of tumor cell binding is because of markedly decreased sialyl-Lewis x/a (sLex/a) carbohydrate ligand- binding epitopes on over-expressed MUC1 and other surface molecules that bind endothelial E-selectin. Decreased sLex/a could result from decreased 3/4-fucosyl transferase activity in MARY-X. The decreased sLex/a fail to confer electrostatic repulsions between tumor cells, which further contributes to the compactness of the MARY-X spheroid by allowing the E-cadherin homodimeric interactions to go unopposed. The exogenous addition of sLex/a caused disadherence of MARY-X spheroids and the disruption of the E- cadherin homodimers mediating cell adhesion.

These results were also observed in actual cases of IBC. The lymphovascular tumor emboli in 25 out of 25 cases of IBC exhibited strong MUC1 immunoreactivity but weak to absent sialyl-Lewis x/a immunoreactivity [94, 95]. Also, this group proposed a concept that tumor cell-endothelial cell aversion contributes to the compactness of the emboli and their passive dissemination (metastasis) in lymphovascular channels by process known as vasculogenic mimicry [96]. This passive dissemination was manifested by a dramatic increase in metastatic pulmonary emboli as a result of palpation of the primary tumor without increase in circulating human tumor cell±derived growth factors (IGF-I, IGF-II, TGF-α and TGF-β) and angiogenic factors (VEGF and bFGF). Increasing the number of circulating tumor cells and resultant distant metastases by increasing intratumoral pressure has been observed for non-breast cancer as well [97]. Therefore, given the anatomy of dermal lymphatic vessels and patterns of metastatic spread in IBC patients, it is doubtful that passive dissemination is the main mode of IBC metastasis.

Schneider and colleagues recently demonstrated that the unique pathogenic properties of IBC result in part from over expression of the translation initiation factor eIF4G1. This over expression leads to a specific increase in the translation of internal ribosomal entry site (IRES) containing mRNAs. Specifically, two such mRNAs, p120 catenin and VEGF, encode key proteins involved in the pathogenesis of IBC. The p120 catenin protein causes retention of E-cadherin at cell surface and VEGF produces angiogenic effects and resistance to hypoxia. Silencing of eIF4G1 caused marked reduction in p120 catenin protein levels and cell surface associated E-cadherin expression in SUM149 cells. Invasion was found to be diminished two-fold by eIF4G1 silencing and three-fold by p120 catenin silencing. Furthermore, ectopic over expression of p120 catenin in eIF4G1 silenced cells was able to restore invasion, E-cadherin cell surface localization, tumor growth and hence ability to generate IBC mammospheres to the levels observed in control [98].

Recently Robertson et al. have examined HDAC inhibitors as an inflammatory breast cancer therapy. Histone deacetylase (HDACs) are involved in the process of epigenetic regulation of gene expression. Epigenetic events are believed to be crucial for the onset and progression of cancer. The acetylation status of histones regulates the organization of chromatin and the access of transcription factors such as eIF4G1 [99–102].

15.3.2 Expression of Pro-angiogenic and Pro-lymphangiogenic Molecules

It has been validated through many studies now that some of the up regulated genes in *in vitro* and *in vivo* IBC models include angiogenic, lymphangiogenic factors and other genes up regulated by hypoxia. One of the initial studies performed by Van der Auwera et al., showed increased mRNA expression of VEGF-C, VEGF-D, KDR, Flt-4, Ang-1, Tie-1, Tie-2, cyclooxygenase-2, fibroblast growth factor-2 (FGF-2), Prox-1, and LYVE-1 in 16 IBC vs. 20 non-IBC specimens. These factors support rapid growth of tumor cells under hypoxic conditions and also promote a venue for dissemination [12–14]. Studies with eIF4G1 also show that IBC cells adapt to the eIF4G1 dependent VEGF protein translation as they encounter hypoxic conditions and thus can survive efficiently in poorly oxygenated tissues. Small lymphatic vessels are freely permeable and experiments have shown that oxygen in lymph is equivalent to the interstitial oxygen found in the surround tissues [103]. However, lymphatic oxygen levels vary due to oxygen consumption by cells in the lymphatic vessels. Colpeart et al. demonstrated an increased level of angiogenesis in IBC versus non-IBC patient samples. By using a marker for hypoxia they concluded that increased angiogenesis in the IBC tumors was, for the most part, not stimulated by hypoxia [104].

15.3.3 IBC Cell Type of Origin

In 2005, Van Laere et al. identified the cell type of origin breast tumor subtypes in IBC. This was carried out using a data set consisting of 16 IBC and 18 non-IBC specimens. Combined HER-2 over expressing and basal like cluster was more expressed in IBC compared to non-IBC. Poor clinical outcome associated with these subtypes can very well explain the fact that IBC is characterized by 3-year survival rate of only 40% compared to 85% in non-IBC. On the other hand, combined luminal A, luminal B and normal-like cluster was more pronounced in non-IBC [105]. A group from M. D. Anderson performed a comparative study on three distinct clinical subtypes of IBC and non-IBC: 1. ER-positive/HER2-normal, 2. HER-2 amplified, and 3. ER-negative/HER2-normal [106]. In contrast to the earlier study by Van Laere, they did not find a significant difference in the gene expression at the individual gene level between stage matched IBC and non-IBC groups, except within HER-2 amplified subset. This could be explained by the differences in the clinical criteria of the groups being compared. Instead, when gene sets were compared for differential expression, they appeared to differentiate IBC from non-IBC in each clinical subtype. This implies a possibility that different biological pathways are involved with the pathogenesis of inflammatory phenotype in different molecular subsets. For example, protein translation and mTOR signaling were found to be over expressed in HER-2 amplified tumors. Rho GTPase activator activity was more in ER negative, HER-2 tumors [107]. These two studies proved to be important from the perspective of designing novel strategies for IBC treatment on case-by-case basis and for understanding how different gene signatures fit into the metastatic profile of the tumor.

15.3.4 The Role of NFκB in IBC Metastasis

Using cDNA microarray analysis on the pre-treatment tumor samples of 16 IBC patients and 18 cell type of origin-matched non-IBC patients, RNA expression of about 10,000 genes was evaluated by Van Laere et al. Among those genes, NFκB target genes and upstream activators of NFκB transcription were found to be over expressed in IBC [108]. Previous studies have documented the role of NFκB activation in regulating invasiveness due to increased cell migration and motility not only in breast cancer, but also in multiple myeloma and pancreatic cancer, two diseases that have a similar etiology as IBC. Activation of NFκB has been shown to be necessary for the induction of IL8 in human breast carcinoma cells, and for the production of IL8 and other pro-angiogenic mediators, such as VEGF, IL6, and IL1, in the SUM149 inflammatory breast cancer cell line. Moreover, NFκB has the ability to stimulate RhoC GTPase. Our laboratory has shown that RhoC GTPase expression and activation is required for expression of VEGF, IL-6, IL-8 and FGF-2 in the SUM149 cells. NFκB activation of RhoC may also provide an explanation for the invasive phenotype of IBC [57].

Biswas et al. reported that NFκB is activated more often in ER- compared with ER+human breast tumors, and most predominantly in ER- and HER2+ breast tumors. This finding gave rise to a thought that there could potentially be an inhibitory cross talk between ER and NF-κB signaling pathway [109]. Recent evidence suggests that all ER+breast tumors arise from ERβ breast tumor cells that stop expressing ERα [110, 111]. One of the reasons for the down regulation of ERα is the over-expression of EGFR and/or HER2 resulting in the hyperactivation of MAPK [112]. This mechanism possibly involves the activation of NFκB and its target genes [113].

15.3.5 Prostoglandins and IBC Spread

Robertson and colleagues have demonstrated the association of elevated Cox-2 mRNA and protein levels in breast tumors with evidence of invasion [6, 114]. Moreover, the presence of Cox-2 directly regulates proliferation, invasion, anchorage independent growth in soft agar and production of VEGF by breast tumor cells *in vitro* [115]. From mRNA expression studies of angiogenic receptors and their receptors Van Laere et al., found elevated levels of Cox-2 in 16 IBC and 20 non-IBC cases (stage matched and nonstage-matched) [14]. But because of the cardiovascular risk involved with Cox-2 inhibitor drugs, alternative approaches to inhibit binding of PGE2 to its G protein coupled receptors, termed as prostanoid receptors (EPs) was proposed [116]. Robertson and colleagues report that PGE2, EP3 and EP4 are all up regulated in IBC cells as opposed to ER positive MCF7 and MDA-MB-231 non-IBC cells. Furthermore, EP4 and EP3 were found to regulate invasion and vasculogenic mimicry associated with MMP-2 activity in SUM149 IBC cells [6, 117].

15.3.6 Stem Cell Markers in Invasive IBC

Because of the resemblance of IBC emboli to the embryonal blastocyst and their resistance to traditional chemotherapy/radiotherapy, Barsky and colleagues investigated the presence of stem cell markers on IBC. Using MARY-X spheroids, they identified embryonal stem cell markers including stellar, rex-1, nestin, H19 and potent transcriptional factors oct-4, nanog and sox-2 expressed. Most importantly, cells making up the MARY-X spheroids expressed CD44 (+)/CD24 (−/low), ALDH1, and CD133 [118]. The invasive gene signature by Liu et al., showed 2 signal transduction pathways: NFκB pathway and RAS/MAPK pathway indicating that these pathways play an important role in the molecular biology of mammary cancer stem cells [119]. Interestingly, Van Laere documented that IBC samples are characterized by more frequent activation of the NF-κB, RAS/MAPK pathway and that RAS/MAPK activation is responsible for NFκB activation in IBC [120].

15.3.7   Growth Factor Signaling and IBC Invasion

Our lab and others have explored the growth factor pathways and signaling cascades that are involved in conferring the IBC invasive phenotype. After treating RhoC GTPase transfected human mammary epithelial (HME) cells and SUM149 IBC cells with either C3 exotransferase (a specific inhibitor of Rho proteins) or a variety of MAPK and PI3K inhibitors at concentrations below cytotoxic levels, we determined that PI3K pathway is involved in the ability of RhoC over expressing cells to grow under anchorage independent conditions and induction of motility and invasion are mediated through activation of the ERK1/2 and p38 arms of the MAPK pathway [121]. Kleer et al., have shown that WISP-3 is a secreted protein and that once in the conditioned media, can effectively modulate IGF-IR activation and its signaling cascade and the cellular growth of IBC cells. This modulation results in the decrease of IGF-1 induced activation of IGF-IR and its downstream signaling molecules IRS-1 and ERK1/2. Also, It was found that addition of WISP-3 containing conditioned media decreased the growth rate of SUM149 cells [122].

Work on the involvement of growth factor and chemokine receptors in IBC biology by Cabioglu et al., demonstrates increased expression of CXCR4, EGFR and HER-2 neu amplification in IBC. Before this particular study, the association between cytoplasmic CCR7 and CXCR4 expression and lymph node positive tumors was demonstrated. Interestingly, Cabioglu et al. observed same pattern in IBC with a significant percentage of tumors (23%) with cytoplasmic CCR7 and CXCR4 expression and exclusively null nuclear expression. Thus, it was determined that increased expression of these growth factor and chemokine receptor appear to be more specific to the IBC phenotype and hence could potentially affect processes of invasion and metastasis [123].

15.3.8   Effect of Farnesyl Transferase Inhibitor on IBC Invasion

Rho proteins get prenylated to get localized in appropriate cellular compartments [124, 125]. RhoC undergoes geranylgeranylation whereas RhoB GTPase can be both geranylgeranylated (gg) and farnesylated (f) [126]. A shift in the balance from ggRhoB to fRhoB is known to occur in transformed cells [127]. Treatment of transformed cells with farnesyl transferase inhibitor (FTI) leads to a shift back to ggRhoB and a reversion of the transformed phenotype [128–130]. van Golen et al. reported that treatment of SUM149 cells with the FTI L-744,832 was able to revert RhoC GTPase induced changes in anchorage independent growth, motility and invasion [131]. One interesting finding of this study was increased expression levels of RhoB GTPase and activity of RhoC GTPase. Moreover, transient transfection of ggRhoB produced similar effects as that of FTI treatment. These findings suggested that FTI treatment increases levels of ggRhoB, which in turn suppresses RhoC function and reverts the aggressive phenotype of IBC.

15.3.9 Akt1/PKBa, Caveolin and PDGFRa

Unlike RhoA, what activates RhoC GTPase is still a mystery. Therefore a main focus of the van Golen laboratory is to study different signaling mechanisms that could potentially activate RhoC GTPase. A current hypothesis is that RhoC-GG gets localized at certain parts of the plasma membrane, which are called 'Caveolae'. These are 80–100 nm invaginations that are made up caveolin protein. In 2006, in collaboration with the Transational Cancer Research Group (TCRG) in Antwerp Belgium, we showed over expression of caveolin-1 and −2 in the IBC cell lines SUM149 and SUM190 as well as in IBC patient samples [132]. Over-expression appears to be due to hypomethylation of the caveolin-1 and −2 promoters that lie proximal to one another. Similar to the findings with E-cadherin, loss of caveolin-1 and 2 are associated with non-IBC progression and provide another example of how IBC has an opposite gene expression pattern from non-IBC [133, 134]. This study also found a correlation between caveolin-1 and −2 with RhoC GTPase. Current work from our lab demonstrates significant reduction in SUM149 cell invasion upon caveolin-1 down regulation or introduction of an exogenous caveolin-1 scaffolding domain, which is shown to assemble various signaling molecules (Joglekar and van Golen, unpublished data).

Several members of Rho GTPase subfamily, including RhoC GTPase, contain a putative site for phosphorylation by Akt/PKB. This site lies within the GTPase switch region, potentially affecting GTPase activation and its interaction with downstream effector molecules. Preliminary data from Lehman et al. demonstrates a significant decrease in SUM149 cell invasion upon pharmacologic inhibition or depletion of Akt1 but not Akt2 or Akt3 (Lehman and van Golen, unpublished data). Conversely, Akt2 affects non-IBC cell migration and invasion and is suggested to play a role in breast cancer metastasis [135, 136].

Again, in collaboration with the TCRG in Antwerp Belgium, we recently performed comparative study between IBC and non-IBC patient samples to look at expression of several molecules involved in PI3K/Akt1 signaling axis. A number of genes were up regulated in the IBC patient samples and when these were segregated by function it was found that PI3K/Akt1 signaling genes associated with cytoskeletal reorganization and motility were the only genes significantly increased in IBC patients.

It was also seen that the platelet derived growth factor receptor α (PDGFRα) was over expressed in IBC compared to non-IBC. It is very well documented that the canonical PDGFRα pathway involves PI3K/Akt activation. Recent work by Huang et al., reports that in a comparison to RhoB null mice, RhoB heterozygous mice show punctate staining of PDGFRβ in the cytoplasm towards the perinuclear region with relatively higher phosphorylated PDGFRβ upon PDGF stimulation [137]. Therefore, it is plausible that increased PDGFRα expression and increased phosphorylation presumably causes aberrant Akt1 activation and hence RhoC GTPase induced invasion and metastasis of IBC. Preliminary immunostaining of IBC cells suggests cytoplasmic localization of PDGFRα. This expression pattern is similar to what is observed for glioblastoma and gastrointestinal stromal tumors (GIST), both of which are treated with Imatinib (a.k.a. Gleevec) [138–140]. Typically, cytoplasmic localization of PDGFRα in glioblastoma and GIST is the result of a deletion mutation leading to loss of an N-linked glycosylation site. Mutation analysis of IBC cells suggests no deletions or mutations in the PDGFRα gene. One possible explanation is the loss of GDP-O-fucosyltransferase (Table 15.1) in IBC cells. Prevention of the addition of O-fucosyl groups results in cytoplasmic localization of PDGFRα, which is still capable of signaling [141].

15.4   Conclusion – Into the Twenty first Century

It appears that in the past decade significant progress in understanding invasion and metastasis of IBC has been made. The journey towards a complete cure of IBC could be envisioned if individual findings are connected to create therapies that would practically impede IBC invasion and metastasis. Figure 15.1 is a comprehensive model of what we believe are key signaling processes in driving IBC invasion and metastasis. Several molecular targets afford themselves for immediate pre-clinical testing. Imatinib is receptor tyrosine kinase inhibitor molecule that specifically acts against the tyrosine kinase domain in abl, c-kit and PDGFRα/β and has the major advantages of low toxicity, 98% bioavailability and an oral route of administration.

   In addition, establishment of new cell lines along with improved *in vitro* and animal models will greatly aid our understanding of the molecular mechanisms underlying IBC metastasis. Increasing evidence indicates that cell shape, cell-cell and cell-microenvironment influences gene transcription and phenotype. To date, most *in vitro* IBC experiments have been performed on cells in monolayer with a few being performed on IBC mammospheres. Mammospheres are formed by growing cells on a layer of Matrigel, a commercially available basement membrane. Although mammospheres are three-dimensional structures, growth on Matrigel is unlike growth and emboli formation in the dermal lymphatics. In an attempt to more accurately study IBC, we have begun to grow cells under conditions that mimic the physical properties of the dermal lymphatic environment. In this system, cells are placed in a medium that is 1.5-fold more viscous than water, at pH 7.52 and under constant oscillatory shear stress. This results in the formation of emboli *in vitro* that resemble those found in patients. Furthermore, non-IBC cells, which have the ability to form mammospheres when grown on Matrigel, do not form emboli in this system. Thus, we believe that this culture system has the potential for an accurate study of the molecular mechanisms of emboli formation and metastasis.

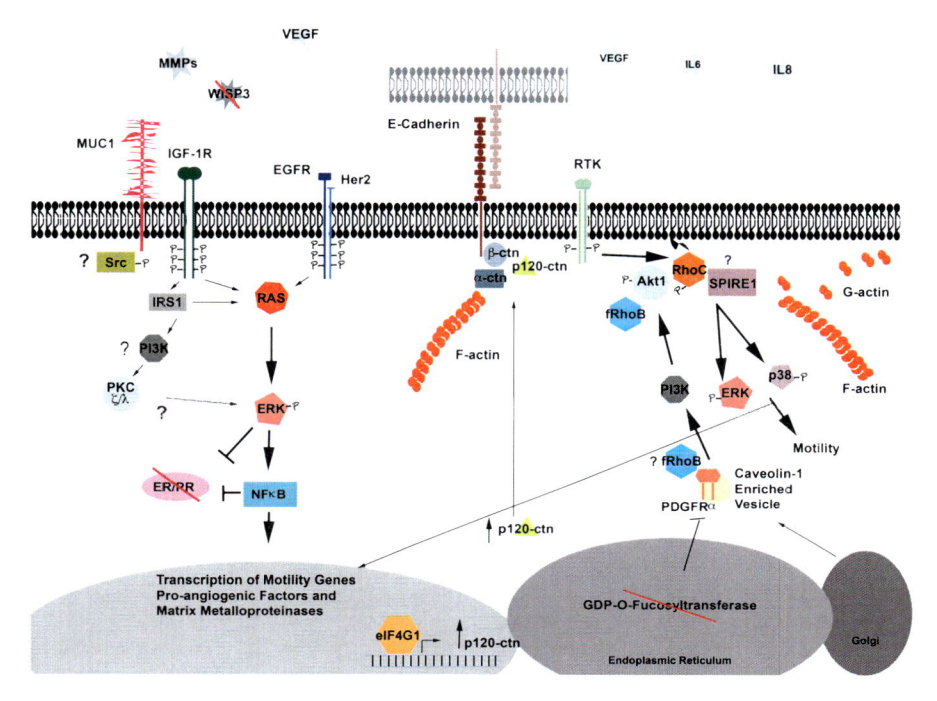

Fig. 15.1 A model of the current knowledge of signaling molecules leading to IBC invasion and metastasis. Loss of WISP3 (a.k.a. LIBC) leads to increased IGF-1 signaling through the scaffolding protein IRS1. IRS1 potentially can lead to the direct activation of MAPK or indirectly through activation of PI3K. Activation of EGFR family members such as EGFR and/or HER2 leads to ERK and NFκB activation leading to the transcription of motility related genes, pro-angiogenic factors and matrix metalloproteinases. Subsequent ERK and NFκB activation also results in the suppression of estrogen and progesterone receptor expression. The transcription factor eIF4G1 drives the expression of p120-catenin, which complexes with and stabilizes E-cadherin at the cell membrane. Included in this complex is the actin binding protein α- and β−catenin. RhoC GTPase is activated by a variety of protein tyrosine kinase receptors including IGF-1R and EGFR. RhoC can also be activated through G-protein coupled receptor activation or integrin ligation (not shown). Active RhoC can signal through downstream effector proteins including SPIRE1, which leads to actin nucleation and reorganization. RhoC signaling also leads to activation of the ERK and p38 arms of the MAPK pathway, which is required for motility. Loss of GDP-O-fucosyltransferase expression may lead to loss of posttranslational glycosylation of the cell surface protein MUC1. MUC1, in some systems can interact with the non-receptor tyrosine kinase Src, although this remains to be tested in IBC. Another protein that may be under glycosylated is PDGFRα. Loss of O-linked fucosylation of PDGFRα results in retention in the cytoplasm, but does not affect signaling capabilities and is able to activate Akt1 via PI3K. PDGFRα associates with caveolin-1 in the cytoplasm and can potentially be shuttled by farnesylated RhoB. Farnesylated RhoB can also shuttle Akt1/PKBα. Phosphorylation of RhoC by Akt1 is required to promote IBC invasion. RhoC driven gene transcription, as well as NFκB mediated gene transcription can drive the production of pro-(lymph)angiogenic molecules and matrix metalloproteinases

References

1. Tabbane F, el May A, Hachiche M, Bahi J et al (1985) Breast cancer in women under 30 years of age. Breast Cancer Res Treat 6(2):137–144
2. Lucas FV, Perez-Mesa C (1978) Inflammatory carcinoma of the breast. Cancer 41(4):1595–1605
3. Kleer CG, van Golen KL, Merajver SD (2000) Molecular biology of breast cancer metastasis. Inflammatory breast cancer: clinical syndrome and molecular determinants. Breast Cancer Res 2(6):423–429
4. Dawood S (2010) Biology and management of inflammatory breast cancer. Expert Rev Anticancer Ther 10(2):209–220. doi:10.1586/era.09.90
5. Dawood S, Merajver SD, Viens P, Vermeulen PB et al (2011) International expert panel on inflammatory breast cancer: consensus statement for standardized diagnosis and treatment. Ann Oncol 22(3):515–523. doi:10.1093/annonc/mdq345
6. Robertson FM, Simeone AM, Lucci A, McMurray JS et al (2010) Differential regulation of the aggressive phenotype of inflammatory breast cancer cells by prostanoid receptors EP3 and EP4. Cancer 116(11 Suppl):2806–2814. doi:10.1002/cncr.25167
7. Piera JM, Alonso MC, Ojeda MB, Biete A (1986) Locally advanced breast cancer with inflammatory component: a clinical entity with a poor prognosis. Radiother Oncol 7(3):199–204
8. Chevallier B, Asselain B, Kunlin A, Veyret C (1987) Inflammatory breast cancer. Determination of prognostic factors by univariate and multivariate analysis. Cancer 60(4):897–902
9. Fields JN, Kuske RR, Perez CA, Fineberg BB et al (1989) Prognostic factors in inflammatory breast cancer. Univariate and multivariate analysis. Cancer 63(6):1225–1232
10. Jaiyesimi IA, Buzdar AU, Hortobagyi G (1992) Inflammatory breast cancer: a review. J Clin Oncol 10(6):1014–1024
11. Gruber G, Ciriolo M, Altermatt HJ, Aebi S et al (2004) Prognosis of dermal lymphatic invasion with or without clinical signs of inflammatory breast cancer. Int J Cancer 109(1):144–148. doi:10.1002/ijc.11684
12. Van der Auwera I, Van den Eynden GG, Colpaert CG, Van Laere SJ et al (2005) Tumor lymphangiogenesis in inflammatory breast carcinoma: a histomorphometric study. Clin Cancer Res 11(21):7637–7642. doi:10.1158/1078-0432.CCR-05-1142
13. Van der Auwera I, Van Laere SJ, Van den Eynden GG, Benoy I et al (2004) Increased angiogenesis and lymphangiogenesis in inflammatory versus noninflammatory breast cancer by real-time reverse transcriptase-PCR gene expression quantification. Clin Cancer Res 10(23):7965–7971. doi:10.1158/1078-0432.CCR-04-0063
14. Vermeulen PB, van Golen KL, Dirix LY (2010) Angiogenesis, lymphangiogenesis, growth pattern, and tumor emboli in inflammatory breast cancer: a review of the current knowledge. Cancer 116(11 Suppl):2748–2754. doi:10.1002/cncr.25169
15. Robertson FM, Bondy M, Yang W, Yamauchi H et al (2010) Inflammatory breast cancer: the disease, the biology, the treatment. CA Cancer J Clin 60(6):351–375. doi:10.3322/caac.20082
16. Radunsky GS, van Golen KL (2005) The current understanding of the molecular determinants of inflammatory breast cancer metastasis. Clin Exp Metastasis 22(8):615–620. doi:10.1007/s10585-006-9000-7
17. Osborne BM (1989) Granulomatous mastitis caused by histoplasma and mimicking inflammatory breast carcinoma. Hum Pathol 20(1):47–52
18. Dahlbeck SW, Donnelly JF, Theriault RL (1995) Differentiating inflammatory breast cancer from acute mastitis. Am Fam Physician 52(3):929–934
19. Chambler AF, Drew PJ, Hill AD, Darzi A et al (1995) Inflammatory breast carcinoma. Surg Oncol 4(5):245–254
20. Dvoretsky PM, Woodard E, Bonfiglio TA, Hempelmann LH et al (1980) The pathology of breast cancer in women irradiated for acute postpartum mastitis. Cancer 46(10):2257–2262
21. Ellis LM, Bland KI, Copeland EM 3rd (1988) Inflammatory breast cancer: advances in therapy. Semin Surg Oncol 4(4):261–267

22. Giordano SH, Hortobagyi GN (2003) Inflammatory breast cancer: clinical progress and the main problems that must be addressed. Breast Cancer Res 5(6):284–288. doi:10.1186/bcr608

23. Burton GV, Cox EB, Leight GS Jr, Prosnitz LR et al (1987) Inflammatory breast carcinoma. Effective multimodal approach. Arch Surg 122(11):1329–1332

24. Maloisel F, Dufour P, Bergerat JP, Herbrecht R et al (1990) Results of initial doxorubicin, 5-fluorouracil, and cyclophosphamide combination chemotherapy for inflammatory carcinoma of the breast. Cancer 65(4):851–855

25. Krutchik AN, Buzdar AU, Blumenschein GR, Hortobagyi GN et al (1979) Combined chemoimmunotherapy and radiation therapy of inflammatory breast carcinoma. J Surg Oncol 11(4):325–332

26. Buzdar AU, Montague ED, Barker JL, Hortobagyi GN et al (1981) Management of inflammatory carcinoma of breast with combined modality approach – an update. Cancer 47(11):2537–2542

27. Pawlicki M, Skolyszewski J, Brandys A (1983) Results of combined treatment of patients with locally advanced breast cancer. Tumori 69(3):249–253

28. Ravaioli A, Gentilini P, Ridolfi R, Amadori D et al (1984) Inflammatory breast carcinoma: results from sixteen patients treated with chemo-radiotherapy and surgery. Chemioterapia 3(2):86–89

29. Attia-Sobol J, Ferriere JP, Cure H, Kwiatkowski F et al (1993) Treatment results, survival and prognostic factors in 109 inflammatory breast cancers: univariate and multivariate analysis. Eur J Cancer 29A(8):1081–1088

30. Rouesse J, Friedman S, Sarrazin D, Mouriesse H et al (1986) Primary chemotherapy in the treatment of inflammatory breast carcinoma: a study of 230 cases from the institut gustave-roussy. J Clin Oncol 4(12):1765–1771

31. Elias EG, Vachon DA, Didolkar MS, Aisner J (1991) Long-term results of a combined modality approach in treating inflammatory carcinoma of the breast. Am J Surg 162(3):231–235

32. Chang S, Parker SL, Pham T, Buzdar AU et al (1998) Inflammatory breast carcinoma incidence and survival: the Surveillance, Epidemiology, and End Results program of the National Cancer Institute, 1975–1992. Cancer 82(12):2366–2372

33. Delarue JC, May-Levin F, Mouriesse H, Contesso G et al (1981) Oestrogen and progesterone cytosolic receptors in clinically inflammatory tumours of the human breast. Br J Cancer 44(6):911–916

34. Harvey HA, Lipton A, Lawrence BV, White DS et al (1982) Estrogen receptor status in inflammatory breast carcinoma. J Surg Oncol 21(1):42–44

35. Paradiso A, Tommasi S, Brandi M, Marzullo F et al (1989) Cell kinetics and hormonal receptor status in inflammatory breast carcinoma. Comparison with locally advanced disease. Cancer 64(9):1922–1927

36. Charpin C, Bonnier P, Khouzami A, Vacheret H et al (1992) Inflammatory breast carcinoma: an immunohistochemical study using monoclonal anti-pHER-2/neu, pS2, cathepsin, ER and PR. Anticancer Res 12(3):591–597

37. Chen RX, Xia YH, Xue TC, Ye SL (2010) Transcription factor c-myb promotes the invasion of hepatocellular carcinoma cells via increasing osteopontin expression. J Exp Clin Cancer Res 29:172. doi:10.1186/1756-9966-29-172

38. Tanno B, Sesti F, Cesi V, Bossi G et al (2010) Expression of slug is regulated by c-myb and is required for invasion and bone marrow homing of cancer cells of different origin. J Biol Chem 285(38):29434–29445. doi:10.1074/jbc.M109.089045

39. Guerin M, Sheng ZM, Andrieu N, Riou G (1990) Strong association between c-myb and oestrogen-receptor expression in human breast cancer. Oncogene 5(1):131–135

40. Guerin M, Gabillot M, Mathieu MC, Travagli JP et al (1989) Structure and expression of c-erbB-2 and EGF receptor genes in inflammatory and non-inflammatory breast cancer: prognostic significance. Int J Cancer 43(2):201–208

41. Gudas JM, Klein RC, Oka M, Cowan KH (1995) Posttranscriptional regulation of the c-myb proto-oncogene in estrogen receptor-positive breast cancer cells. Clin Cancer Res 1(2):235–243

42. Guerin M, Barrois M, Riou G (1988) The expression of c-myb is strongly associated with the presence of estrogen and progesterone receptors in breast cancer]. C R Acad Sci III 307(20):855–861

43. Cox LA, Chen G, Lee EY (1994) Tumor suppressor genes and their roles in breast cancer. Breast Cancer Res Treat 32(1):19–38

44. Michalovitz D, Halevy O, Oren M (1990) Conditional inhibition of transformation and of cell proliferation by a temperature-sensitive mutant of p53. Cell 62(4):671–680

45. Diller L, Kassel J, Nelson CE, Gryka MA et al (1990) P53 functions as a cell cycle control protein in osteosarcomas. Mol Cell Biol 10(11):5772–5781

46. Martinez J, Georgoff I, Martinez J, Levine AJ (1991) Cellular localization and cell cycle regulation by a temperature-sensitive p53 protein. Genes Dev 5(2):151–159

47. Nigro JM, Baker SJ, Preisinger AC, Jessup JM et al (1989) Mutations in the p53 gene occur in diverse human tumour types. Nature 342(6250):705–708. doi:10.1038/342705a0

48. Moll UM, Riou G, Levine AJ (1992) Two distinct mechanisms alter p53 in breast cancer: mutation and nuclear exclusion. Proc Natl Acad Sci U S A 89(15):7262–7266

49. Riou G, Le MG, Travagli JP, Levine AJ et al (1993) Poor prognosis of p53 gene mutation and nuclear overexpression of p53 protein in inflammatory breast carcinoma. J Natl Cancer Inst 85(21):1765–1767

50. Zheng WQ, Lu J, Zheng JM, Hu FX et al (2001) Variation of ER status between primary and metastatic breast cancer and relationship to p53 expression*. Steroids 66(12):905–910

51. Sezgin C, Gokmen E, Kapkac M, Zekioglu O et al (2011) P53 protein accumulation and presence of visceral metastasis are independent prognostic factors for survival in patients with metastatic inflammatory breast carcinoma. Med Princ Pract 20(2):159–164. doi:10.1159/000319916

52. Turpin E, Bieche I, Bertheau P, Plassa LF et al (2002) Increased incidence of ERBB2 overexpression and TP53 mutation in inflammatory breast cancer. Oncogene 21(49):7593–7597. doi:10.1038/sj.onc.1205932

53. Gonzalez-Angulo AM, Sneige N, Buzdar AU, Valero V et al (2004) P53 expression as a prognostic marker in inflammatory breast cancer. Clin Cancer Res 10(18 Pt 1):6215–6221. doi:10.1158/1078-0432.CCR-04-0202

54. Yang CH, Cristofanilli M (2006) The role of p53 mutations as a prognostic factor and therapeutic target in inflammatory breast cancer. Future Oncol 2(2):247–255. doi:10.2217/14796694.2.2.247

55. van Golen KL, Davies S, Wu ZF, Wang Y et al (1999) A novel putative low-affinity insulin-like growth factor-binding protein, LIBC (lost in inflammatory breast cancer), and RhoC GTPase correlate with the inflammatory breast cancer phenotype. Clin Cancer Res 5(9): 2511–2519

56. Van den Eynden GG, Van der Auwera I, Van Laere S, Colpaert CG et al (2004) Validation of a tissue microarray to study differential protein expression in inflammatory and non-inflammatory breast cancer. Breast Cancer Res Treat 85(1):13–22. doi:10.1023/B:BREA.0000021028.33926.a8

57. Van Laere S, Van der Auwera I, Van den Eynden GG, Fox SB et al (2005) Distinct molecular signature of inflammatory breast cancer by cDNA microarray analysis. Breast Cancer Res Treat 93(3):237–246. doi:10.1007/s10549-005-5157-z

58. Hwa V, Oh Y, Rosenfeld RG (1999) The insulin-like growth factor-binding protein (IGFBP) superfamily. Endocr Rev 20(6):761–787

59. Thorstensen L, Diep CB, Meling GI, Aagesen TH et al (2001) WNT1 inducible signaling pathway protein 3, WISP-3, a novel target gene in colorectal carcinomas with microsatellite instability. Gastroenterology 121(6):1275–1280

60. Brigstock DR (2003) The CCN family: a new stimulus package. J Endocrinol 178(2): 169–175

61. Jaffe AB, Hall A (2005) Rho GTPases: biochemistry and biology. Annu Rev Cell Dev Biol 21:247–269. doi:10.1146/annurev.cellbio.21.020604.150721

62. Ridley AJ, Hall A (1992) The small GTP-binding protein rho regulates the assembly of focal adhesions and actin stress fibers in response to growth factors. Cell 70(3):389–399

63. Hall A, Paterson HF, Adamson P, Ridley AJ (1993) Cellular responses regulated by rho-related small GTP-binding proteins. Philos Trans R Soc Lond B Biol Sci 340(1293):267–271. doi:10.1098/rstb.1993.0067
64. Takai Y, Kaibuchi K, Sasaki T, Tanaka K et al (1994) Rho small G protein and cytoskeletal control. Princess Takamatsu Symp 24:338–350
65. Nobes CD, Hall A (1995) Rho, rac and cdc42 GTPases: regulators of actin structures, cell adhesion and motility. Biochem Soc Trans 23(3):456–459
66. Ridley AJ (2001) Rho GTPases and cell migration. J Cell Sci 114(Pt 15):2713–2722
67. Sahai E, Marshall CJ (2002) RHO-GTPases and cancer. Nat Rev Cancer 2(2):133–142. doi:10.1038/nrc725
68. Rossman KL, Der CJ, Sondek J (2005) GEF means go: turning on RHO GTPases with guanine nucleotide-exchange factors. Nat Rev Mol Cell Biol 6(2):167–180. doi:10.1038/nrm1587
69. Moon SY, Zheng Y (2003) Rho GTPase-activating proteins in cell regulation. Trends Cell Biol 13(1):13–22
70. DerMardirossian C, Bokoch GM (2005) GDIs: central regulatory molecules in rho GTPase activation. Trends Cell Biol 15(7):356–363. doi:10.1016/j.tcb.2005.05.001
71. Fukumoto Y, Kaibuchi K, Hori Y, Fujioka H et al (1990) Molecular cloning and characterization of a novel type of regulatory protein (GDI) for the rho proteins, ras p21-like small GTP-binding proteins. Oncogene 5(9):1321–1328
72. Schmidt A, Hall A (2002) Guanine nucleotide exchange factors for rho GTPases: turning on the switch. Genes Dev 16(13):1587–1609. doi:10.1101/gad.1003302
73. Garrett MD, Self AJ, van Oers C, Hall A (1989) Identification of distinct cytoplasmic targets for ras/R-ras and rho regulatory proteins. J Biol Chem 264(1):10–13
74. Madaule P, Axel R (1985) A novel ras-related gene family. Cell 41(1):31–40
75. Wennerberg K, Der CJ (2004) Rho-family GTPases: It's not only rac and rho (and I like it). J Cell Sci 117(Pt 8):1301–1312. doi:10.1242/jcs.01118
76. Takai Y, Sasaki T, Matozaki T (2001) Small GTP-binding proteins. Physiol Rev 81(1): 153–208
77. Fritz G, Just I, Kaina B (1999) Rho GTPases are over-expressed in human tumors. Int J Cancer 81(5):682–687
78. Moscow JA, He R, Gnarra JR, Knutsen T et al (1994) Examination of human tumors for rhoA mutations. Oncogene 9(1):189–194
79. Hall A, Marshall CJ, Spurr NK, Weiss RA (1983) Identification of transforming gene in two human sarcoma cell lines as a new member of the ras gene family located on chromosome 1. Nature 303(5916):396–400
80. Hall A (1990) The cellular functions of small GTP-binding proteins. Science 249(4969): 635–640
81. Hall A (1998) Rho GTPases and the actin cytoskeleton. Science 279(5350):509–514
82. van Golen KL, Wu ZF, Qiao XT, Bao LW et al (2000) RhoC GTPase, a novel transforming oncogene for human mammary epithelial cells that partially recapitulates the inflammatory breast cancer phenotype. Cancer Res 60(20):5832–5838
83. van Golen KL, Wu ZF, Qiao XT, Bao L et al (2000) RhoC GTPase overexpression modulates induction of angiogenic factors in breast cells. Neoplasia 2(5):418–425
84. Larsson O (1994) Effects of isoprenoids on growth of normal human mammary epithelial cells and breast cancer cells in vitro. Anticancer Res 14(1A):123–128
85. Wejde J, Carlberg M, Hjertman M, Larsson O (1993) Isoprenoid regulation of cell growth: identification of mevalonate-labelled compounds inducing DNA synthesis in human breast cancer cells depleted of serum and mevalonate. J Cell Physiol 155(3):539–548. doi:10.1002/jcp.1041550312
86. Addeo R, Altucci L, Battista T, Bonapace IM et al (1996) Stimulation of human breast cancer MCF-7 cells with estrogen prevents cell cycle arrest by HMG-CoA reductase inhibitors. Biochem Biophys Res Commun 220(3):864–870. doi:10.1006/bbrc.1996.0494
87. Park HJ, Kong D, Iruela-Arispe L, Begley U et al (2002) 3-hydroxy-3-methylglutaryl coenzyme a reductase inhibitors interfere with angiogenesis by inhibiting the geranylgeranylation of RhoA. Circ Res 91(2):143–150

88. Alpaugh ML, Tomlinson JS, Shao ZM, Barsky SH (1999) A novel human xenograft model of inflammatory breast cancer. Cancer Res 59(20):5079–5084

89. Kleer CG, van Golen KL, Braun T, Merajver SD (2001) Persistent E-cadherin expression in inflammatory breast cancer. Mod Pathol 14(5):458–464. doi:10.1038/modpathol.3880334

90. Blick T, Widodo E, Hugo H, Waltham M et al (2008) Epithelial mesenchymal transition traits in human breast cancer cell lines. Clin Exp Metastasis 25(6):629–642. doi:10.1007/s10585-008-9170-6

91. De Leeuw WJ, Berx G, Vos CB, Peterse JL et al (1997) Simultaneous loss of E-cadherin and catenins in invasive lobular breast cancer and lobular carcinoma in situ. J Pathol 183(4):404–411. doi:2-9

92. Yoshida R, Kimura N, Harada Y, Ohuchi N (2001) The loss of E-cadherin, alpha- and beta-catenin expression is associated with metastasis and poor prognosis in invasive breast cancer. Int J Oncol 18(3):513–520

93. Tomlinson JS, Alpaugh ML, Barsky SH (2001) An intact overexpressed E-cadherin/alpha, beta-catenin axis characterizes the lymphovascular emboli of inflammatory breast carcinoma. Cancer Res 61(13):5231–5241

94. Alpaugh ML, Tomlinson JS, Ye Y, Barsky SH (2002) Relationship of sialyl-lewis(x/a) under-expression and E-cadherin overexpression in the lymphovascular embolus of inflammatory breast carcinoma. Am J Pathol 161(2):619–628. doi:10.1016/S0002-9440(10)64217-4

95. Alpaugh ML, Tomlinson JS, Kasraeian S, Barsky SH (2002) Cooperative role of E-cadherin and sialyl-lewis X/A-deficient MUC1 in the passive dissemination of tumor emboli in inflammatory breast carcinoma. Oncogene 21(22):3631–3643. doi:10.1038/sj.onc.1205389

96. Mahooti S, Porter K, Alpaugh ML, Ye Y et al (2010) Breast carcinomatous tumoral emboli can result from encircling lymphovasculogenesis rather than lymphovascular invasion. Oncotarget 1(2):131–147

97. Price JE, Carr D, Tarin D (1984) Spontaneous and induced metastasis of naturally occurring tumors in mice: analysis of cell shedding into the blood. J Natl Cancer Inst 73(6):1319–1326

98. Silvera D, Arju R, Darvishian F, Levine PH et al (2009) Essential role for eIF4GI overexpression in the pathogenesis of inflammatory breast cancer. Nat Cell Biol 11(7):903–908. doi:10.1038/ncb1900

99. Wanczyk M, Roszczenko K, Marcinkiewicz K, Bojarczuk K et al (2011) HDACi–going through the mechanisms. Front Biosci 16:340–359

100. Robertson FM, Woodward WA, Pickei R, Ye Z et al (2010) Suberoylanilide hydroxamic acid blocks self-renewal and homotypic aggregation of inflammatory breast cancer spheroids. Cancer 116(11 Suppl):2760–2767. doi:10.1002/cncr.25176

101. Atadja PW (2011) HDAC inhibitors and cancer therapy. Prog Drug Res 67:175–195

102. Mani S, Herceg Z (2010) DNA demethylating agents and epigenetic therapy of cancer. Adv Genet 70:327–340. doi:10.1016/B978-0-12-380866-0.60012-5

103. Silvera D, Schneider RJ (2009) Inflammatory breast cancer cells are constitutively adapted to hypoxia. Cell Cycle 8(19):3091–3096

104. Colpaert CG, Vermeulen PB, Benoy I, Soubry A et al (2003) Inflammatory breast cancer shows angiogenesis with high endothelial proliferation rate and strong E-cadherin expression. Br J Cancer 88(5):718–725. doi:10.1038/sj.bjc.6600807

105. Van Laere SJ, Van den Eynden GG, Van der Auwera I, Vandenberghe M et al (2006) Identification of cell-of-origin breast tumor subtypes in inflammatory breast cancer by gene expression profiling. Breast Cancer Res Treat 95(3):243–255. doi:10.1007/s10549-005-9015-9

106. Bertucci F, Finetti P, Rougemont J, Charafe-Jauffret E et al (2005) Gene expression profiling identifies molecular subtypes of inflammatory breast cancer. Cancer Res 65(6):2170–2178. doi:10.1158/0008-5472.CAN-04-4115

107. Iwamoto T, Bianchini G, Qi Y, Cristofanilli M et al (2011) Different gene expressions are associated with the different molecular subtypes of inflammatory breast cancer. Breast Cancer Res Treat 125(3):785–795. doi:10.1007/s10549-010-1280-6

108. Van Laere SJ, Van der Auwera I, Van den Eynden GG, Elst HJ et al (2006) Nuclear factor-kappaB signature of inflammatory breast cancer by cDNA microarray validated by quantitative real-time reverse transcription-PCR, immunohistochemistry, and nuclear factor-kappaB DNA-binding. Clin Cancer Res 12(11 Pt 1):3249–3256. doi:10.1158/1078-0432.CCR-05-2800

109. Biswas DK, Shi Q, Baily S, Strickland I et al (2004) NF-kappa B activation in human breast cancer specimens and its role in cell proliferation and apoptosis. Proc Natl Acad Sci U S A 101(27):10137–10142. doi:10.1073/pnas.0403621101

110. Van Laere SJ, Van der Auwera I, Van den Eynden GG, van Dam P et al (2007) NF-kappaB activation in inflammatory breast cancer is associated with oestrogen receptor downregulation, secondary to EGFR and/or ErbB2 overexpression and MAPK hyperactivation. Br J Cancer 97(5):659–669. doi:10.1038/sj.bjc.6603906

111. Creighton CJ, Hilger AM, Murthy S, Rae JM et al (2006) Activation of mitogen-activated protein kinase in estrogen receptor alpha-positive breast cancer cells in vitro induces an in vivo molecular phenotype of estrogen receptor alpha-negative human breast tumors. Cancer Res 66(7):3903–3911. doi:10.1158/0008-5472.CAN-05-4363

112. Oh AS, Lorant LA, Holloway JN, Miller DL et al (2001) Hyperactivation of MAPK induces loss of ERalpha expression in breast cancer cells. Mol Endocrinol 15(8):1344–1359

113. Holloway JN, Murthy S, El-Ashry D (2004) A cytoplasmic substrate of mitogen-activated protein kinase is responsible for estrogen receptor-alpha down-regulation in breast cancer cells: the role of nuclear factor-kappaB. Mol Endocrinol 18(6):1396–1410. doi:10.1210/me.2004-0048

114. Brueggemeier RW, Quinn AL, Parrett ML, Joarder FS et al (1999) Correlation of aromatase and cyclooxygenase gene expression in human breast cancer specimens. Cancer Lett 140(1–2):27–35

115. Prosperi JR, Mallery SR, Kigerl KA, Erfurt AA et al (2004) Invasive and angiogenic phenotype of MCF-7 human breast tumor cells expressing human cyclooxygenase-2. Prostaglandins Other Lipid Mediat 73(3–4):249–264

116. Mukherjee D, Nissen SE, Topol EJ (2001) Risk of cardiovascular events associated with selective COX-2 inhibitors. JAMA 286(8):954–959

117. Robertson FM, Simeone AM, Mazumdar A, Shah AH et al (2008) Molecular and pharmacological blockade of the EP4 receptor selectively inhibits both proliferation and invasion of human inflammatory breast cancer cells. J Exp Ther Oncol 7(4):299–312

118. Xiao Y, Ye Y, Yearsley K, Jones S et al (2008) The lymphovascular embolus of inflammatory breast cancer expresses a stem cell-like phenotype. Am J Pathol 173(2):561–574. doi:10.2353/ajpath.2008.071214

119. Liu R, Wang X, Chen GY, Dalerba P et al (2007) The prognostic role of a gene signature from tumorigenic breast-cancer cells. N Engl J Med 356(3):217–226. doi:10.1056/NEJMoa063994

120. Van Laere S, Limame R, Van Marck EA, Vermeulen PB et al (2010) Is there a role for mammary stem cells in inflammatory breast carcinoma? A review of evidence from cell line, animal model, and human tissue sample experiments. Cancer 116(11 Suppl):2794–2805. doi:10.1002/cncr.25180

121. van Golen KL, Bao LW, Pan Q, Miller FR et al (2002) Mitogen activated protein kinase pathway is involved in RhoC GTPase induced motility, invasion and angiogenesis in inflammatory breast cancer. Clin Exp Metastasis 19(4):301–311

122. Kleer CG, Zhang Y, Pan Q, Merajver SD (2004) WISP3 (CCN6) is a secreted tumor-suppressor protein that modulates IGF signaling in inflammatory breast cancer. Neoplasia 6(2):179–185. doi:10.1593/neo.03316

123. Cabioglu N, Gong Y, Islam R, Broglio KR et al (2007) Expression of growth factor and chemokine receptors: new insights in the biology of inflammatory breast cancer. Ann Oncol 18(6):1021–1029. doi:10.1093/annonc/mdm060

124. Cox AD, Der CJ (1992) Protein prenylation: more than just glue? Curr Opin Cell Biol 4(6):1008–1016

125. Zhang FL, Casey PJ (1996) Protein prenylation: molecular mechanisms and functional consequences. Annu Rev Biochem 65:241–269. doi:10.1146/annurev.bi.65.070196.001325
126. Adamson P, Marshall CJ, Hall A, Tilbrook PA (1992) Post-translational modifications of p21rho proteins. J Biol Chem 267(28):20033–20038
127. Mazieres J, Tillement V, Allal C, Clanet C et al (2005) Geranylgeranylated, but not farnesylated, RhoB suppresses ras transformation of NIH-3T3 cells. Exp Cell Res 304(2):354–364. doi:10.1016/j.yexcr.2004.10.019
128. Lebowitz PF, Casey PJ, Prendergast GC, Thissen JA (1997) Farnesyltransferase inhibitors alter the prenylation and growth-stimulating function of RhoB. J Biol Chem 272(25):15591–15594
129. Du W, Lebowitz PF, Prendergast GC (1999) Cell growth inhibition by farnesyltransferase inhibitors is mediated by gain of geranylgeranylated RhoB. Mol Cell Biol 19(3):1831–1840
130. Du W, Prendergast GC (1999) Geranylgeranylated RhoB mediates suppression of human tumor cell growth by farnesyltransferase inhibitors. Cancer Res 59(21):5492–5496
131. van Golen KL, Bao L, DiVito MM, Wu Z et al (2002) Reversion of RhoC GTPase-induced inflammatory breast cancer phenotype by treatment with a farnesyl transferase inhibitor. Mol Cancer Ther 1(8):575–583
132. Van den Eynden GG, Van Laere SJ, Van der Auwera I, Merajver SD et al (2006) Overexpression of caveolin-1 and-2 in cell lines and in human samples of inflammatory breast cancer. Breast Cancer Res Treat 95(3):219–228. doi:10.1007/s10549-005-9002-1
133. Sloan EK, Stanley KL, Anderson RL (2004) Caveolin-1 inhibits breast cancer growth and metastasis. Oncogene 23(47):7893–7897. doi:10.1038/sj.onc.1208062
134. Williams TM, Lisanti MP (2004) The caveolin proteins. Genome Biol 5(3):214. doi:10.1186/gb-2004-5-3-214
135. Arboleda MJ, Lyons JF, Kabbinavar FF, Bray MR et al (2003) Overexpression of AKT2/protein kinase bbeta leads to up-regulation of beta1 integrins, increased invasion, and metastasis of human breast and ovarian cancer cells. Cancer Res 63(1):196–206
136. Cheng GZ, Chan J, Wang Q, Zhang W et al (2007) Twist transcriptionally up-regulates AKT2 in breast cancer cells leading to increased migration, invasion, and resistance to paclitaxel. Cancer Res 67(5):1979–1987. doi:10.1158/0008-5472.CAN-06-1479
137. Huang M, Duhadaway JB, Prendergast GC, Laury-Kleintop LD (2007) RhoB regulates PDGFR-beta trafficking and signaling in vascular smooth muscle cells. Arterioscler Thromb Vasc Biol 27(12):2597–2605. doi:10.1161/ATVBAHA.107.154211
138. Orsenigo M, Brich S, Riva C, Conca E et al (2010) Fluorescence in situ hybridization analysis and immunophenotyping of c-Kit/PDGFRA and bcl-2 expression in gastrointestinal stromal tumors. Anal Quant Cytol Histol 32(4):225–233
139. Clarke ID, Dirks PB (2003) A human brain tumor-derived PDGFR-alpha deletion mutant is transforming. Oncogene 22(5):722–733. doi:10.1038/sj.onc.1206160
140. Ganjoo KN, Patel S (2011) Current and emerging pharmacological treatments for gastrointestinal stromal tumour. Drugs 71(3):321–330. doi:10.2165/11585370-000000000-00000
141. Keating MT, Harryman CC, Williams LT (1989) Platelet-derived growth factor receptor inducibility is acquired immediately after translation and does not require glycosylation. J Biol Chem 264(16):9129–9132

Chapter 16
Inflammatory Mediators as Therapeutic Targets for Inflammatory Breast Cancer

Fredika M. Robertson, Khoi Chu, Rita Circo, Julia Wulfkuhle, Lance Liotta, Annie Z. Luo, Kimberly M. Boley, Erik M. Freiter, Hui Liu, Pijus K. Mandal, John S. McMurray, Massimo Cristofanilli, and Emanuel F. Petricoin

Abstract The molecular signature of inflammatory breast cancer (IBC) includes activation of target genes of the nuclear factor-kappa B (NF-κB) transcription factor. These NF-κB target genes are differentially activated in IBC tumors and primarily produce pro-inflammatory mediators such as the chemokine interleukin-8 (IL-8), the lipid mediator prostaglandin E2, the chemokine receptor CXCR4 and its ligand partner CXCL12, and the axis defined by IL-6/Janus kinases and signal transducer and activator of transcription 3 (STAT3). While these genes are known to regulate

F.M. Robertson, Ph.D. (✉)
The Department of Experimental Therapeutics and The Center for Targeted Therapy, Unit 1950,
The University of Texas MD Anderson Cancer Center, P.O. Box 301429,
South Campus Research Building 4, 3.1009, Houston, TX 77230-1429, USA

The Morgan Welch Inflammatory Breast Cancer Research Program,
The University of Texas MD Anderson Cancer Center, Houston, TX, USA
e-mail: frobertson@mdanderson.org

K. Chu, Ph.D. • A.Z. Luo, M.D. • K.M. Boley • E.M. Freiter, B.S. • H. Liu, Ph.D.
• P.K. Mandal, Ph.D. • J.S. McMurray, Ph.D.
The Department of Experimental Therapeutics and The Center for Targeted Therapy, Unit 1950,
The University of Texas MD Anderson Cancer Center, P.O. Box 301429,
South Campus Research Building 4, Houston, TX 77230-1429, USA

R. Circo, Ph.D.
Istituto Superiore di Sanità, Rome, Italy

The Center for Applied Proteomics and Molecular Medicine, George Mason University,
Manassas, VA, USA

J. Wulfkuhle, Ph.D. • L. Liotta, M.D., Ph.D. • E.F. Petricoin, Ph.D.
The Center for Applied Proteomics and Molecular Medicine, George Mason University,
Manassas, VA, USA

M. Cristofanilli
Department of Medical Oncology, Fox Chase Cancer Center,
Cottman Avenue, Room C315 333, Philadelphia, PA, USA

N.T. Ueno and M. Cristofanilli (eds.), *Inflammatory Breast Cancer: An Update*,
DOI 10.1007/978-94-007-3907-9_16, © Springer Science+Business Media B.V. 2012

innate immune responses, they also are critically important to survival of tumor cells and to metastatic progression. Ongoing research is defining the roles of these inflammatory mediators and associated signaling pathways in breast cancer, in general, and in IBC. Some of these studies have evaluated pharmacological and biological agents that effectively target these pro-inflammatory mediators and have led to development of new therapeutics that may effectively abrogate IBC growth and metastasis. In summary, this chapter reviews the inflammatory mediators that have been identified as part of the molecular fingerprint of IBC and describes new evidence for the potential for inhibitors of these mediators to target specific populations of cells within IBC tumors that contribute to tumor initiation and metastatic progression.

Keywords Inflammatory breast cancer • Cancer stem cells • Metastasis • NF-κB • Cox-2 • CXCR4 • Interleukin-8 • Interleukin-6 • JAK • STAT3

Abbreviations

bFGF	basic fibroblast growth factor
Cox-2	cyclooxygenase-2
CXCL	chemokine (C-X-C motif) ligand
CXCR	C-X-C chemokine receptor
EGFR	epidermal growth factor receptor
EP	prostanoid receptor
ER	estrogen receptor
GROα	growth-related oncogene alpha
IBC	inflammatory breast cancer
IL	interleukin
JAK	Janus kinase
MAPK	mitogen-activated protein kinase
NF-κB	nuclear factor kappa B
PGE_2	prostaglandin E_2
PI3K	phosphatidylinositol 3 kinase
RANKL	receptor activator of nuclear factor kappa B
sIL-6R	soluble interleukin-6 receptor
STAT3	signal transducers and activators of transcription 3
VEGF	vascular endothelial growth factor

16.1 Introduction

Inflammatory breast cancer (IBC) is not associated with a true inflammatory process, and patients with an IBC diagnosis have no fever, leukocytosis, or noticeable infiltration of inflammatory leukocytes or lymphocytes. Rather, as first described by

Haagensen [1], this lethal variant of locally advanced breast cancer was designated as "inflammatory" on the basis of specific characteristics including "rapid enlargement of the breast, induration with or without the presence of a breast mass, rapid development of erythema involving at least one third of the breast, diffuse swelling, redness of the skin and a characteristic orange-peel appearance of the skin of the breast, sometimes accompanied by tenderness and pain within the breast and axilla," which are the first signs of this type of breast cancer [2–4]. The changes in the skin overlying the involved breast, which develop with rapid onset, have been attributed primarily to blockage of lymphatic drainage due to invasion of tumor cell aggregates, defined as IBC tumor emboli [5]. Other factors that may be associated with the erythema and edema of the skin of IBC patients include production of inflammatory mediators that have been reported to be expressed abundantly in IBC tumors; these have recently become the focus of intense study because of their potential importance as therapeutic targets in the development of more effective treatments for IBC.

Investigators using molecular approaches to elucidate the genomic and proteomic changes in IBC reported that IBC tumors, as well as IBC cell lines and xenograft tissues from preclinical models of IBC, have increased expression of certain genes encoding inflammatory mediators, cytokines, and chemokines, with concomitant activation of signaling pathways and receptor tyrosine kinases that are involved in regulation of innate immune responses and play central roles in tumorigenesis and metastasis. As a starting point, we have defined the molecular fingerprint of genes that produce inflammatory mediators, receptors, and other relevant signaling pathways that have been reported to be differentially expressed in IBC (Fig. 16.1). This chapter reviews the published studies, explores newly emerging concepts about the role of these inflammatory signatures of IBC, and discusses their potential as therapeutic targets in the development of novel treatments for IBC.

16.2 NF-κB Target Genes as Therapeutic Targets in IBC

Although IBC tumors, like other breast tumors, have been categorized on the basis of hormone receptor and *Her-2* oncogene status [6], IBC differs from other breast cancers in important ways. Our understanding of the distinct biology of IBC comes in part from studies evaluating the molecular signature of IBC tumors. Studies using cDNA microarrays for genome-wide expression profiling, validated by quantitative polymerase chain reaction and immunochemistry, were the first to report that IBC tumors had differentially increased expression of nuclear factor-kappaB (NF-κB) target genes and upstream activators of the NF-κB signaling pathway [7, 8]. These same studies reported a negative association between estrogen receptor (ER) and activation of the NF-κB pathway, which was linked to overexpression of epidermal growth factor receptor (EGFR) and/or Her2 [8]. While NF-κB can regulate the expression of multiple genes involved in immune and inflammatory responses, inflammatory mediators can, in turn, induce activation of the NF-κB pathway, setting

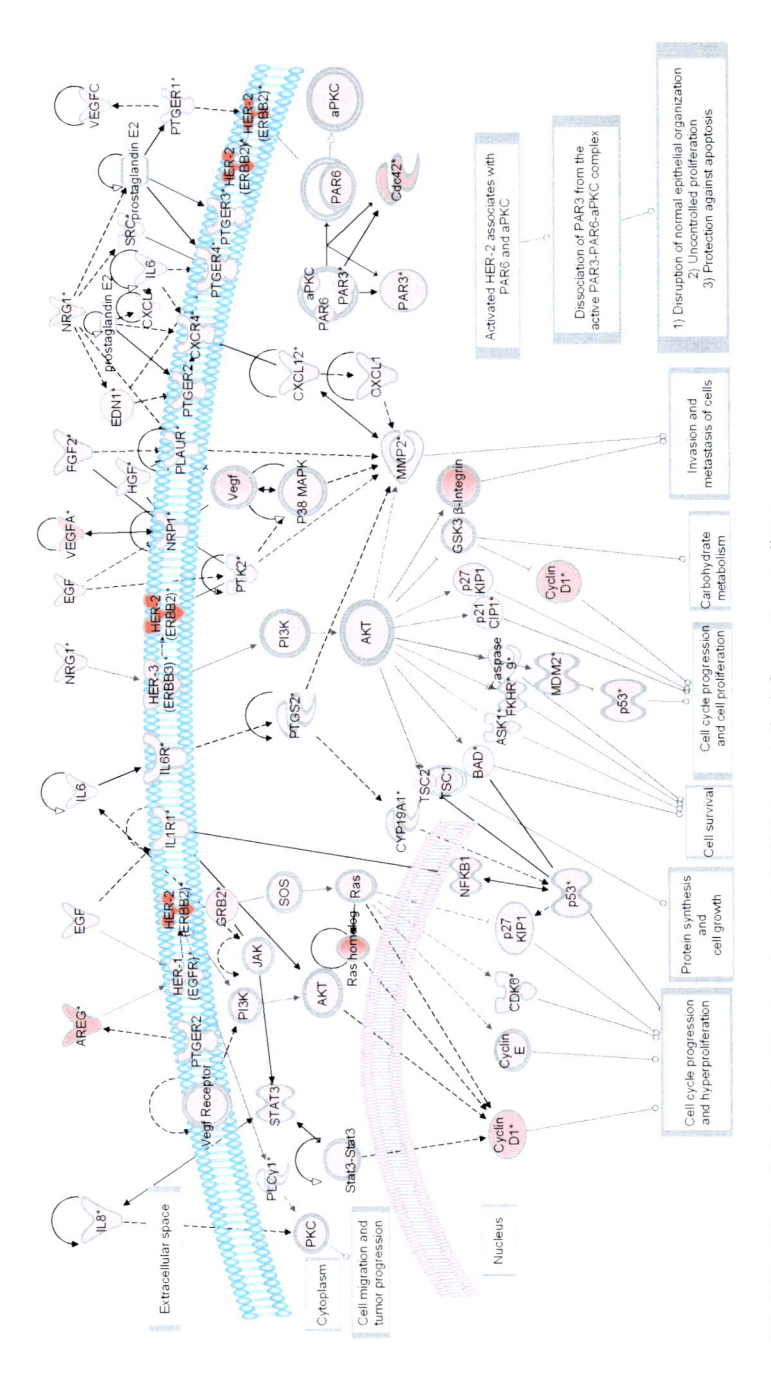

Fig. 16.1 Schematic illustration of activated genes in IBC that encode for inflammatory mediators

up a positive regulatory loop that perpetuates inflammatory responses [reviewed in 9]. These studies identified NF-κB target genes that were differentially upregulated in IBC tumors compared to non-IBC; these genes were categorized as NF-κB genes, immune response genes, inflammatory response genes, proliferation genes, chemotaxis and cell-matrix adhesion genes, tumor-promoting genes, or angiogenesis genes. Of these genes, only two, *PTGS2/COX2*, which encodes for the cyclooxygenase-2 (Cox-2) enzyme, and *CXCL1/GRO1*, which encodes for chemokine ligand 1 and the closely related chemokine and receptor pair, interleukin-8/C-X-C receptor 1 and 2 (IL-8/CXCR1/2), were found to be upregulated both in primary IBC tumors and in IBC metastases. Based on these studies, a five-gene molecular signature was developed that matched patient outcomes, and included *IL-8*, angiogenic growth factor vascular endothelial growth factor (*VEGF*), and three other genes unrelated to NF-κB. Taken together, these studies suggest that the NF-κB pathway contributes to the distinct phenotype and metastatic progression of IBC. These studies also suggested that NF-κB target genes encoding for inflammatory mediators and chemokines may be novel therapeutic targets for effective treatment of IBC.

The natural product curcumin (diferuloylmethane), a member of the ginger family, is a yellow substance from the root of the plant *Curcuma longa* Linn and is the principal component of the dietary spice turmeric [10]. It has been shown to inhibit NF-κB activation. Turmeric has historically been used as a component of Indian Ayurvedic medicine, and there is significant interest in this agent as a potential chemopreventive and as a therapeutic for a wide variety of illnesses associated with chronic inflammation. Curcumin not only downregulates gene targets of NF-κB, but also directly inhibits other genes and signaling pathways, including COX-2, signal transducer and activator of transcription 3 (STAT3), Akt, antiapoptotic proteins, growth factor receptors, and multidrug-resistance proteins. Clinical trials, primarily in precancerous lesions such as oral leukoplakia and intestinal metaplasia, have shown that curcumin has no toxicity, even at very high doses, and has clinically relevant activity as a chemopreventive agent with a demonstrated ability to prevent disease progression in early preneoplastic lesions [11]. The therapeutic efficacy of curcumin has been improved by liposomal nano-encapsulation technology, resulting in demonstration that curcumin sensitizes tumor cells to the effects of paclitaxel [12] and has enhanced activity in metastatic disease [13]. Numerous studies have reported that curcumin can act as a chemosensitizer and radiosensitizer for multiple organ types while protecting normal cells from the toxic effects of a wide variety of chemotherapies and radiation [10]. A phase II clinical trial now in progress at The University of Texas MD Anderson Cancer Center is evaluating the effects of curcumin in advanced pancreatic cancer [14]. To date, there have been no studies evaluating the effects of curcumin or curcumin analogs in preclinical models of IBC.

The proteosomal degradation inhibitor bortezomib (Velcade; Millenium Pharmaceuticals, Inc., and Johnson & Johnson Pharmaceutical Research & Development, LLC) has also been shown to inhibit NF-κB – mediated events. The effects of bortezomib as a single agent were evaluated in a phase II study in patients with metastatic breast cancer [15]. Although bortezomib effectively inhibited levels of circulating IL-6, no objective responses were observed in this study. These results suggest that future development of bortezomib for the treatment of metastatic breast cancer should be guided by studies using preclinical *in vivo* models that optimize the activity of bortezomib in combination with other antitumor agents.

Another agent shown to suppress the NF-κB signaling cascade is the copper chelator tetrathiomolybdate, which has been shown to effectively inhibit angiogenesis and metastasis in the SUM149 preclinical model of IBC [16, 17]. Interestingly, the inhibition of NF-κB transcriptional activity by this agent was associated with decreased production of IL-8, IL-6, VEGF, basic fibroblast growth factor (bFGF), and IL-1α and was shown to inhibit motility and invasion of SUM149 IBC tumor cells. Studies in the SUM149 IBC xenograft model demonstrated that tetrathiomolybdate significantly inhibited increases in tumor volume and had antiangiogenic activity as illustrated by significantly decreased CD-31 staining and associated loss of mean vessel density [17].

New approaches such as high-throughput screening will likely identify a number of novel agents that inhibit the NF-κB signaling that is a prominent feature of IBC. A recent study screened a chemical library of 2,800 known small molecule inhibitors and identified 19 agents that potently inhibit NF-κB signaling [18]. The agents identified by this study are being evaluated in preclinical models of IBC for their ability to inhibit NF-κB activation as well as proliferation and invasion of IBC tumor cells.

A number of other agents that have been identified as inhibitors of NF-κB may undergo evaluation for their ability to inhibit the aggressive phenotype of IBC. Compounds that have been reported to inhibit NF-κB include parthenolide, pyrrolidinedithiocarbamate, and its analog diethyldithiocarbamate [19]. Interestingly, these agents have been reported to inhibit proliferation and colony formation of breast cancer cell lines that have characteristics of cancer stem cells. *In vivo* studies demonstrate that pyrrolidinedithiocarbamate, when combined with paclitaxel, effectively inhibits breast tumor xenograft growth *in vivo*. Taken together, these findings suggest that NF-κB signaling plays a role in survival of breast cancer stem cells and that inhibitors of NF-κB have potential utility in targeting this subpopulation of cells, which are believed to be responsible for tumor initiation and metastasis. Together with reports that IBC and preclinical models of IBC are enriched in cells with a cancer stem cell phenotype that are resistant to chemotherapy [20–23], these observations suggest that agents that block NF-κB activation may be especially potent inhibitors of IBC tumor progression.

A newly identified protease inhibitor, nafamostat mesilate, has been reported to effectively inhibit downstream target genes of NF-κB, including *IL-8* and *VEGF*, resulting in inhibition of cell adhesion, angiogenesis, invasion, and metastasis [24]. Initial studies evaluating nafamostat mesilate were performed in a preclinical model of pancreatic cancer, and its use was associated with prolonged survival in a preclinical model of peritoneal metastasis. Nafamostat mesilate is now available commercially and is a candidate for evaluation as a therapy for IBC.

Overall, these studies demonstrate that the molecular signature of IBC includes activation of NF-κB target genes and that agents that target NF-κB signaling pathways may represent advances in treatment strategies for IBC. Further investigation of these agents in IBC is particularly important in light of reports that NF-κB is involved in conferring resistance to chemotherapy [25–27] and that NF-κB inhibitors target specific subpopulations of breast cancer cells that exhibit cancer stem cell characteristics [19, 28].

16.3 Multiple Roles of Interleukin-8 in IBC

The studies that defined the molecular signature of IBC identified *IL-8/CXCL1/2* as an NF-κB target gene that was differentially expressed in IBC tumors [7, 8]. IL-8 was initially identified as a potent chemokine that recruits and activates immune and inflammatory cells. It has a role in both innate immune and inflammatory responses as well as in the pathophysiological processes associated with chronic inflammation [29]. IL-8 has been shown to be a key effector in breast tumor cell invasion, tumor-associated angiogenesis, and tumor progression, and was found to be overexpressed in metastatic breast cancer lesions [30–33]. The production of IL-8 was inversely correlated with ER status, and its presence was also associated with shorter relapse-free survival in patients with ER-positive breast cancers treated with tamoxifen [32–34].

Other roles for IL-8 are suggested by recent evidence that IL-8 regulates, at least in part, the survival of breast cancer stem cells [20]. This may be of importance since IBC tumors as well as the Mary-X preclinical model of IBC, which recapitulates the human disease; and the SUM149 IBC cell line have all been shown to be enriched for populations of cells with characteristics of tumor-initiating cells or cancer stem cells, including surface expression of CD44$^+$/CD24$^{low/-}$ and production of the aldehyde dehydrogenase enzyme, as assessed by the ALDEFLUOR assay [21–23]. IL-8 was also demonstrated to support mammosphere formation by breast cancer cells *in vitro* under non-adherent culture conditions and to increase the number of putative cancer stem cells, based on detection of increased numbers of ALDEFLUOR-positive cells [20]. Mammospheres serve as *in vitro* surrogates for IBC tumor emboli, the metastatic lesion of IBC, and we, and others, have used mammospheres to determine the response of IBC cells to specific therapeutic agents and to evaluate the effects of manipulation of genes potentially important in IBC [35–38].

Although IL-8 is of interest for its role in IBC, its importance as a therapeutic target remains to be determined because of the lack of potent agents that inhibit IL-8 as their primary mechanism of action, with the exception of anti-IL-8 antibodies. A few IL-8 inhibitors have recently emerged and must be evaluated for their activity in preclinical models of IBC before advancing to clinical trial. A recent study identified pigment epithelium-derived factor as a suppressor of IL-8 through its ability to upregulate peroxisome proliferator-activated receptor–gamma and to suppress NF-κB – mediated transcriptional activation, ultimately resulting in inhibition of proliferation of prostate cancer cells [39]. Other recent studies reported that small molecular inhibitors of the oncogene *cMet* effectively inhibited IL-8, growth-regulated oncogene alpha (GROα) and urokinase plasminogen activator receptor [40]. Because of their inhibitory activity, small molecular inhibitors of cMET may be of interest for their potential to induce apoptosis in populations of cells that exhibit stem cell characteristics in preclinical models of IBC.

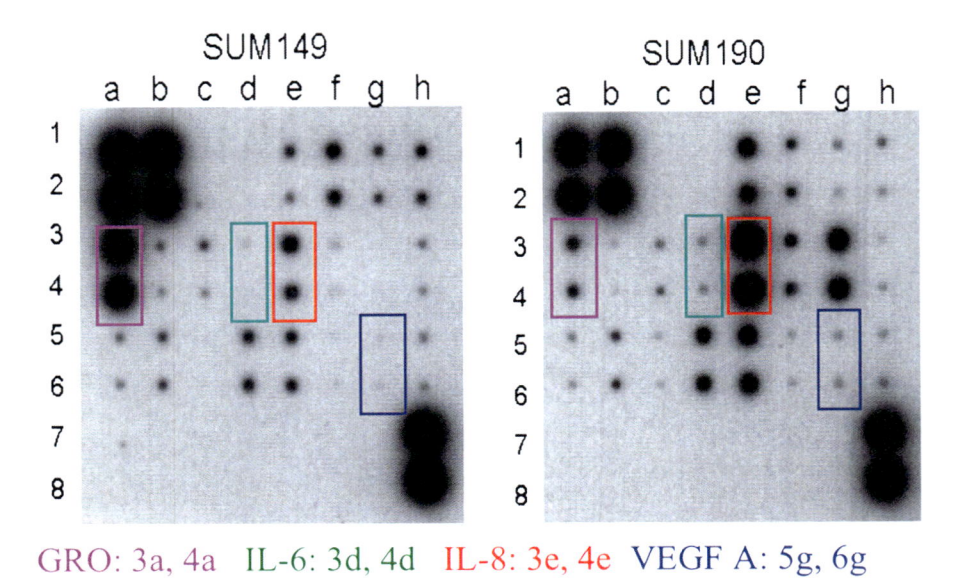

Fig. 16.2 Protein array analysis of proteins secreted by IBC cell lines SUM149 and SUM190 reveals the comparative levels of production of IL-8, GROα, IL-6, and VEGF

Our studies have demonstrated that the IBC cell lines SUM149 and SUM190 produce high levels of secreted IL-8 as well as GROα, suggesting that studies evaluating the effects of inhibition of IL-8 in models of IBC may shed light on the specific functions of IL-8 in mediating growth, invasion, and metastasis of IBC (Fig. 16.2).

Taken together, the findings of the studies described here suggest that IL-8 has multiple roles in tumor development and disease progression, including a newly identified role in survival of cancer stem cells. Historically, few effective IL-8 inhibitors were available, but several agents have now been identified that target the multiple and complex roles of IL-8 in the angiogenesis and metastasis of IBC tumors. Potentially, inhibitors of IL-8 may effectively target the important populations of cancer stem cells, providing very useful therapeutic approaches for IBC as well as other tumor types that are highly enriched in cancer stem cells.

16.4 Cyclooxygenase-2, Prostaglandin E$_2$, and the Prostaglandin Receptors as Therapeutic Targets in IBC

Studies that initially defined the molecular signature of IBC identified *PTGS2/COX2* as a critical gene in IBC that was differentially upregulated in IBC compared to non-IBC tumors (Fig. 16.1) [7, 8, 41]. Since *COX-2* and its primary product, prostaglandin E$_2$ (PGE$_2$), as well as the PGE$_2$ receptors EP1, EP2, EP3, and EP4, encoded for by the *PTGER 1, 2, 3, and 4* genes (Fig. 16.1), have been reported to be involved in regulating breast tumor proliferation, invasion, angiogenesis, metastasis, and colonization at distinct organ sites, *COX-2* is a key component of the molecular signature of IBC. Furthermore, Cox-2, PGE$_2$, and the associated EP receptors are attractive therapeutic targets for inhibiting these activities of IBC tumors. This section provides a general overview of the biology of Cox-2, PGE$_2$, and the EP receptors and reviews the known and newly emerging agents that target this inflammatory mediator and associated receptors. This section also reviews ongoing evaluations of these agents' activities in breast cancer metastasis and outlines the studies in IBC.

The cyclooxygenase (Cox) enzymes, also known as prostaglandin H synthases, catalyze the rate-limiting step in the formation of inflammatory prostaglandins [42, 43]. Cox-1 is constitutively produced, and PGE$_2$, derived from this enzyme, is associated with survival of crypt stem cells in the gastrointestinal tract [44]. *Cox-2* is an inducible immediate early gene primarily responsible for production of PGE$_2$. Since *Cox-2* was first cloned and sequenced in 1992 [45], numerous studies have documented the association between elevated expression of this gene and proliferation, invasion, angiogenesis, and metastasis in human tumors from different organ sites, including breast cancer, and the potential of Cox-2 as a therapeutic target [46, 47]. Our studies were the first to report that *Cox-2* mRNA and protein are elevated in invasive breast cancer regardless of hormone receptor status or *Her-2/neu* status [48], a finding subsequently confirmed by other investigators [49, 50]. Additional studies from our laboratory demonstrated that Cox-2 directly regulates the activity of the CYP19 1A1 enzyme aromatase, which is responsible for biotransformation of androgens to produce estrogens, through switching in usage of specific promoter regions [51–53]. Interestingly, the direct regulation of the aromatase enzyme by Cox-2 has also been shown to link interactions with both the *Her-2/neu* oncogene and *EGFR*. These studies suggested that Cox-2 inhibitors could be effectively combined with aromatase inhibitors, which has been demonstrated to be the case [53, 54].

While selective Cox-2 inhibitors, such as celecoxib (Celebrex, Pfizer, Inc), showed great promise as inhibitors of tumor growth and angiogenesis [55, 56], their use has been limited because of their unacceptably high rate of cardiovascular side effects [57, 58]. The selective Cox-2 inhibitor rofexocib (Vioxx, Merck, Inc) was removed from the U.S. market on September 30, 2004, and a black box warning issued for celecoxib. Following disclosure of the cardiovascular risks associated with rofexocib, interest turned from development of selective Cox-2 inhibitors to evaluation of the effects of antagonists and agonists of the EP receptors, which differentially regulate the cellular responses following binding of PGE$_2$ to one or more of four prostanoid receptors [59].

EP1, EP2, EP3, and EP4, members of the superfamily of G-protein – coupled receptors, are the receptors for the PGE$_2$ ligand [60]. One study in a mammary carcinoma model of metastasis reported that EP4 antagonists AH23848 or ONO-AE3-208 significantly inhibited pulmonary metastasis [61], suggesting that the EP4 receptor is involved in mediating functions of mammary tumor cells associated with invasion and metastasis. Our studies identified EP4 as the primary EP receptor involved in mediating these activities in IBC tumor cells [62, 63], with a role for EP3 in suppressing vasculogenic mimicry and vasculogenesis, which are predominant features of the distinct signature of angiogenesis exhibited by IBC tumors [62]. Our studies also demonstrated that inhibition of EP4, either by knockdown of *EP4* or by administration of EP4 antagonist GW627368, effectively blocked invasion by IBC tumor cells [63]. While these studies indicate that EP4 antagonists may have therapeutic activity in IBC, no suitable EP4 antagonist is available for a clinical trial.

In the search for alternative Cox-2 – targeted compounds to evaluate for their potential effect in IBC, our recent studies have identified an interesting compound, tranilast (N-[3,4-dimethoxycinnamonyl]-anthranilic acid; SB 252218; Rizaben, Kissei Pharmaceutical Co, Ltd), an orally active agent used clinically as an antiallergy and antifibrotic agent that potently inhibits production of PGE_2 ($IC_{50} = \sim 1-20\,\mu M$) and pro-inflammatory cytokines [64, 65]. Tranilast was shown to inhibit proliferation and migration/invasion of both mouse mammary tumor cells and triple-negative human breast tumor cells [66–68]. While tranilast inhibited the growth of mouse mammary carcinoma cells by as much as 50%, it significantly (>90%) inhibited both pulmonary and liver metastasis *in vivo* [66]. Interestingly, a recent study demonstrated that tranilast effectively blocks colony-forming efficiency and mammosphere formation by triple-negative human breast cancer cells that exhibit a cancer stem cell phenotype [69]. These studies reported that tranilast has a unique mechanism of action as an agonist for the aryl hydrocarbon hydroxylase receptor, AHR, which is a member of the basic helix-loop-helix/Per-Arnt-Sim family of transcription factors. Other studies have reported that tranilast inhibits IL-8 [70] and has antiangiogenic properties [71–73]. Taken together, these findings suggest that tranilast should be evaluated for its ability to block the invasive and metastatic activities of IBC tumors, which have been reported to be enriched in cancer stem cells [24, 25].

In addition to tranilast, we have identified a new selective coxib analog, apricoxib (Capoxigem; Tragara Pharmaceuticals, Inc.), currently being evaluated in clinical trials for non-small cell lung cancer and metastatic pancreatic carcinoma [74, 75]. When used in combination with other chemotherapeutic agents such as erlotinib, gemcitabine, or 5-fluorouracil, apricoxib has demonstrated synergistic antitumor activities [76, 77]. The findings thus far suggest that apricoxib may have antitumor, antiangiogenic, and antimetastatic activities in IBC.

Despite the initial enthusiasm for the potential anticancer activities of selective Cox-2 inhibitors, loss of the coxibs from widespread clinical use dampened enthusiasm for Cox-2 and PGE_2 as therapeutic targets. With agents such as tranilast and apricoxib emerging from pharmaceutical development, there is increased interest in exploring their effects on the Cox-2 – mediated events that regulate the aggressive phenotype exhibited in IBC tumors.

16.5   The CXCR4/CXCL12 Axis in IBC

Although breast tumor cells are known to preferentially "home" to specific organ sites such as bone, the mechanisms that regulate the interactions between tumor cells and the organ microenvironment that are critical to organ-specific metastasis are only now being elucidated. Once the ligands and receptors that mediate organ-specific metastasis are identified, these molecules and the signaling pathways they activate will be important targets for development of effective antimetastasis therapeutics. This is especially critical in IBC, which is characterized by very rapid disease progression with metastasis to bone as well as other organ sites [3]. One receptor that has been identified as being highly expressed in IBC is the seven-transmembrane G-protein – coupled C-X-C chemokine receptor type 4 (CXCR4; CD184) [78]. The ligand for CXCR4 is the C-X-C motif chemokine 12 (CXCL12), also known as stromal cell – derived factor-1 alpha, which is involved in tumor-stroma crosstalk that mediates interactions between the tumor and microenvironment that are critical to metastatic progression. As an example, CXCL12, produced by bone-forming osteoblasts, regulates survival and recruitment to the bone of CXCR4-expressing breast cancer cells [79]. Once breast tumor cells are recruited to the bone, they modify the functions of both the osteoblasts and the bone-resorbing osteoclasts, resulting in skeletal complications such as pathological fractures and pain that commonly occur in breast cancer patients with bone metastases. In addition to a demonstrated role in mediating bone metastasis in breast cancer in general and in IBC specifically [78], the CXCR4/CXCL12 axis has multiple other roles, including stimulation of a positive autocrine loop with VEGF during neoangiogenesis [80] and transactivation of both the *Her2/neu* oncogene and *EGFR* [81].

The CXCR4/CXCL12 receptor-ligand pair has been demonstrated to regulate survival of cells with a cancer stem cell phenotype, to recruit stromal cells that support metastasis, and to promote angiogenesis through both autocrine and paracrine mechanisms [82]. As an example, CXCL12 is stimulated by activation of hypoxia-inducible factor-1 following radiation treatment. It activates the CXCR4 receptor present on bone marrow cells, which are then recruited to form new blood vessels [83]. Taken together, these functions suggest that CXCR4 antagonists and/or antagonists of the signaling pathways activated by the CXCR4/CXCL12 axis are potential therapeutic targets that would be important to evaluate for their ability to inhibit the metastasis of IBC to specific organ sites such as bone and to inhibit tumor-associated angiogenesis and neoangiogenesis that occur following radiation therapy.

On the basis of the observations suggesting that CXCR4 could be an important therapeutic target in IBC, the effects of a combination of CTCE 9908, a peptide-based antagonist of CXCR4, and paclitaxel on primary tumor growth and development of visceral and skeletal metastasis were evaluated in the SUM149 preclinical model of triple-negative IBC [84]. While CTCE 9908, either alone or in combination with paclitaxel, did not effectively inhibit either primary tumor growth or pulmonary metastasis as compared to control groups, single-agent CTCE-9908 significantly inhibited skeletal metastases. In a preclinical model of triple-negative non-IBC breast cancer that used both parental MDA-MB-231 cells and clones selected for their propensity to develop skeletal metastasis, the CXCR4 peptide antagonist inhibited both primary tumor growth and development of skeletal metastasis by the "bone seeking" clones [85]. Interestingly, the disparity between the results of these two studies suggests that the role of CXCR4/CXCL12 in tumorigenesis and metastasis of IBC is significantly different than that in non-IBC metastasis. These findings suggest, moreover, that agents identified as having antitumor and/or antimetastatic efficacy in preclinical models of non-IBC breast cancer cannot necessarily be assumed to have similar activity in primary or metastatic IBC. These studies also suggest the importance of evaluating the specific underlying mechanisms by which CXCR4 antagonists block metastatic progression of IBC to the bone.

Collectively, these studies demonstrate the potential importance of continued evaluation of the role of CXCR4/CXCL12 in organ-specific metastasis exhibited by IBC and of the multiple new CXCR4/CXCL12 antagonists that are showing promise as inhibitors of disease progression.

16.6 Interleukin-6 and JAK/STAT3 Pathway Activation as Therapeutic Targets in IBC

Levels of inflammatory cytokine IL-6 have been shown to be elevated in the serum of breast cancer patients, and this elevation is associated with advanced tumor stage, greater numbers of metastatic sites, and poor prognosis [86–88]. Levels of both IL-6 and IL-8 have been reported to be elevated in the SUM149 preclinical model of IBC, and this elevation was shown to be directly regulated by *RhoC* GTPase, one of only a few genes identified as having a regulatory role in the angiogenic and invasive phenotype of IBC [89]. Interestingly, recent evidence demonstrates that IL-6 is a central regulator of survival of cells with a cancer stem cell phenotype [90–92], suggesting that IL-6 may be an important therapeutic target in IBC, which has been reported to be enriched in cancer stem cells.

The IL-6 (or gp130) family of cytokines activates multiple downstream effectors that collectively regulate proliferation and survival/resistance to apoptosis, and are involved in invasion and metastasis [93, 94]. IL-6 production is stimulated by PGE_2 synthesized by Cox-2, which has been demonstrated to be upregulated in IBC [7, 8, 41, 63, 64], by transforming growth factor – beta, or by IL-1. IL-6 activates downstream effectors using both canonical and noncanonical signaling pathways. In the canonical pathway, the IL-6 ligand binds to the membrane-bound IL-6 receptor, forming a heterotrimer with gp130, resulting in activation of Janus kinases (JAK), with subsequent recruitment and phosphorylation of transcription factors within the STAT3 protein family. Activation of STAT3 in a JAK-dependent fashion leads to increased expression of receptor activator of nuclear factor-κB ligand. IL-6 also activates AKT through JAK-dependent stimulation of the phosphatidylinositol 3-kinase (PI3K) pathway. Simultaneously, mitogen-activated protein kinase (MAPK) is stimulated following JAK activation by IL-6. There is also a trans-IL-6 signaling pathway, in which IL-6 binds to a truncated soluble IL-6 receptor, forming an IL-6/sIL-6R complex. This complex binds to membrane-bound gp130 dimers, forming IL-6 trans-signaling complexes, which then activate the JAK/STAT3, PI3K/Akt, and MAPK signaling pathways [92, 93].

Strategies to block the effects of IL-6 in tumorigenesis and metastasis have targeted both the IL-6–receptor interaction as well as the JAK/STAT3 pathway.

This section reviews the current status of the various therapeutic agents that target IL-6/JAK/STAT3 signaling pathways and are being generally evaluated in solid tumors and hematologic malignancies and specifically in IBC.

One biological agent that has been developed to selectively target IL-6 and the interactions of the ligand/receptor pairs is a monoclonal antibody directed against IL-6, siltuximab (CNTO 328) [95–97]. The results of clinical trials of siltuximab in metastatic renal cell cancer [98, 99], castration-resistant prostate cancer [100], and Castelman's disease, an atypical lymphoproliferative disorder [101], have recently been reported. Overall, siltuximab has been well tolerated, with no maximum tolerated dose or immune response observed, and is showing promise for treatment of renal cell cancer and Castelman's disease [98, 99, 101]; however, siltuximab failed to block serum IL-6 levels in castration-resistant prostate cancer, with continued high serum levels of IL-6 associated with a poor prognosis [100]. Based on the production of IL-6 by IBC tumor cells [89] as well as the association between IL-6 signaling activation and cancer stem cells [90–92], studies are currently underway to evaluate the effectiveness of siltuximab in preclinical models of IBC as a prelude to potential clinical trials in IBC patients.

Due to the central role of the JAK/STAT3 signaling pathway in regulating the activities of inflammatory cytokines such as IL-6 [92, 93], there has been significant effort by both academic laboratories and pharmaceutical companies to develop inhibitors of phospho-Stat3 activation as well as inhibitors of the JAK kinase enzymes. Interestingly, recent reports suggest that the JAK2/STAT3 signaling pathway is required for growth and survival of tumor cells that express $CD44^+/CD24^{-/low}$ and have a cancer stem cell phenotype [102], indicating that targeting this pathway may be an effective means of eliminating these tumor-initiating populations of cells.

Using reverse-phase microarray-based proteomics approaches [103–105], our studies mapped the signaling pathways activated in preclinical models of IBC. We found that a number of biochemically linked signaling proteins within the JAK/STAT signaling pathway, including JAK1, STAT3, PDK1, and AKT, are activated (e.g., phosphorylated) in IBC cell lines compared to non-IBC cell lines (Fig. 16.3). From a panel of newly developed novel STAT3-targeted peptidomimetics [106], we found that the lead compound, designated PM-73G, inhibited phospho-STAT3, and this inhibition was associated with blockade of the robust invasion, anchorage-independent growth in soft agar, and vasculogenic mimicry exhibited by IBC tumor cells without a significant antiproliferative effect [107]. Taken together, these findings suggest that STAT3 serves both as a molecular signature and as a potential target for new, more effective therapeutics for IBC. Recent evidence also demonstrates that a novel JAK2 inhibitor, LY2784544, effectively inhibited STAT3 activation in a dose-dependent manner and that this blockade induced cell death in SUM149 IBC tumor spheres [108].

These studies indicate that preclinical models of IBC are characterized by activation of the IL-6/JAK/STAT3 axis. Given the studies demonstrating that IBC is enriched with cancer stem cells that are responsible for tumor initiation and disease progression [21–23], combined with the emerging evidence for the role of the IL-6/JAK/STAT3 axis in supporting cancer stem cell development and survival [90–92, 102],

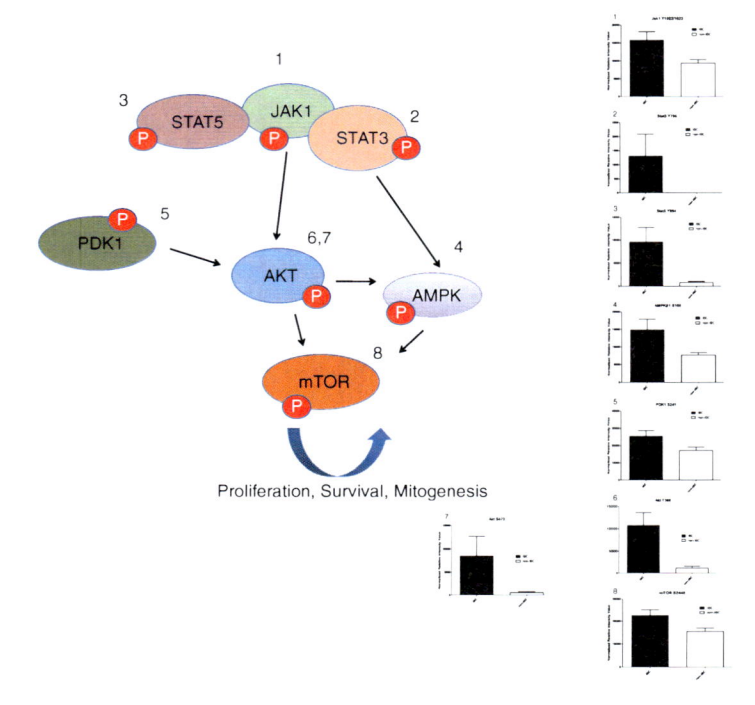

Fig. 16.3 Reverse-phase microarray analysis demonstrates that specific signal transduction pathways are activated in IBC, including the JAK/STAT3 and P13K/pathways. For each histogram, reverse phase microarray analysis was used to generate relative intensity values for IBC tumor cells, shown by black bars (*left*) compared with non-IBC tumor cells by white bars (*right*) which are shown with error bars are shown

it appears that studies using preclinical models of IBC to evaluate therapeutics that target these signaling pathways to block IBC metastasis are warranted.

16.7 Summary

The molecular signature of IBC includes pro-inflammatory mediators that regulate the characteristic rapid growth and accelerated metastasis observed in IBC. Progress in identifying and evaluating therapeutics that selectively target these pro-inflammatory mediators and the associated receptors and signal transduction pathways that are activated in IBC has been slow over the past 15 years. The improved molecular platforms, new models of IBC combined with new approaches that allow us to refine our understanding of the molecular fingerprint of IBC and to carefully map the signaling pathways that are differentially activated in IBC offer multiple new opportunities to accelerate the development of effective treatment strategies to impact the overall survival of patients with an IBC diagnosis.

Acknowledgments Supported by the American Airlines-Komen For the Cure Foundation Promise Grant KGO81287 (FMR, MC) and The State of Texas Fund for Rare and Aggressive Breast Tumors (FMR). The authors appreciate the generous support of Dr. Vikas Chandhoke and the College of Life Sciences at George Mason University. This work was partially supported by the Italian Istituto Superiore di Sanità within the framework Italy/USA cooperation agreement between the U.S. Department of Health and Human Services, George Mason University, and the Italian Ministry of Public Health.

References

1. Haagansen CD (1973) Inflammatory carcinoma. In: Haagensen CD (ed) Diseases of the breast, 2nd edn. Saunders, Philadelphia
2. Resetkova E (2008) Pathologic aspects of inflammatory breast carcinoma: part 1. Histomorphology and differential diagnosis. Semin Oncol 35(1):25–32
3. Robertson FM, Bondy M, Yang W, Yamauchi H, Wiggins S, Kamrudin S, Krishnamurthy S, Le-Petross H, Bidaut L, Player AN, Barsky SH, Woodward WA, Buchholz T, Lucci A, Ueno Naoto T, Cristofanilli M (2010) Inflammatory breast cancer: the disease, the biology, the treatment. CA Cancer J Clin 60(6):351–375
4. Singletary SE, Cristofanilli M (2008) Defining the clinical diagnosis of inflammatory breast cancer. Semin Oncol 35(1):7–10
5. Vermeulen PB, van Golen KL, Dirix LY (2010) Angiogenesis, lymphangiogenesis, growth pattern, and tumor emboli in inflammatory breast cancer: a review of the current knowledge. Cancer 116(11 Suppl):2748–2754
6. Bertucci F, Finetti P, Rougemont J, Charafe-Jauffret E, Cervera N, Tarpin C, Nguyen C, Xerri L, Houlgatte R, Jacquemier J, Viens P, Birnbaum D (2005) Gene expression profiling identifies molecular subtypes of inflammatory breast cancer. Cancer Res 65(6): 2170–2178
7. Van Laere SJ, Van der Auwera I, Van den Eynden GG et al (2005) Distinct molecular signature of inflammatory breast cancer by cDNA microarray analysis. Breast Cancer ResTreat 3:237–246
8. Van Laere SJ, Van der Auwera I, Van den Eynden GG, van Dam P, Van Marck EA, Vermeulen PB, Dirix LY (2007) NF-kappaB activation in inflammatory breast cancer is associated with oestrogen receptor downregulation, secondary to EGFR and/or ErbB2 overexpression and MAPK hyperactivation. Br J Cancer 97(5):659–669
9. Barnes PJ, Karin M (1997) Nuclear factor-kappaB: a pivotal transcription factor in chronic inflammatory diseases. N Engl J Med 336(15):1066–1071
10. Goel A, Aggarwal BB (2010) Curcumin, the golden spice from Indian saffron, is a chemosensitizer and radiosensitizer for tumors and chemoprotector and radioprotector for normal organs. Nutr Cancer 62(7):919–930
11. Cheng AL, Hsu CH, Lin JK, Hsu MM, Ho YF, Shen TS, Ko JY, Lin JT, Lin BR, Ming-Shiang W, Yu HS, Jee SH, Chen GS, Chen TM, Chen CA, Lai MK, Pu YS, Pan MH, Wang YJ, Tsai CC, Hsieh CY (2001) Phase I clinical trial of curcumin, a chemopreventive agent, in patients with high-risk or pre-malignant lesions. Anticancer Res 21(4B):2895–2900
12. Yallapu MM, Gupta BK, Jaggi M, Chauhan SC (2010) Fabrication of curcumin encapsulated PLGA nanoparticles for improved therapeutic effects in metastatic cancer cells. J Colloid Interface Sci 351(1):19–29
13. Sreekanth CN, Bava SV, Sreekumar E, Anto RJ (2011) Molecular evidences for the chemosensitizing efficacy of liposomal curcumin in paclitaxel chemotherapy in mouse models of cervical cancer. Oncogene 30(28):3139–3152. doi: 10.1038/onc.2011.23. Epub 2011 Feb 14.
14. National Institutes of Health. Trial of curcumin in advanced pancreatic cancer. ClinicalTrials. gov. http://clinicaltrials.gov/ct2/show/NCT00094445. Accessed Dec 15, 2011

15. Yang CH, Gonzalez-Angulo AM, Reuben JM, Booser DJ, Pusztai L, Krishnamurthy S, Esseltine D, Stec J, Broglio KR, Islam R, Hortobagyi GN, Cristofanilli M (2006) Bortezomib (VELCADE) in metastatic breast cancer: pharmacodynamics, biological effects, and prediction of clinical benefits. Ann Oncol 17(5):813–817
16. Pan Q, Bao LW, Merajver SD (2003) Tetrathiomolybdate inhibits angiogenesis and metastasis through suppression of the NFkappaB signaling cascade. Mol Cancer Res 1(10):701–706
17. Pan Q, Kleer CG, van Golen KL, Irani J, Bottema KM, Bias C, De Carvalho M, Mesri EA, Robins DM, Dick RD, Brewer GJ, Merajver SD (2002) Copper deficiency induced by tetrathiomolybdate suppresses tumor growth and angiogenesis. Cancer Res 62(17):4854–4859
18. Miller SC, Huang R, Sakamuru S, Shukla SJ, Attene-Ramos MS, Shinn P, Van Leer D, Leister W, Austin CP, Xia M (2010) Identification of known drugs that act as inhibitors of NF-kappaB signaling and their mechanism of action. Biochem Pharmacol 79(9):1272–1280
19. Zhou J, Zhang H, Gu P, Bai J, Margolick JB, Zhang Y (2008) NF-kappaB pathway inhibitors preferentially inhibit breast cancer stem-like cells. Breast Cancer Res Treat 111(3):419–427
20. Charafe-Jauffret E, Ginestier C, Iovino F, Wicinski J, Cervera N, Finetti P, Hur MH, Diebel ME, Monville F, Dutcher J, Brown M, Viens P, Xerri L, Bertucci F, Stassi G, Dontu G, Birnbaum D, Wicha MS (2009) Breast cancer cell lines contain functional cancer stem cells with metastatic capacity and a distinct molecular signature. Cancer Res 69(4):1302–1313
21. Charafe-Jauffret E, Ginestier C, Iovino F, Tarpin C, Diebel M, Esterni B, Houvenaeghel G, Extra JM, Bertucci F, Jacquemier J, Xerri L, Dontu G, Stassi G, Xiao Y, Barsky SH, Birnbaum D, Viens P, Wicha MS (2010) Aldehyde dehydrogenase 1-positive cancer stem cells mediate metastasis and poor clinical outcome in inflammatory breast cancer. Clin Cancer Res 16(1):45–55
22. Fillmore CM, Kuperwasser C (2008) Human breast cancer cell lines contain stem-like cells that self-renew, give rise to phenotypically diverse progeny and survive chemotherapy. Breast Cancer Res 10(2):R25
23. Xiao Y, Ye Y, Yearsley K, Jones S, Barsky SH (2008) The lymphovascular embolus of inflammatory breast cancer expresses a stem cell-like phenotype. Am J Pathol 173(2):561–574
24. Fujiwara Y, Furukawa K, Haruki K, Shimada Y, Iida T, Shiba H, Uwagawa T, Ohashi T, Yanaga K (2011) Nafamostat mesilate can prevent adhesion, invasion and peritoneal dissemination of pancreatic cancer thorough nuclear factor kappa-B inhibition. J Hepatobiliary Pancreat Sci 18(5):731–739
25. Wang CY, Cusack JC Jr, Liu R, Baldwin AS Jr (1999) Control of inducible chemoresistance: enhanced anti-tumor therapy through increased apoptosis by inhibition of NF-KB. Nat Med 5:412–417
26. Wang CY, Mayo MW, Baldwin AS Jr (1996) TNF- and cancer therapy-induced apoptosis: potentiation by inhibition of NF-KB. Science (Wash DC) 274:784–787
27. Arlt A, Schäfer H (2002) NFkappaB-dependent chemoresistance in solid tumors. Int J Clin Pharmacol Ther 40(8):336–347
28. Liu M, Sakamaki T, Casimiro MC, Willmarth NE, Quong AA, Ju X, Ojeifo J, Jiao X, Yeow WS, Katiyar S, Shirley LA, Joyce D, Lisanti MP, Albanese C, Pestell RG (2010) The canonical NF-kappaB pathway governs mammary tumorigenesis in transgenic mice and tumor stem cell expansion. Cancer Res 70(24):10464–10473
29. Moser B, Wolf M, Walz A, Loetscher P (2004) Chemokines: multiple levels of leukocyte migration control. Trends Immunol 25(2):75–84
30. Bièche I, Chavey C, Andrieu C, Busson M, Vacher S, Le Corre L, Guinebretière JM, Burlinchon S, Lidereau R, Lazennec G (2007) CXC chemokines located in the 4q21 region are up-regulated in breast cancer. Endocr Relat Cancer 14(4):1039–1052
31. Freund A, Jolivel V, Durand S, Kersual N, Chalbos D, Chavey C, Vignon F, Lazennec G (2004) Mechanisms underlying differential expression of interleukin-8 in breast cancer cells. Oncogene 23(36):6105–6114
32. Yao C, Lin Y, Chua MS, Ye CS, Bi J, Li W, Zhu YF, Wang SM (2007) Interleukin-8 modulates growth and invasiveness of estrogen receptor-negative breast cancer cells. Int J Cancer 121(9):1949–1957

33. Lin Y, Huang R, Chen L, Li S, Shi Q, Jordan C, Huang RP (2004) Identification of interleukin-8 as estrogen receptor-regulated factor involved in breast cancer invasion and angiogenesis by protein arrays. Int J Cancer 109(4):507–515

34. Freund A, Chauveau C, Brouillet JP, Lucas A, Lacroix M, Licznar A, Vignon F, Lazennec G (2003) IL-8 expression and its possible relationship with estrogen-receptor-negative status of breast cancer cells. Oncogene 22(2):256–265

35. Robertson FM, Ogasawara MA, Ye Z, Chu K, Pickei R, Debeb BG, Woodward WA, Hittelman WN, Cristofanilli M, Barsky SH (2010) Imaging and analysis of 3D tumor spheroids enriched for a cancer stem cell phenotype. J Biomol Screen 15(7):820–829

36. Robertson FM, Woodward WA, Pickei R, Ye Z, Bornmann W, Pal A, Peng Z, Hall CS, Cristofanilli M (2010) Suberoylanilide hydroxamic acid blocks self-renewal and homotypic aggregation of inflammatory breast cancer spheroids. Cancer 116(11 Suppl):2760–2767

37. Debeb BG, Xu W, Mok H, Li L, Robertson F, Ueno NT, Reuben J, Lucci A, Cristofanilli M, Woodward WA (2010) Differential radiosensitizing effect of valproic acid in differentiation versus self-renewal promoting culture conditions. Int J Radiat Oncol Biol Phys 76(3): 889–895

38. Alpaugh ML, Barsky SH (2002) Reversible model of spheroid formation allows for high efficiency of gene delivery ex vivo and accurate gene assessment in vivo. Hum Gene Ther 13(10):1245–1258

39. Hirsch J, Johnson CL, Nelius T, Kennedy R, Riese WD, Filleur S (2011) PEDF inhibits IL8 production in prostate cancer cells through PEDF receptor/phospholipase A2 and regulation of NFκB and PPARγ. Cytokine 55(2):202–210. Epub 2011 May 13

40. Torti D, Sassi F, Galimi F, Gastaldi S, Perera T, Comoglio PM, Trusolino L, Bertotti A (2012) A preclinical algorithm of soluble surrogate biomarkers that correlate with therapeutic inhibition of the MET oncogene in gastric tumors. Int J Cancer 130(6):1357–1366. doi: 10.1002/ijc.26137. Epub 2011 May 30

41. Van der Auwera I, Van Laere SJ, Van den Eynden GG, Benoy I, van Dam P, Colpaert CG, Fox SB, Turley H, Harris AL, Van Marck EA, Vermeulen PB, Dirix LY (2004) Increased angiogenesis and lymphangiogenesis in inflammatory versus noninflammatory breast cancer by real-time reverse transcriptase-PCR gene expression quantification. Clin Cancer Res 10(23):7965–7971

42. Rouzer CA, Marnett LJ (2009) Cyclooxygenases: structural and functional insights. J Lipid Res 50(Suppl):S29–S34

43. Hla T, Bishop-Bailey D, Liu CH, Schaefers HJ, Trifan OC (1999) Cyclooxygenase-1 and -2 isoenzymes. Int J Biochem Cell Biol 31(5):551–557

44. Cohn SMZ, Schloemann S, Tessner T, Seibert K, Stenson WF (1997) Crypt stem cell survival in the mouse intestinal epithelium is regulated by prostaglandins synthesized through cyclooxygenase-1. J Clin Invest 99(6):1367–1379

45. Hla T, Neilson K (1992) Human cyclooxygenase-2 cDNA. Proc Natl Acad Sci USA 89(16):7384–7388

46. Wang D, Dubois RN (2004) Cyclooxygenase-2: a potential target in breast cancer. Semin Oncol 31(1 Suppl 3):64–73

47. Menter DG, Schilsky RL, DuBois RN (2010) Cyclooxygenase-2 and cancer treatment: understanding the risk should be worth the reward. Clin Cancer Res 16(5):1384–1390

48. Parrett M, Harris R, Joarder F, Ross M, Clausen K, Robertson F (1997) Cyclooxygenase-2 gene expression in human breast cancer. Int J Oncol 10(3):503–507

49. Hwang D, Scollard D, Byrne J, Levine E (1998) Expression of cyclooxygenase-1 and cyclooxygenase-2 in human breast cancer. J Natl Cancer Inst 90(6):455–460

50. Soslow RA, Dannenberg AJ, Rush D, Woerner BM, Khan KN, Masferrer J, Koki AT (2000) COX-2 is expressed in human pulmonary, colonic, and mammary tumors. Cancer 89(12):2637–2645

51. Brueggemeier RW, Quinn AL, Parrett ML, Joarder FS, Harris RE, Robertson FM (1999) Correlation of aromatase and cyclooxygenase gene expression in human breast cancer specimens. Cancer Lett 140(1–2):27–35

52. Robertson FM (2001) Regulation of aromatase in breast cancer and correlation of aromatase and cyclooxygenase gene expression. In: Li JJ, Daling JR, Li SA (eds) Hormonal carcinogenesis III. Springer, New York

53. Prosperi JR, Robertson FM (2006) Cyclooxygenase-2 directly regulates gene expression of P450 Cyp19 aromatase promoter regions pII, pI.3 and pI.7 and estradiol production in human breast tumor cells. Prostaglandins Other Lipid Mediat 81(1–2):55–70

54. Brodie AM, Lu Q, Long BJ, Fulton A, Chen T, Macpherson N, DeJong PC, Blankenstein MA, Nortier JW, Slee PH, van de Ven J, van Gorp JM, Elbers JR, Schipper ME, Blijham GH, Thijssen JH (2001) Aromatase and COX-2 expression in human breast cancers. J Steroid Biochem Mol Biol 79(1–5):41–47

55. Masferrer JL, Leahy KM, Koki AT, Zweifel BS, Settle SL, Woerner BM, Edwards DA, Flickinger AG, Moore RJ, Seibert K (2000) Antiangiogenic and antitumor activities of cyclooxygenase-2 inhibitors. Cancer Res 60(5):1306–1311

56. Abou-Issa HM, Alshafie GA, Seibert K, Koki AT, Masferrer JL, Harris RE (2001) Dose-response effects of the COX-2 inhibitor, celecoxib, on the chemoprevention of mammary carcinogenesis. Anticancer Res 21(5):3425–3432

57. Psaty BM, Furberg CD (2005) COX-2 inhibitors–lessons in drug safety. N Engl J Med 352(11):1133–1135

58. Graham DJ, Campen D, Hui R, Spence M, Cheetham C, Levy G, Shoor S, Ray WA (2005) Risk of acute myocardial infarction and sudden cardiac death in patients treated with cyclooxygenase 2 selective and non-selective non-steroidal anti-inflammatory drugs: nested case-control study. Lancet 365(9458):475–481

59. Jones RL, Giembycz MA, Woodward DF (2009) Prostanoid receptor antagonists: development strategies and therapeutic applications. Br J Pharmacol 158(1):104–145

60. Narumiya S, Furuyashiki T (2011) Fever, inflammation, pain and beyond: prostanoid receptor research during these 25 years. FASEB J 25(3):813–818

61. Ma X, Kundu N, Rifat S, Walser T, Fulton AM (2006) Prostaglandin E receptor EP4 antagonism inhibits breast cancer metastasis. Cancer Res 66(6):2923–2927

62. Robertson FM, Simeone AM, Lucci A, McMurray JS, Ghosh S, Cristofanilli M (2010) Differential regulation of the aggressive phenotype of inflammatory breast cancer cells by prostanoid receptors EP3 and EP4. Cancer 116(11 Suppl):2806–2814

63. Robertson FM, Simeone AM, Mazumdar A, Shah AH, McMurray JS, Ghosh S, Cristofanilli M (2008) Molecular and pharmacological blockade of the EP4 receptor selectively inhibits both proliferation and invasion of human inflammatory breast cancer cells. J Exp Ther Oncol 7(4):299–312

64. Suzawa H, Kikuchi S, Ichikawa K, Koda A (1992) Inhibitory action of tranilast, an anti-allergic drug, on the release of cytokines and PGE2 from human monocytes-macrophages. Jpn J Pharmacol 60(2):85–90

65. Pae HO, Jeong SO, Koo BS, Ha HY, Lee KM, Chung HT (2008) Tranilast, an orally active anti-allergic drug, up-regulates the anti-inflammatory heme oxygenase-1 expression but down-regulates the pro-inflammatory cyclooxygenase-2 and inducible nitric oxide synthase expression in RAW264.7 macrophages. Biochem Biophys Res Commun 371(3):361–365

66. Chakrabarti R, Subramaniam V, Abdalla S, Jothy S, Prud'homme GJ (2009) Tranilast inhibits the growth and metastasis of mammary carcinoma. Anticancer Drugs 20(5):334–345

67. Subramaniam V, Chakrabarti R, Prud'homme GJ, Jothy S (2010) Tranilast inhibits cell proliferation and migration and promotes apoptosis in murine breast cancer. Anticancer Drugs 21(4):351–361

68. Subramaniam V, Ace O, Prud'homme GJ, Jothy S (2011) Tranilast treatment decreases cell growth, migration and inhibits colony formation of human breast cancer cells. Exp Mol Pathol 90(1):116–122

69. Prud'homme GJ, Glinka Y, Toulina A, Ace O, Subramaniam V, Jothy S (2010) Breast cancer stem-like cells are inhibited by a non-toxic aryl hydrocarbon receptor agonist. PLoS One 5(11):e13831

70. Capper EA, Roshak AK, Bolognese BJ, Podolin PL, Smith T, Dewitt DL, Anderson KM, Marshall LA (2000) Modulation of human monocyte activities by tranilast, SB 252218, a compound demonstrating efficacy in restenosis. J Pharmacol Exp Ther 295(3):1061–1069

71. Koyama S, Takagi H, Otani A, Suzuma K, Nishimura K, Honda Y (1999) Tranilast inhibits protein kinase C-dependent signalling pathway linked to angiogenic activities and gene expression of retinal microcapillary endothelial cells. Br J Pharmacol 127(2):537–545

72. Isaji M, Miyata H, Ajisawa Y, Yoshimura N (1998) Inhibition by tranilast of vascular endothelial growth factor (VEGF)/vascular permeability factor (VPF)-induced increase in vascular permeability in rats. Life Sci 63(4):PL71–PL74

73. Isaji M, Miyata H, Ajisawa Y, Takehana Y, Yoshimura N (1997) Tranilast inhibits the proliferation, chemotaxis and tube formation of human microvascular endothelial cells in vitro and angiogenesis in vivo. Br J Pharmacol 122(6):1061–1066

74. National Institutes of Health. APRiCOT-P: Study to evaluate the safety and efficacy of apricoxib with gemcitabine and erlotinib in the treatment of patients with advanced pancreatic cancer (TP2001-203). ClinicalTrials.gov. http://clinicaltrials.gov/ct2/show/NCT00709826. Accessed Oct 27, 2012

75. National Institutes of Health. APRiCOT-L: Study to evaluate efficacy and safety of apricoxib with erlotinib in patients with non-small cell lung cancer (TP2001-201). ClinicalTrials.gov. http://clinicaltrials.gov/ct2/show/NCT00652340. Accessed Mar 16 2010

76. Senzaki M, Ishida S, Yada A, Hanai M, Fujiwara K, Inoue S, Kimura T, Kurakata S (2008) CS-706, a novel cyclooxygenase-2 selective inhibitor, prolonged the survival of tumor-bearing mice when treated alone or in combination with anti-tumor chemotherapeutic agents. Int J Cancer 122(6):1384–1390

77. Reckamp K, Gitlitz B, Chen LC, Patel R, Milne G, Syto M, Jezior D, Zaknoen S (2011) Biomarker-based phase I dose-escalation, pharmacokinetic, and pharmacodynamic study of oral apricoxib in combination with erlotinib in advanced nonsmall cell lung cancer. Cancer 117(4):809–818

78. Cabioglu N, Gong Y, Islam R, Broglio KR, Sneige N, Sahin A, Gonzalez-Angulo AM, Morandi P, Bucana C, Hortobagyi GN, Cristofanilli M (2007) Expression of growth factor and chemokine receptors: new insights in the biology of inflammatory breast cancer. Ann Oncol 18(6):1021–1029

79. Clézardin P (2011) Therapeutic targets for bone metastases in breast cancer. Breast Cancer Res 13(2):207

80. Liekens S, Schols D, Hatse S (2010) CXCL12-CXCR4 axis in angiogenesis, metastasis and stem cell mobilization. Curr Pharm Des 16(35):3903–3920

81. Li YM, Pan Y, Wei Y, Cheng X, Zhou BP, Tan M, Zhou X, Xia W, Hortobagyi GN, Yu D, Hung MC (2004) Upregulation of CXCR4 is essential for HER2-mediated tumor metastasis. Cancer Cell 6(5):459–469

82. Duda DG, Kozin SV, Kirkpatrick ND, Xu L, Fukumura D, Jain RK (2011) CXCL12 (SDF1alpha)-CXCR4/CXCR7 pathway inhibition: an emerging sensitizer for anticancer therapies? Clin Cancer Res 17(8):2074–2080

83. Greenfield JP, Cobb WS, Lyden D (2010) Resisting arrest: a switch from angiogenesis to vasculogenesis in recurrent malignant gliomas. J Clin Invest 120(3):663–667

84. Singh B, Cook KR, Martin C, Huang EH, Mosalpuria K, Krishnamurthy S, Cristofanilli M, Lucci A (2010) Evaluation of a CXCR4 antagonist in a xenograft mouse model of inflammatory breast cancer. Clin Exp Metastasis 27(4):233–240

85. Huang EH, Singh B, Cristofanilli M, Gelovani J, Wei C, Vincent L, Cook KR, Lucci A (2009) A CXCR4 antagonist CTCE-9908 inhibits primary tumor growth and metastasis of breast cancer. J Surg Res 155(2):231–236

86. Ravishankaran P, Karunanithi R (2011) Clinical significance of preoperative serum interleukin-6 and C-reactive protein level in breast cancer patients. World J Surg Oncol 9(1):18

87. Carpi A, Nicolini A, Antonelli A, Ferrari P, Rossi G (2009) Cytokines in the management of high risk or advanced breast cancer: an update and expectation. Curr Cancer Drug Targets 9(8):888–903

88. Goldberg JE, Schwertfeger KL (2010) Proinflammatory cytokines in breast cancer: mechanisms of action and potential targets for therapeutics. Curr Drug Targets 11(9): 1133–1146

89. van Golen KL, Wu ZF, Qiao XT, Bao L, Merajver SD (2000) RhoC GTPase overexpression modulates induction of angiogenic factors in breast cells. Neoplasia 2(5):418–425

90. Iliopoulos D, Hirsch HA, Wang G, Struhl K (2011) Inducible formation of breast cancer stem cells and their dynamic equilibrium with non-stem cancer cells via IL6 secretion. Proc Natl Acad Sci USA 108(4):1397–1402

91. Hinohara K, Gotoh N (2010) Inflammatory signaling pathways in self-renewing breast cancer stem cells. Curr Opin Pharmacol 10(6):650–654

92. Murohashi M, Hinohara K, Kuroda M, Isagawa T, Tsuji S, Kobayashi S, Umezawa K, Tojo A, Aburatani H, Gotoh N (2010) Gene set enrichment analysis provides insight into novel signaling pathways in breast cancer stem cells. Br J Cancer 102:206–212

93. Heinrich PC, Behrmann I, Haan S, Hermanns HM, Müller-Newen G, Schaper F (2003) Principles of interleukin (IL)-6-type cytokine signalling and its regulation. Biochem J 374 (Pt 1):1–20

94. Tawara K, Oxford JT, Jorcyk CL (2011) Clinical significance of interleukin (IL)-6 in cancer metastasis to bone: potential of anti-IL-6 therapies. Cancer Manag Res 3:177–189

95. Li J, Hu XF, Xing PX (2005) CNTO-328 (Centocor). Curr Opin Investig Drugs 6(6):639–645

96. Zaki MH, Nemeth JA, Trikha M (2004) CNTO 328, a monoclonal antibody to IL-6, inhibits human tumor-induced cachexia in nude mice. Int J Cancer 111(4):592–595

97. Trikha M, Corringham R, Klein B, Rossi JF (2003) Targeted anti-interleukin-6 monoclonal antibody therapy for cancer: a review of the rationale and clinical evidence. Clin Cancer Res 9(13):4653–4665

98. Rossi JF, Négrier S, James ND, Kocak I, Hawkins R, Davis H, Prabhakar U, Qin X, Mulders P, Berns B (2010) A phase I/II study of siltuximab (CNTO 328), an anti-interleukin-6 monoclonal antibody, in metastatic renal cell cancer. Br J Cancer 103(8):1154–1162

99. Puchalski T, Prabhakar U, Jiao Q, Berns B, Davis HM (2010) Pharmacokinetic and pharmacodynamic modeling of an anti-interleukin-6 chimeric monoclonal antibody (siltuximab) in patients with metastatic renal cell carcinoma. Clin Cancer Res 16(5):1652–1661

100. Dorff TB, Goldman B, Pinski JK, Mack PC, Lara PN Jr, Van Veldhuizen PJ, DI Jr Q, Vogelzang NJ, Thompson IM Jr, Hussain MH (2010) Clinical and correlative results of SWOG S0354: a phase II trial of CNTO328 (siltuximab), a monoclonal antibody against interleukin-6, in chemotherapy-pretreated patients with castration-resistant prostate cancer. Clin Cancer Res 16(11):3028–3034

101. van Rhee F, Fayad L, Voorhees P, Furman R, Lonial S, Borghaei H, Sokol L, Crawford J, Cornfeld M, Qi M, Qin X, Herring J, Casper C, Kurzrock R (2010) Siltuximab, a novel anti-interleukin-6 monoclonal antibody, for Castleman's disease. J Clin Oncol 28(23): 3701–3708

102. Marotta LL, Almendro V, Marusyk A, Shipitsin M, Schemme J, Walker SR, Bloushtain-Qimron N, Kim JJ, Choudhury SA, Maruyama R, Wu Z, Gönen M, Mulvey LA, Bessarabova MO, Huh SJ, Silver SJ, Kim SY, Park SY, Lee HE, Anderson KS, Richardson AL, Nikolskaya T, Nikolsky Y, Liu XS, Root DE, Hahn WC, Frank DA, Polyak K (2011) The JAK2/STAT3 signaling pathway is required for growth of CD44 + CD24- stem cell-like breast cancer cells in human tumors. J Clin Invest 121(7):2723–2735. doi: 10.1172/JCI44745

103. Speer R, Wulfkuhle J, Espina V, Aurajo R, Edmiston KH, Liotta LA, Petricoin EF 3rd (2008) Molecular network analysis using reverse phase protein microarrays for patient tailored therapy. Adv Exp Med Biol 610:177–186

104. Wilson B, Liotta LA, Petricoin E 3 rd (2010) Monitoring proteins and protein networks using reverse phase protein arrays. Dis Markers 28(4):225–232

105. Espina V, Liotta LA, Petricoin EF 3 rd (2009) Reverse-phase protein microarrays for theranostics and patient tailored therapy. Methods Mol Biol 520:89–105

106. Mandal PK, Gao F, Lu Z, Ren Z, Ramesh R, Birtwistle JS, Kaluarachchi KK, Chen X, Bast RC, Liao WS, McMurray JS (2011) Potent and selective phosphopeptide mimetic prodrugs

targeted to the Src homology 2 (SH2) domain of signal transducer and activator of transcription 3. J Med Chem 54(10):3549–3563

107. Thudi N, Mandal P, McMurray JS, Robertson, FM (2009) STAT3 as a molecular signature and therapeutic target in inflammatory breast cancer. In: Proceedings of the annual meeting of the American Association for Cancer Research 2009, Washington, DC, Apr 17–21. AACR 2009, Philadelphia. Abstract nr. 653

108. Ma L, Zhao B, Walgren RA, Clayton JR, Burkholder TP (2011) LY2784544, a small molecule JAK2 inhibitor, induces apoptosis in inflammatory breast cancer spheres through targeting IL-6-JAK-STAT3 pathway. In: Proceedings of the annual meeting of the American Association for Cancer Research 2011, Orlando, FL, Apr 2–6. AACR 2011, Philadelphia. Abstract nr.2820

Chapter 17
Immunology of Inflammatory Breast Cancer

James M. Reuben and Bang-Ning Lee

Abstract It was shown several decades ago that IBC patients were immunocompetent as demonstrated by their ability to develop normal delayed-type hypersensitivity responses to common recall microbial antigens. However, studies of larger numbers of patients were needed to establish an immune profile that is unique to IBC patients and to determine whether the immune system plays a role in the pathogenesis of the disease.

In this chapter, we present data on the immune profiles of IBC patients and compare these data with those of healthy women and of locally advanced or metastatic breast cancer patients without IBC features. The data show that patients with early-stage IBC have a normal immune profile, as demonstrated by the normal immunophenotypes of their peripheral blood leukocytes and T-cell function. However, IBC patients with metastasis have pronounced immunosuppression, characterized by extreme lymphopenia and severely suppressed function of T cells. Nevertheless, it is unclear if these immune defects are the cause of rapid disease progression or the results of aggressive treatment.

Keywords Delayed-type hypersensitivity • Leukocyte immunophenotypes • T-cell function • Dendritic cell • Cell-mediated immunity • Antibody-dependent cellular cytotoxicity • Cytotoxic T lymphocytes • Inflammatory cytokines • Regulatory T (TR) lymphocytes • Natural killer (NK) T • Th1-Th2-Th17-Tc17 lymphocytes • Locally advanced breast cancer • Inflammatory breast cancer • Metastatic breast cancer

J.M. Reuben, Ph.D., M.B.A. (✉)
Department of Hematopathology, Diagnostic and Immunology Core, Morgan Welch Inflammatory Breast Cancer Research Program and Clinic, The University of Texas MD Anderson Cancer Center, Houston, TX, USA
e-mail: jreuben@mdanderson.org

B.-N. Lee, Ph.D.
Department of Hematopathology, The University of Texas MD Anderson Cancer Center, Houston, TX, USA
e-mail: blee@mdanderson.org

N.T. Ueno and M. Cristofanilli (eds.), *Inflammatory Breast Cancer: An Update*, DOI 10.1007/978-94-007-3907-9_17, © Springer Science+Business Media B.V. 2012

17.1   Introduction

Inflammatory breast cancer (IBC) is a rare, aggressive type of locally advanced breast cancer (LABC). It was first considered a distinct clinical phase of carcinoma of the breast by Lee and Tannenbaum in 1924 [1]. IBC accounts for about 2–5% of all cases of breast cancer. Patients with IBC typically are younger, are more likely to have metastatic disease at diagnosis, have more rapidly progressive disease, and have poorer overall survival rates than non-IBC breast cancer patients [2]. The American Joint Committee on Cancer classifies IBC as T4d disease, and IBC falls into stages IIIB, IIIC, or IV, depending on the nodal status and distant metastasis [3]. The unique clinical characteristics of IBC are edema (*peau d'orange*), warmth, and erythema in the invaded tissue. The pathologic hallmark of IBC is the presence of tumor emboli in dermal lymphatic vessels [4].

The extensive invasion of lymphatic vessels by tumor emboli in IBC patients suggests that the host immune surveillance system is suboptimal or that the tumor cells have lowered their immunogenicity through immunoediting to avoid detection by the host. In the immunocompetent host, tumor cells must overcome both innate and adaptive immunologic defenses of the host. Cell-mediated immunity (CMI) is essential for maintaining immune surveillance against tumor progression [5]. CD4+ T lymphocytes, in particular, enhance tumor antigen-specific immune responses by activating cytotoxic T lymphocytes through cytokines or by directly interacting with costimulatory molecules and major histocompatibility complex class II antigens expressed on the surface of cytotoxic T lymphocytes [6]. In addition to lowered immunogenicity through immunoediting, tumor cells may develop strategies to avoid antigen processing and presentation by lowering the expression of costimulatory molecules [7]. Tumor cells may also modify the microenvironment by overproducing immunosuppressive cytokines, such as transforming growth factor-beta or interleukin (IL)-10 [8], to inhibit the function of immune cells.

Tumor cells may produce inflammatory cytokines, such as IL-1β, IL-6, or tumor necrosis factor (TNF)-α, to facilitate their survival [9–11]. Furthermore, tumor cells can selectively recruit and/or induce immunosuppressive cells such as regulatory T (TR) lymphocytes [12], natural killer T (NKT) lymphocytes [13], and myeloid-derived suppressor cells [14]. TR lymphocytes, in particular, have been shown to play a critical role in inhibiting naturally or therapeutically induced antitumor immunity [15–17].

As early as 1978, the rapid disease progression seen in a group of IBC patients in Tunisia prompted studies to identify differences between IBC patients with and without rapid progression. The studies included patient immune evaluation that assessed delayed-type hypersensitivity (DTH) to a battery of common recall microbial antigens and tumor lysates [18, 19], lymphocyte immunophenotyping, and mitogen-induced lymphocyte proliferation [19]. These studies showed that patients with rapidly progressing IBC and those without rapidly progressing IBC had comparable responses to the battery of common recall microbial antigens [18, 19]. Furthermore, it was reported that the patients with rapidly progressing IBC had a stronger response to breast-tumor-related antigens than did other breast cancer patients [19]. Together, these studies lessened the possibility that the rapid progression of disease in IBC patients was due to the impairment of cellular immunity.

Although DTH is one of the best tools to assess CMI *in vivo*, the measurement of DTH to assess the immune status of cancer patients [20] may not represent the complete repertoire of host responses to antigens associated with less immunogenic tumors. In immunocompetent IBC patients, it is possible that surviving tumor clones have undergone selective immunoediting to decrease their immunogenicity, thus allowing them to invade the lymphatic system with minimal scrutiny by the host immune system.

Although IBC is known for its aggressive clinical presentation [21], there is a paucity of information on peripheral blood leukocyte immunophenotypes and their function in IBC patients. To investigate immune parameters of IBC patients, we initiated a study in which peripheral blood was collected from breast cancer patients prior to their starting a new therapy, as well as from healthy female donors (HFD), and the blood was analyzed to determine the immunophenotype and function of dendritic cells (DC), T cells, B cells, TR cells, and NK lymphocytes [22, 23]. Some early results based on a smaller subset of patients (n = 87) were presented at the 2009 annual meeting of the San Antonio Breast Cancer Symposium [24] and the 2010 Annual Meeting of the American Association for Cancer Research [25, 26]. In this chapter, we provide information on some of the basic immune parameters of IBC patients and contrast them with those of HFDs and non-IBC patients with locally advanced and metastatic disease.

17.2 Immune Characteristics of IBC

17.2.1 Population Studied

We conducted a prospective, laboratory-based study that was approved by the Institutional Review Board of The University of Texas MD Anderson Cancer Center. Patients were eligible to enroll if they were starting a new line of therapy and had a diagnosis of IBC, LABC (stage II-III non-IBC), non-IBC metastatic breast cancer (MBC), or IBC with metastatic disease (MIBC). To date, 115 breast cancer patients and 31 age-matched HFDs have been recruited for this ongoing study. However, complete sets of data are available for only 87 of the 115 patients, including 26 patients with LABC, 22 with IBC, 15 with MBC, and 24 with MIBC. The median age of the patient population was 54 years (range, 34–76 years). Immunohistochemical staining of the primary tumor for estrogen receptor (ER)/progesterone receptor (PR) and HER2/neu status in each patient revealed that 37 patients had luminal A (ER/PR-positive, HER2 normal), 18 had luminal B (ER/PR-positive, HER2-positive), 10 had HER2-amplified (HER2-positive, ER/PR-negative), and 22 had triple-negative breast cancer tumor subtypes.

All patients provided a blood sample on the same day as starting a new therapy, and HFDs provided a blood sample upon enrollment in the study. We used the blood of patients to determine total and differential counts of leukocytes and to identify lymphocyte subpopulations according to a standardized protocol of immunophenotyping by flow cytometry [27]. We used Kruskal-Wallis and Mann-Whitney tests to assess the differences between patients and HFDs, as well as between the following groups of patients: (1) LABC vs IBC (clinical presentation of non-metastatic disease); (2) LABC vs MBC, IBC vs MIBC, and LABC and IBC vs MBC and MIBC (severity of disease); and (3) IBC vs non-IBC, regardless of metastasis (unique clinical presentation).

17.2.2 Total and Differential Leukocyte Counts in IBC

Peripheral blood samples were examined for complete blood counts and leukocyte differential analysis by an automated system (Table 17.1). The data showed that hematological parameters were similar for patients with LABC, patients with IBC, and HFDs. MBC patients had significantly lower mean leukocyte counts than did non-MBC patients, which is consistent with prior reports [18, 21, 28]. We also found no differences in mean leukocyte counts or percentages between LABC and IBC patients, which is similar to findings reported by Levine and colleagues in Tunisian patients [18].

However, we found that LABC patients had a significantly higher mean leukocyte count (p = 0.007), higher mean absolute lymphocyte count (p = 0.001), higher mean absolute neutrophil count (p = 0.001), and lower mean percentage of monocytes (p = 0.023) than did MBC patients. Of particular interest is our observation that IBC patients with non-metastatic disease had a significantly higher mean leukocyte count, percentage of lymphocytes, percentage of monocytes, and mean absolute lymphocyte count than did IBC patients with metastatic disease. Furthermore, IBC patients with metastatic disease had a significantly lower mean absolute neutrophil count and mean percentages of lymphocytes, monocytes, and neutrophils than did MBC patients without IBC.

IBC patients with non-metastatic disease had a significantly higher mean (± standard error of the mean [SEM]) percentage of lymphocytes than did IBC patients with metastatic disease (27.2% ± 1.9% vs 20.6% ± 1.8%; p = 0.009) and a significantly lower mean percentage of lymphocytes than did non-IBC patients (27.2% ± 1.9% vs 29.1% ± 1.3%; p = 0.010). With respect to mean (± SEM) leukocyte counts, significant differences were observed in the following paired groups. MBC patients had a significantly lower mean leukocyte count ($5.3 \pm 0.5 \times 10^9/\mu L$) than did either LABC patients ($6.7 \pm 0.4 \times 10^9/\mu L$; p = 0.022) or HFDs ($6.6 \pm 0.4 \times 10^9/\mu L$; p = 0.042). Additionally, LABC patients had a significantly higher mean lymphocyte count than did MBC patients (p = 0.001) and MIBC patients (p = 0.007).

In summary, these results indicate that hematological parameters are normal in patients with non-metastatic disease but deteriorate with the development of metastatic disease and further worsen with a diagnosis of metastatic IBC.

Table 17.1 Complete blood counts and differential counts

| Hematologic parameter | Mean ± SEM by patient group | | | | | Significant differences[a] |
	LABC	IBC	MBC	MIBC	HFD	
No. patients	23	24	21	43	37	
Leukocytes, ×10³/μL	7.2±0.7	7.2±0.4	5.3±0.4*	6.3±0.4	7±0.4	a, c, e, g
% Lymphocytes	29.9±2	27.4±1.6*	26.9±2.1*	20.6±1.4*	32.1±1.2	a, b, c, f, g
Lymphocytes/μL	2,085±127	1,937±138	1,380±131*	1,260±102*	2,194±117	a, c, e, g
% Monocytes	6.6±0.4	6.4±0.4	8.5±0.7*	9.4±0.5*	6.9±0.3	a, c, e, g
Monocytes/μL	49±4	47±4	44±4	58±4*	48±3	f, g
% Neutrophils	61±2.4	63.7±1.7*	60.9±2.1	67±1.4*	58.4±1.3	b, f, g
Neutrophils/μL	479±58	463±27	325±32*	432±35	418±30	a, e, f, g
% Eosinophils	1.8±0.2	1.9±0.3	2.7±0.4	2.4±0.4	1.9±0.2	n.s.
Eosinophils/μL	13±2	15±3	14±3	14±3	13±2	n.s.
% Basophils	0.5±0.1	0.4±0*	0.7±0.2	0.5±0.1	0.6±0.1	g
Basophils/μL	3±0	3±0	4±2	3±0*	4±1	g
% Other leukocytes	0.1±0	0.2±0*	0.2±0.1	0.2±0	0.1±0	g

SEM standard error of the mean, *LABC* locally advanced breast cancer, *IBC* inflammatory breast cancer, *MBC* metastatic breast cancer, *MIBC* IBC with metastasis, *HFD* healthy female donors

[a]Significant ($p<0.05$) pairwise comparisons: a, metastatic (MBC+MIBC) vs non-metastatic (LABC+IBC); b, IBC (IBC+MIBC) vs non-IBC (LABC+MBC); c, IBC vs MIBC; d, LABC vs IBC; e, LABC vs MBC; f, MBC vs MIBC; g, *indicates significantly different from HFD. n.s., no significant differences

17.2.3   Leukocyte Immunophenotypes

Leukocyte immunophenotypes have been useful in the laboratory assessment of patients with immunodeficiency. Immune leukocytes comprise several subtypes including T and non-T lymphocytes namely, B cells and natural killer (NK) cells, and dendritic cells (DC) or antigen-presenting cells. T lymphocytes play a major moderating role in cellular immunity [29] and are comprised of T-helper (Th), T-cytotoxic (Tc) and regulatory T (TR) cells. The Th lymphocytes recognize tumor antigens expressed on the surface of tumor cells or tumor antigens that may be shed by tumor cells and internalized, processed, and presented in association with major histocompatibility complex class II on antigen-presenting cells. There are two subsets of Th lymphocytes that can be distinguished from each other based on their mutually exclusive cytokine production profiles. T-helper type 1 (Th1) lymphocytes produce IL-2 and IFN-γ to provide help to tumor-specific cytotoxic T lymphocytes by inducing their proliferation and differentiation with elaboration of a cellular immune response. T-helper type 2 (Th2) lymphocytes produce IL-4 to help B cells produce antibodies that represent the humoral immune response. An imbalance of the normal ratio of Th1 to Th2 is consistent with the immune dysregulation that is frequently associated with impaired host immunity in advanced stages of cancer [30, 31]. On the other hand, immunity to intracellular pathogens is often dependent upon the generation of CD8+ memory T lymphocytes, which provide long-lasting cellular immunity and effective protection [32].

CD8+ Tc lymphocytes are a major defense against tumor targets, and their production of IFN-γ and cytolytic activity is a key element in the host immune response to tumor cells. CD8+ Tc lymphocytes are composed of 2 subsets, Tc1 and Tc2, based on their cytokine production profiles [33]. Tc1 lymphocytes produce the Th1 cytokine IFN-γ, and Tc2 lymphocytes produce the Th2 cytokines IL-4 and IL-5 during the DTH reaction [34].

To study the immune cells in IBC, we measured the percentages and counts of CD3+ total T, Th, Tc, CD3^{neg}CD56+CD16+ NK, CD3+CD4+CD25^{hi}CD127^{neg} TR, and CD19+ B lymphocytes, as well as myeloid-derived (mDC) and lymphoid- or plasmacytoid-derived (pDC) DC subsets, in the peripheral blood of patients and HFDs (Table 17.2). Among all patient groups (LABC, IBC, MBC, and MIBC), only the non-metastatic IBC patients had a significantly higher mean (±SEM) percentage of CD3+ T lymphocytes than did HFDs (79.1% ± 1.6% vs 75.7% ± 1.8%; p = 0.025). This contradicts an earlier study that reported significantly fewer CD3+ T lymphocytes in LABC patients than in HFDs [35].

We also measured the percentages and counts of total number of total T (CD3+), Th (CD4+), and Tc (CD8+) lymphocytes in the peripheral blood and found that patients with metastatic disease had a lower mean percentage of Th lymphocytes than did patients without metastatic disease [25]. For example, the mean percentage of Th lymphocytes differed significantly between patients with metastatic disease (MBC) and those with non-metastatic disease (LABC) (46.2% ± 1.7% vs 8.5% ± 1.5%; p = 0.002) and between IBC patients without metastatic disease and IBC patients

Table 17.2 Distribution of leukocytes, including T-cell subsets, NK cells, and DC subsets

Measurement	Mean ± SEM by patient group					Significant differences[a]
	LABC	IBC	MBC	MIBC	HFD	
No. patients	25	22	14	24	20	
% CD3 T	76.5 ± 1.3	79.1 ± 1.6*	74.7 ± 3.2	78.7 ± 1.8	75.7 ± 1	g
CD3+ T/µL	1,532 ± 98	1,477 ± 154	978 ± 106*	978 ± 108*	1,577 ± 84	a, c, e, g
% CD3+ CD4+ Th	53.1 ± 1.7	52.1 ± 1.6	49 ± 2.9	45.1 ± 2.3	50.4 ± 1.7	a, c
CD3+CD4+ Th/µL	1,069 ± 78	995 ± 113	645 ± 78*	579 ± 80*	1,051 ± 66	a, c, e, g
% CD3+CD8+ Tc	19.3 ± 1.2	21.6 ± 1.8	20.7 ± 1.2	29 ± 2.9*	19.4 ± 1.3	a, c, g
CD3+CD8+ Tc/µL	383 ± 32	380 ± 40	269 ± 32*	348 ± 57*	404 ± 35	a, e, g
%CD56+CD16+ NK	12.2 ± 2.6	15.5 ± 2.5	17.9 ± 2.8	18 ± 2.4	13.5 ± 2.1	a, e
CD56+CD16+ NK/µL	99 ± 17	98 ± 15	98 ± 23	69 ± 12	99 ± 12	n.s.
%TR in CD4	6.9 ± 0.4	6.9 ± 0.5	9 ± 0.6*	7.8 ± 0.4*	6.4 ± 0.3	a, e, g
TR/µL	73 ± 6	65 ± 8	55 ± 6	46 ± 8*	67 ± 6	a, b, c, g
%CD19+ B	10.4 ± 0.8	9.3 ± 0.8*	11.7 ± 1.6	7.1 ± 1.2*	12.7 ± 1.2	b, c, f, g
CD19+ B/µL	206 ± 19	170 ± 21*	156 ± 26*	103 ± 31*	283 ± 43	a, b, c, f, g
%DC in lin[neg] HLA-DR+	0.35 ± 0.04	0.39 ± 0.04	0.43 ± 0.05	0.36 ± 0.03	0.36 ± 0.04	n.s.
DC/mL	13,670 ± 1,755	12,581 ± 1,982	12,194 ± 2,880	7,869 ± 1,020*	15,815 ± 2,224	g
%mDC subset	48.4 ± 2	45.2 ± 3	40.6 ± 5.1	43.8 ± 3.2	50.4 ± 2.2	n.s.
mDC/mL subset	6,514 ± 697	5,199 ± 733	5,344 ± 1,385	3,591 ± 534*	7,895 ± 1,159*	a, g
%pDC subset	21.3 ± 2.2	18.4 ± 1.4	17.7 ± 2.1	22.7 ± 1.9	20.6 ± 2.1	n.s.
pDC/mL subset	3,494 ± 992	2,079 ± 321	2,267 ± 625	1,814 ± 253*	3,346 ± 532	g

Data available on only 85 of 115 patients of this ongoing study. *NK* indicates natural killer cells, *DC* dendritic cells

SEM standard error of the mean, *LABC* locally advanced breast cancer, *IBC* inflammatory breast cancer, *MBC* metastatic breast cancer, *MIBC* IBC with metastasis, *HFD* healthy female donors, *Th* T helper, *Tc* T cytotoxic, *TR* T regulatory cells, *lin[neg] HLA-DR+* lineage-negative HLA-positive DC+, *mDC* myeloid-derived DC, *pDC* plasmacytoid-derived DC

[a]Significant (p < 0.05) pairwise comparisons: a, metastatic (MBC + MIBC) vs non-metastatic (LABC + IBC); b, IBC (IBC + MIBC) vs non-IBC (LABC + MBC); c, IBC vs MIBC; d, LABC vs IBC; e, LABC vs MBC; f, MBC vs MIBC; g, * indicates significantly different from HFD. n.s., no significant differences

with metastatic disease (MIBC) ($52.1\% \pm 1.6\%$ vs $45.1\% \pm 2.3\%$; p = 0.027) [25]. By contrast, others have reported that breast cancer patients who were either treatment-naïve or not receiving therapy at the time of immunologic assessment were likely to have normal values for CD4+ T lymphocytes [35, 36].

In previous reports, we showed that the mean percentage of CD8+ Tc lymphocytes was higher in IBC patients than in non-IBC patients ($25.5\% \pm 1.8\%$ vs $19.8 \pm 0.0\%$; p = 0.028), in patients with metastasis (M1) than in those with non-metastatic disease (M0; $26.1\% \pm 1.9\%$ vs $19.7\% \pm 1.0\%$; p < 0.001), and in MIBC patients than in HFDs ($29.0\% \pm 2.9\%$ vs $19.3\% \pm 1.2\%$; p = 0.015) [24, 25]. Because it has been reported that IBC patients had normal DTH responses [18], one can speculate that the CD8+ Tc lymphocytes of IBC patients preferentially produce Tc1 and not Tc2 cytokines in DTH reactions. Indeed we were able to affirm this speculation by demonstrating that IBC patients had a higher mean percentage of CD8+ Tc1 lymphocytes that produced IFN-γ than did MIBC patients ($14.4\% \pm 2.1\%$ vs $8.9\% \pm 1.3\%$; p = 0.033) without a significant difference in the mean percentage of CD8+ Tc2 lymphocytes that synthesized IL-4 using a method to determine *de novo* synthesis of cytokines [37].

Because non-metastatic IBC patients had a significantly higher mean percentage of CD4+ Th lymphocytes than did IBC patients with metastasis ($52.1\% \pm 1.6\%$ vs $45.1\% \pm 2.3\%$; p = 0.027) and a similar mean percentage of CD8+ Tc lymphocytes, the CD4/CD8 ratio of non-metastatic IBC patients was significantly higher than the CD4/CD8 ratio of IBC patients with metastasis ($2.9\% \pm 0.4\%$ vs $2.0\% \pm 0.2\%$; p = 0.035). Others have reported that the CD4/CD8 ratio is related to the stage of breast cancer and to clinical evolution of the disease [37, 38]. Imbalance in the CD4/CD8 ratio may be related to prior exposure to therapy. Patients who have received multiple lines of therapy are more likely to have undergone unsuccessful prior treatments and, as a result, are more likely to have a smaller proportion of CD4+ Th lymphocytes to CD8+ Tc lymphocytes than patients who have not undergone multiple unsuccessful treatments [35, 39].

17.2.4 TR Lymphocytes

In humans, TR lymphocytes, which make up about 1–2% of circulating Th lymphocytes that co-express a very high density of IL-2 receptor-alpha (CD25^{hi}), inhibit cytokine production and proliferation of activated CD4+CD25^{neg} T lymphocytes in a contact-dependent manner [40, 41]. TR lymphocytes are a subset of T lymphocytes that can inhibit both cell-mediated and humoral immune responses [42, 43]. TR lymphocytes both are controlled by and express the transcription factor FoxP3 [44, 45].

In the early stages of cancer, chronic stimulation and interactions with tumor cells may cause T lymphocytes to become suppressive TR lymphocytes, leading to immune tolerance and promoting tumor growth that can result in disease progression [46]. In general, cancer patients have been reported to have a significantly higher frequency of TR lymphocytes in their peripheral blood than do healthy controls [16].

In accordance with this, we found that M1 (MBC plus MIBC) patients had more TR lymphocytes than did M0 (LABC plus IBC) patients ($8.3\% \pm 0.3\%$ vs $6.8\% \pm 0.3\%$ [mean $\pm$ SEM]; $p = 0.003$) and that both MBC and MIBC patients had higher percentages of TR lymphocytes than did HFDs. LABC patients had a significantly lower mean percentage of TR lymphocytes than did MBC patients ($6.9\% \pm 0.4\%$ vs $9.0\% \pm 0.6\%$; $p = 0.006$). There were no other significant differences in mean percentages of TR lymphocytes among the groups studied [25]. Thus, these data suggest that patients with metastatic disease are more likely to exhibit immunosuppression than patients with non-metastatic disease. However, it is unclear whether the immunosuppression induces metastasis or the metastasis induces the immunosuppression.

17.2.5 CD19+ B Cells

Non-T B cells are important because they are the only cell-type capable of producing immunoglobulin that mediates the humoral immune response. Patients with metastatic breast cancer have significantly lower proportions of CD19+ B cells and significantly fewer CD19+ B cells than do HFDs [35]. Neoadjuvant therapy has been shown to reduce the proportion and absolute number of CD19+ B cells [35, 47]. In our study, the mean percentage of CD19+ B cells was significantly lower in both MIBC and locally advanced IBC patients than in HFDs (Fig. 17.1). MIBC patients had a significantly lower mean percentage of CD19+ B cells than did MBC and IBC patients. Moreover, all breast cancer patient groups except the LABC group had significantly fewer CD19+ B cells than did HFDs. HFDs had significantly more CD19+ B lymphocytes than did IBC, MBC, and MIBC patients. These findings are consistent with our previous report showing that MIBC patients had significantly fewer CD19+ B cells than did LABC, MBC, and IBC patients [25]. Some reports have indicated that host inflammatory cell infiltration is rare in the tumor field in IBC [48, 49], but this observation may be limited by the lack of sufficient tumor tissue for analysis.

17.2.6 NK Cells

NK cells are another subset of non-T cells that have been shown to play an important role in early and metastatic cancers. As many as five subpopulations of NK cells have been identified in human peripheral blood based on the expression of CD56 (neural cell adhesion molecule 1) and CD16 ($Fc\gamma RIIIA$, low-affinity receptor for the Fc portion of IgG) [50]. During NK cell differentiation, CD56+ lymphocytes acquire CD16, and the amount of CD16 expression correlates with the level of NK cell maturation [51]. It is generally accepted that the NK cells in the $CD56^{bright}CD16^{neg}$ subpopulation have a high proliferation potential and give rise to the $CD56^{dim}$ subset of NK lymphocytes [52]. NK lymphocytes in this subset show high expression of CD16 and contain perforin, granzyme, and cytolytic granules but have a low

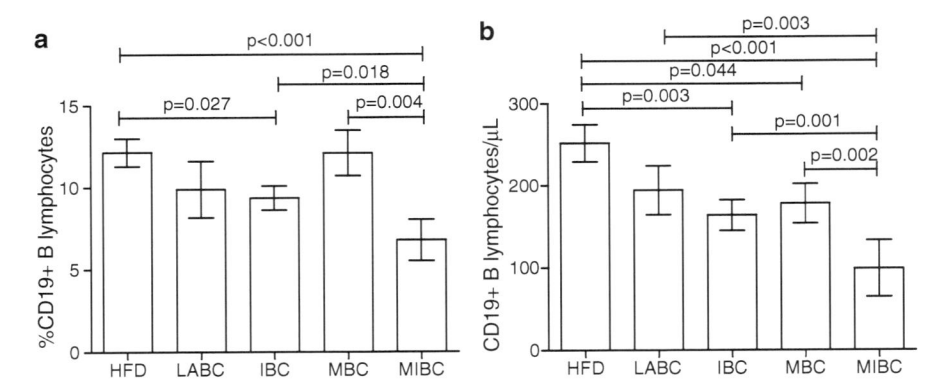

Fig. 17.1 Distribution of mean CD19+ B-lymphocyte percentages (**a**) and counts (**b**) in breast cancer patient groups: *HFD* indicates healthy female donors, *LABC* locally advanced breast cancer, *IBC* inflammatory breast cancer, *MBC* metastatic breast cancer, and *MIBC* metastatic inflammatory breast cancer. *Horizontal lines* indicate significant differences between patient groups. *Vertical bars* within histograms indicate standard error of the mean

proliferation potential [52]. Most NK lymphocytes in the peripheral circulation coexpress CD56 and CD16 and possess potent antibody-dependent cellular cytotoxicity (ADCC) [53] Our results showed that M1 patients had a significantly lower mean percentage of CD56+CD16+ NK cells than did M0 patients (Table 17.3) and therefore would have less ADCC activity than M0 patients. In addition, there were no differences in the mean percentages of CD56+CD16^{neg} NK lymphocytes among patient groups or between all patients and HFDs.

17.2.7 Cytokine Synthesis by Activated T Lymphocytes

T lymphocytes produce several cytokines that can either augment or suppress host immune function. It is generally accepted that Th1 cytokines such as IL-2, IFN-γ, and TNF-α favor a robust host CMI response, whereas Th2 cytokines such as IL-4, IL-6, and IL-10 are responsible for attenuating that response. The results of many studies measuring Th1 and Th2 cytokine levels in the plasma, serum, and body fluids of breast cancer patients are consistent with this concept [54, 55]. In a study with a population of treatment-naïve, early stage (I-III) breast cancer patients, Campbell et al reported significantly fewer T lymphocytes that were capable of *de novo* synthesis of Th1 cytokines than did control subjects [56]. They concluded that immune dysfunction was discernible at early stages of breast cancer even though they failed to demonstrate a relationship between immune dysregulation and clinicopathologic characteristics such as stage or nodal status.

Despite the numerous studies illustrating cytokine profiles of breast cancer patients with different stages of disease and the effects of treatment on those cytokine

Table 17.3 Distribution of NK cell subsets

NK subset	Mean ± SEM by patient group					Significant differences[a]
	LABC	IBC	MBC	MIBC	HFD	
No. patients	25	22	14	24	20	
CD56+ CD16+	12.2 ± 2.6	15.5 ± 2.5	17.9 ± 2.8	18 ± 2.4	13.5 ± 2.1	a, c
CD56+ CD16-	2.0 ± 0.3	2.8 ± 0.4	2.2 ± 0.3	5.1 ± 1	3.6 ± 0.9	a, b, c, d

Data available on only 85 of 115 patients of this ongoing study. *NK* indicates natural killer cells, *SEM* standard error of the mean, *LABC* locally advanced breast cancer, *IBC* inflammatory breast cancer, *MBC* metastatic breast cancer, *MIBC* IBC with metastasis, *HFD* healthy female donors
[a]Significant (p < 0.05) pairwise comparisons: a, metastatic (MBC + MIBC) vs non-metastatic (LABC + IBC); b, IBC (IBC + MIBC) vs non-IBC (LABC + MBC); c, LABC vs MBC; d, MBC vs MIBC

profiles [57], to our knowledge there are no previous studies of cytokine profiles of IBC patients. In our study, we examined the ability of activated T-lymphocyte subsets in IBC patients to synthesize Th1 and Th2 cytokines as previously described [58]. Our results suggest that the majority of significant differences among patient groups were within the CD8+ Tc lymphocyte population and not in the CD4+ Th lymphocytes (Table 17.4). Compared with the induced cytokine responses of M0 patients, M1 patients had significantly lower mean percentages of CD8+ Tc1 lymphocytes that synthesized TNF-α (p = 0.008) and IFN-γ (p = 0.009), CD8+ Tc2 lymphocytes that synthesized IL-10 (p = 0.04), and CD8+ Tc17 lymphocytes that synthesized IL-17 (p = 0.001) [26]. There were no significant differences between M0 patients and M1 patients with respect to CD8+ Tc1 lymphocytes that synthesized IL-2. There were also no significant differences in the proportion of cytokine-producing CD4+ Th lymphocytes between M1 patients and M0 patients, even though M1 patients had fewer CD4+ Th1 lymphocytes that synthesized IL-2, TNF-α, and IFN-γ and Th2 lymphocytes that synthesized IL-4 and IL-10 than did M0 patients [26].

In the study by Campbell et al, both CD4+ and CD8+ T-lymphocyte subsets from early-stage breast cancer patients were unable to synthesize *de novo* Th1 and Th2 cytokines following activation [56]. By contrast, we found no differences in CD4+ Th lymphocyte responses between LABC patients and HFDs. Moreover, the CD8+ Tc1 lymphocyte responses in LABC patients with respect to the synthesis of IL-2, TNF-α, IFN-γ, Tc2 lymphocytes that synthesized IL-4 and IL-10, and CD4+ T lymphocytes that synthesized IL-17 were comparable to the responses of Th lymphocyte subsets in HFDs. Hence, we did not observe any immune dysfunction or immunosuppression in LABC patients as assessed by the ability of TCR-activated CD4+ and CD8+ T lymphocytes to synthesize *de novo* cytokines [26].

Previous studies of the correlation between immune dysregulation and the expression of hormone receptors on the primary breast tumor have had conflicting results. Some have reported inverse correlations between immune dysregulation and Th1 cytokine responses [56] and lymphocyte proliferation [59] in breast cancer patients with hormone-receptor-positive tumors compared with lymphocyte function in patients with hormone-receptor-negative tumors [60].

Table 17.4 Intracellular cytokine syntheses by T-cell receptor-activated T-cell subsets

Cell type	Cytokine	Mean±SEM by patient group					Significant differences[a]
		LABC	IBC	MBC	MIBC	HFD	
No. patients		25	22	14	24	20	
%CD4+	IL-2	14.1±1.4	15.8±1.9	13.4±2.7	15.3±2.7	14.3±1.7	n.s.
	TNF-α	23.4±2.1	24.3±2.6	17.9±3.7	21.3±3	23.3±2.4	n.s.
	IFN-γ	10.4±1.2	11.2±1.6	8.5±2	9.8±1.4	9.1±1.2	n.s.
	IL-4	2.7±0.3	2.3±0.3	2.5±0.5	2.1±0.3	2.8±0.3	n.s.
	IL-10	4.9±0.7	5.6±1.1	3.7±0.5	6.3±0.9	6±1	n.s.
	IL-17	2.7±0.3	2.7±0.3	2.3±0.5	2.6±0.4	2.5±0.3	n.s.
%CD8+	IL-2	7.7±1.1	5.9±1.2	6.2±1.6	5.3±1.5	6.2±1.3	n.s.
	TNF-α	17.9±1.9	13.2±2	11.1±2.7	9.9±1.9	13.4±1.9	a, e
	IFN-γ	14±1.5	14.4±2.1	9.3±2	8.9±1.3	12.2±1.8	a, c
	IL-4	2.2±0.3*	1.3±0.3	1.2±0.2	0.9±0.1	1.4±0.2*	a, b, c, d, e, f
	IL-10	5±0.7	4.9±0.9	2.6±0.3*	4.2±0.8	5.2±0.8*	a, e, f
	IL-17	2.5±0.3*	1.8±0.4	1.3±0.3	0.9±0.1	1.1±0.2*	a, b, d, e, f

Data available on only 85 of 115 patients of this ongoing study. *SEM* standard error of the mean, *LABC* locally advanced breast cancer, *IBC* inflammatory breast cancer, *MBC* metastatic breast cancer, *MIBC* IBC with metastasis, *HFD* healthy female donors, *IL* interleukin, *TNF* tumor necrosis factor, *IFN* interferon

[a]Significant (p<0.05) pairwise comparisons: a, metastatic (MBC+MIBC) vs non-metastatic (LABC+IBC); b, IBC (IBC+MIBC) vs non-IBC (LABC+MBC); c, IBC vs MIBC; d, LABC vs IBC; e, LABC vs MBC; f, * indicates significantly different from HFD. n.s., no significant differences

17.2.8 Phenotypes of DC Subsets

DCs are the most potent antigen-presenting cells that are responsible for immune surveillance. When DCs detect a pathogen, they prime and regulate the adoptive immune response [61, 62]. There are at least two subsets of DCs in human peripheral blood, mDCs and pDCs [63]. The DC subsets do not express leukocyte-lineage-specific markers (lin-negative) and can be distinguished from one another based on their mutually exclusive expression of surface markers CD11c (mDC) and CD123 (pDC) using flow cytometry as previously reported [23, 64]. Generally, mDCs support the generation of Th1 responses, while pDCs prime predominantly Th2 responses.

Whereas pDCs in the peripheral blood are important for defense against viruses, mDCs are involved in the induction and maintenance of peripheral immune responses [65]. Upon encountering a virus, pDCs produce copious amounts of IFN-α to inactivate the virus, thereby playing a crucial role in innate immunity by providing a danger signal to the effector cells [66, 67]. pDCs also induce TR cells to produce IL-10 [68] and an immunosuppressive Th2 cytokine microenvironment, which in turn down-regulates the expression of the major histocompatibility complex class-I antigens and β2-microglobulin [69, 70], resulting in impaired function of intraepithelial antigen-presenting cells [71].

Ferrari et al examined the effects of chemotherapy on mDC and pDC subsets in the peripheral blood of advanced breast cancer patients [72]. They reported that the percentage of mDC and the mDC/pDC ratios in these patients before treatment were similar to those in HFDs but were significantly lower after chemotherapy. In our study, we examined the distribution of mDCs and pDCs in LABC, IBC, MBC, and MIBC patients and compared the results with those in HFDs. Our results were consistent with those of Ferrari et al [72], showing that the mean percentages of mDCs and pDCs in LABC, IBC, MBC, and MIBC patients were similar to those of HFDs. Hence, the stage of disease does not seem to affect the proportion of either DC subset.

However, previous studies indicate that there are differences in the mean number of mDCs and pDCs among different breast cancer patient subgroups and between patients and HFDs [24]. In our study, the median number of DC precursors was significantly lower in breast cancer patients than in HFDs (Fig. 17.2a). Moreover, the median number of mDCs in the peripheral blood of LABC, IBC, and MIBC patients was lower than the number of mDCs in the peripheral blood of HFDs (Fig. 17.2b). Because mDC and pDC subsets determine the type of Th1/Th2 or Tc1/Tc2 responses, our data suggest that Th1 and Tc1 responses would be compromised in patients with LABC, IBC, and MIBC. We observed a significantly lower median number of pDCs in IBC and MIBC patients than in HFDs, but the same was not true for the median number of pDCs in LABC and MBC patients compared with the number of pDCs in HFDs (Fig. 17.2c). These data suggest that Th2 and Tc2 responses may be lower in IBC and MIBC patients than in HFDs [24].

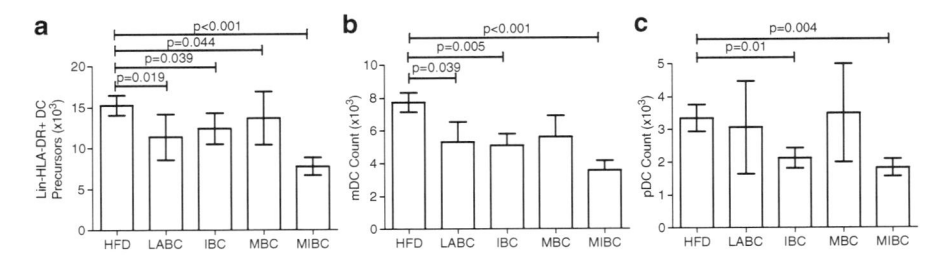

Fig. 17.2 Distribution of mean dendritic cell (DC) subset counts in breast cancer patient groups: *HFD* indicates healthy female donors, *LABC* locally advanced breast cancer, *IBC* inflammatory breast cancer; MBC, metastatic breast cancer, and *MIBC* metastatic inflammatory breast cancer. (**a**) Lin^neg^HLA-DR+DC precursors. (**b**) Myeloid-derived DCs (mDC). (**c**) Lymphoid- or plasmacytoid-derived DCs (pDC). *Horizontal lines* indicate significant differences between patient groups. *Vertical bars* within histograms indicate standard error of the mean

17.3 Summary and Future Direction

The most current data from this ongoing study suggest that patients with locally advanced IBC are immunocompetent, as evidenced by the normal distribution and function of T-lymphocyte subsets in their peripheral blood. However, in IBC patients who had developed metastasis, we found that the immunophenotype of the T-lymphocyte subsets had changed from a Th1 phenotype to a Th2 phenotype and that the T-lymphocyte response profile had deteriorated, as exemplified by the switch from the Th1 to the Th2 cytokine profile.

Using modern cellular techniques to assess different compartments of the immune system, we were able to produce a snapshot of the cellular immune parameters in IBC patients. In this chapter, we focused on the enumeration of leukocyte subsets, including T-lymphocyte subsets of the Th1/Tc1 and Th2/Tc2 phenotype, NK lymphocytes, and mDC and pDC subsets. We also evaluated the function of Th1/Tc1 and Th2/Tc2 T lymphocyte subsets *in vitro* using a flow cytometry technique of cellular cytokine staining and analysis that determines the phenotype and function at the single-cell level. We have confirmed earlier reports that IBC patients with locally advanced disease are not immunocompromised. We also demonstrated that IBC patients with metastasis have severe lymphopenia, signified by a reduction in the number of CD4+ Th lymphocytes; an inverted CD4/CD8 ratio; a reduction in the number of CD4+ Th lymphocytes that produce Th1 (IL-2, IFN-γ, TNF-α) cytokines; a reduction in IFN-γ+CD8+ Tc1 lymphocytes, resulting in a predominant Th2/Tc2 profile; and a significant decrease in CD19+ B lymphocytes. These results indicate that IBC with metastatic disease would be severely immunocompromised and thus would be susceptible to infection and a lower level of immune surveillance could facilitate additional metastasis.

Although the clinical and biologic features of IBC and LABC are quite different, the immunologic features are similar, except that IBC patients have lower percentages of TCR-activated CD8+ Tc2 and Tc17 lymphocytes than do LABC patients.

Overall, patients with IBC are immunologically competent, at least until they develop metastatic disease. It is unclear if the immune defects in IBC patients with metastatic disease contributed to the spread of disease or was the result of metastasis. Moreover, as patients with metastatic disease are likely to have been treated more extensively and more aggressively than patients with localized disease, the effect of treatment needs to be evaluated for its effect(s) on the immune system. This current study provided valuable information and suggested that monitoring and preserving immune function may be considered when giving therapeutic regimens to IBC patients. In addition, a longitudinal study to assess the natural history of immune responses in IBC patients is warranted to better understand the role of host immunity in disease progression of IBC.

References

1. Lee BJ, Tannenbaum NE (1924) Inflammatory carcinoma of the breast: a report of twenty-eight cases from the breast clinic of the Memorial Hospital. Surg Gynecol Obstet 39:580–595
2. Levine PH et al (1985) Inflammatory breast cancer: the experience of the Surveillance, Epidemiology, and End Results (SEER) program. J Natl Cancer Inst 74(2):291–297
3. Singletary SE et al (2002) Revision of the American Joint Committee on Cancer staging system for breast cancer. J Clin Oncol 20(17):3628–3636
4. Taylor G, Meltzer A (1938) Inflammatory carcinoma of the breast. Am J Cancer 33:33–49
5. Standish LJ et al (2008) Breast cancer and the immune system. J Soc Integr Onco 6(4):158–168
6. Zhang S, Zhang H, Zhao J (2009) The role of CD4 T cell help for CD8 CTL activation. Biochem Biophys Res Commun 384:405–408
7. Wolfram RM et al (2000) Defective antigen presentation resulting from impaired expression of costimulatory molecules in breast cancer. Int J Cancer 88(2):239–244
8. Khong HT, Restifo NP (2002) Natural selection of tumor variants in the generation of "tumor escape" phenotypes. Nat Immunol 3(11):999–1005
9. Voronov E et al (2003) IL-1 is required for tumor invasiveness and angiogenesis. Proc Natl Acad Sci USA 100(5):2645–2650
10. Grivennikov S, Karin M (2008) Autocrine IL-6 signaling: a key event in tumorigenesis? Cancer Cell 13(1):7–9
11. Szlosarek PW, Balkwill FR (2003) Tumour necrosis factor alpha: a potential target for the therapy of solid tumours. Lancet Oncol 4(9):565–573
12. Allan SE et al (2008) CD4+ T-regulatory cells: toward therapy for human diseases. Immunol Rev 223:391–421
13. Terabe M, Berzofsky JA (2008) The role of NKT cells in tumor immunity. Adv Cancer Res 101:277–348
14. Naiditch H, Shurin MR, Shurin GV (2011) Targeting myeloid regulatory cells in cancer by chemotherapeutic agents. Immunol Res 50(2–3):276–285
15. Liyanage UK et al (2002) Prevalence of regulatory T cells is increased in peripheral blood and tumor microenvironment of patients with pancreas or breast adenocarcinoma. J Immunol 169(5):2756–2761
16. Liu L et al (2008) CD4+CD25high regulatory cells in peripheral blood of cancer patients. Neuro Endocrinol Lett 29(2):240–245
17. Bates GJ et al (2006) Quantification of regulatory T cells enables the identification of high-risk breast cancer patients and those at risk of late relapse. J Clin Oncol 24(34):5373–5380

18. Levine PH et al (1981) Studies on the role of cellular immunity and genetics in the etiology of rapidly progressing breast cancer in Tunisia. Int J Cancer 27(5):611–615
19. Mourali N et al (1978) Rapidly progressing breast cancer (poussee evolutive) in Tunisia: studies on delayed hypersensitivity. Int J Cancer 22(1):1–3
20. Mosca PJ et al (2005) Immune monitoring. Cancer Treat Res 123:369–388
21. Cristofanilli M et al (2007) Inflammatory breast cancer (IBC) and patterns of recurrence: understanding the biology of a unique disease. Cancer Immunol Immunother 110:1436–1444
22. Jain N et al (2009) Synthetic tumor-specific breakpoint peptide vaccine in patients with chronic myeloid leukemia and minimal residual disease. A phase 2 trial. Cancer 115: 3924–3934
23. Naing A et al (2011) Phase I Dose Escalation Study of Sodium Stibogluconate (SSG), a Protein Tyrosine Phosphatase Inhibitor, Combined with Interferon Alpha for Patients with Solid Tumors. J Cancer 2:81–89
24. Gao H et al (2009) Immune profile of inflammatory breast cancer patients. In: Proc 32nd Annual San Antonio Breast Cancer Symposium, 2009, San Antonio, TX, Abstract # 4129
25. Cohen EN et al (2010) Innate immune profile of inflammatory breast cancer patients. In: Proc Am Assoc Cancer Res 101st Annual Meeting, Washington, DC, Abstract # 5583
26. Gao H et al (2010) T-cell cytokine production profile of breast cancer patients. In: Proc Am Assoc Cancer Res 101st Annual Meeting, 2010, Washington, DC, Abstract # 5589
27. Mandy FF, Nicholson JK, McDougal JS (2003) Guidelines for performing single-platform absolute CD4+ T-cell determinations with CD45 gating for persons infected with human immunodeficiency virus. Centers for Disease Control and Prevention. MMWR Recomm Rep 52(RR-2):1–13
28. McCluskey D et al (1983) T lymphocyte subsets in the peripheral blood of patients with benign and malignant breast disease. Br J Cancer 47:307–309
29. Lewinsohn DA, Gold MC, Lewinsohn DM (2011) Views of immunology: effector T cells. Immunol Rev 240:25–39
30. Sato M et al (1998) Impaired production of Th1 cytokines and increased frequency of Th2 subsets in PBMC from advanced cancer patients. Anticancer Res 18:3951–3955
31. Goto S et al (1999) Analysis of Th1 and Th2 cytokine production by peripheral blood mononuclear cells as a parameter of immunological dysfunction in advanced cancer patients. Cancer Immunol Immunother 48:435–442
32. Huster KM, Stemberger C, Busch DH (2006) Protective immunity towards intracellular pathogens. Curr Opin Immunol 18:458–464
33. Mosmann TR, Li L, Sad S (1997) Functions of CD8 T-cell subsets secreting different cytokine patterns. Semin Immunol 9:87–92
34. Mosmann TR et al (1997) Differentiation and functions of T cell subsets. Ciba Found Symp 204:148–154
35. Murta EF et al (2000) Lymphocyte subpopulations in patients with advanced breast cancer submitted to neoadjuvant chemotherapy. Tumori 86:403–407
36. Sewell HF et al (1993) Chemotherapy-induced differential changes in lymphocyte subsets and natural-killer-cell function in patients with advanced breast cancer. Int J Cancer 55: 735–738
37. Lissoni P et al (1990) Correlation of serum interleukin-2 levels, soluble interleukin-2 receptors and T lymphocyte subsets in cancer patients. Tumori 76:14–17
38. Lissoni P et al (1990) Changes in T lymphocyte subsets after single dose epirubicin. Eur J Cancer 26:767–768
39. Melichar B et al (2001) The peripheral blood leukocyte phenotype in patients with breast cancer: effect of doxorubicin/paclitaxel combination chemotherapy. Immunopharmacol Immunotoxicol 23:163–173
40. Baecher-Allan C et al (2001) CD4+CD25high regulatory cells in human peripheral blood. J Immunol 167(3):1245–1253
41. Shevach EM et al (2003) Control of T cell activation by CD4+CD25+ suppressor T cells. Novartis Found Symp 252:24–36

42. Suri-Payer E et al (1998) CD4+CD25+ T cells inhibit both the induction and effector function of autoreactive T cells and represent a unique lineage of immunoregulatory cells. J Immunol 160(3):1212–1218
43. Thornton AM, Shevach EM (1998) CD4+CD25+ immunoregulatory T cells suppress polyclonal T cell activation in vitro by inhibiting interleukin 2 production. J Exp Med 188(2):287–296
44. Hori S, Nomura T, Sakaguchi S (2003) Control of regulatory T cell development by the transcription factor Foxp3. Science 299(5609):1057–1061
45. Feuerer M et al (2009) Foxp3+ regulatory T cells: differentiation, specification, subphenotypes. Nat Immunol 10(7):689–695
46. Wang HY, Wang RF (2007) Regulatory T cells and cancer. Curr Opin Immunol 19(2):217–223
47. Mellios T, Ko HL, Beuth J (2010) Impact of adjuvant chemo- and radiotherapy on the cellular immune system of breast cancer patients. In Vivo 24(2):227–230
48. Gong Y (2008) Pathologic aspects of inflammatory breast cancer: part 2. Biologic insights into its aggressive phenotype. Semin Oncol 35(1):33–40
49. Resetkova E (2008) Pathologic aspects of inflammatory breast carcinoma: part 1. Histomorphology and differential diagnosis. Semin Oncol 35(1):25–32
50. Caligiuri MA (2008) Human natural killer cells. Blood 112(3):461–469
51. Cooper MA, Fehniger TA, Caligiuri MA (2001) The biology of human natural killer-cell subsets. Trends Immunol 22(11):633–640
52. Jacobs R et al (2001) CD56bright cells differ in their KIR repertoire and cytotoxic features from CD56dim NK cells. Eur J Immunol 31(10):3121–3127
53. Nagler A et al (1989) Comparative studies of human FcRIII-positive and negative natural killer cells. J Immunol 143(10):3183–3191
54. Nicolini A, Carpi A, Rossi G (2006) Cytokines in breast cancer. Cytokine Growth Factor Rev 17:325–337
55. Carpi A et al (2009) Cytokines in the management of high risk or advanced breast cancer: an update and expectation. Curr Cancer Drug Targets 9:888–903
56. Campbell MJ et al (2005) Immune dysfunction and micrometastases in women with breast cancer. Breast Cancer Res Treat 91:163–171
57. Goldberg JE, Schwertfeger KL (2010) Proinflammatory cytokines in breast cancer: mechanisms of action and potential targets for therapeutics. Curr Drug Targets 11(9):1133–1146
58. Gao H et al (2005) Imatinib mesylate suppresses cytokine synthesis by activated CD4 T cells of patients with chronic myelogenous leukemia. Leukemia 19(11):1905–1911
59. Kastelan M et al (1985) Lymphocyte reactivity to mitogens and tumor sex steroid receptors in breast cancer patients. Biomed Pharmacother 39(8):442–444
60. Elliott RL, Head JF, McCoy JL (1994) Comparison of estrogen and progesterone receptor status to lymphocyte immunity against tumor antigens in breast cancer patients. Breast Cancer Res Treat 30(3):299–304
61. Banchereau J, Steinman RM (1998) Dendritic cells and the control of immunity. Nature 392:245–252
62. Banchereau J et al (2000) Immunobiology of dendritic cells. Annu Rev Immunol 18:767–811
63. Rissoan MC et al (1999) Reciprocal control of T helper cell and dendritic cell differentiation. Science 283(5405):1183–1186
64. Ida JA et al (2006) A whole blood assay to assess peripheral blood dendritic cell function in response to Toll-like receptor stimulation. J Immunol Methods 310:86–99
65. Arpinati M et al (2003) Role of plasmacytoid dendritic cells in immunity and tolerance after allogeneic hematopoietic stem cell transplantation. Transpl Immunol 11(3–4):345–356
66. Cella M et al (1999) Plasmacytoid monocytes migrate to inflamed lymph nodes and produce large amounts of type I interferon. Nat Med 5(8):919–923
67. Siegal FP et al (1999) The nature of the principal type 1 interferon-producing cells in human blood. Science 284:1835–1837
68. Gilliet M, Liu YJ (2002) Human plasmacytoid-derived dendritic cells and the induction of T-regulatory cells. Hum Immunol 63:1149–1155

69. Cromme FV et al (1993) MHC class I expression in HPV 16-positive cervical carcinomas is post-transcriptionally controlled and independent from c-myc overexpression. Oncogene 8:2969–2975
70. Torres LM et al (1993) HLA class I expression and HPV-16 sequences in premalignant and malignant lesions of the cervix. Tissue Antigens 41:65–71
71. Rosini S et al (1996) Depletion of stromal and intraepithelial antigen-presenting cells in cervical neoplasia in human immunodeficiency virus infection. Hum Pathol 27:834–838
72. Ferrari S et al (2005) Flow cytometric analysis of circulating dendritic cell subsets and intracellular cytokine production in advanced breast cancer patients. Oncol Rep 14:113–120

Chapter 18
Angiogenesis and Lymphangiogenesis in IBC: Insights from a Genome-Wide Gene Expression Profiling Study

Peter B. Vermeulen, Gert Van den Eynden, Pascal Finetti, Daniel Birnbaum, Naoto T. Ueno, Patrice Viens, François Bertucci, Luc Y. Dirix, and Steven J. Van Laere

Abstract Inflammatory breast cancer (IBC) is an aggressive form of locally advanced breast cancer. Past molecular and morphological studies on cell lines, animal models and human tissue samples have unambiguously demonstrated that IBC is highly (lymph)angiogenic. Nevertheless, two vital questions remain unanswered: A. what is the role of the differential distribution of the molecular subtypes (particularly Luminal A) between IBC and nIBC in determining the observed difference in (lymph)angiogenesis and B. what are the exact molecular mechanisms that support angiogenesis in IBC? In this study, we aim to provide a clue for both questions by analyzing a gene expression data set of 137 IBC samples and 252 nIBC samples. In order to resolve the first question, a Gene Ontology analysis focusing

P.B. Vermeulen (✉) • G. Van den Eynden • L.Y. Dirix
Translational Cancer Research Unit, Oncology Center, General Hospital Sint-Augustinus, Wilrijk, Belgium

World IBC Consortium
e-mail: Peter.Vermeulen@GZA.be

S.J. Van Laere
Translational Cancer Research Unit, Oncology Center, General Hospital Sint-Augustinus, Wilrijk, Belgium

Department of Oncology, Catholic University Leuven, Leuven, Belgium

P. Finetti • D. Birnbaum • P. Viens • F. Bertucci
Département d'Oncologie Moléculaire, Centre de Recherche en Cancérologie de Marseille, UMR891 Inserm, Institut Paoli-Calmettes (IPC), Marseille, France

World IBC Consortium

N.T. Ueno, M.D., Ph.D., F.A.C.P.
Morgan Welch Inflammatory Breast Cancer Program and Clinic, Department of Breast Medical Oncology, The University of Texas, MD Anderson Cancer Center, Unit 1354, Holcombe Blvd. 1515, Houston, TX, USA

World IBC Consortium

N.T. Ueno and M. Cristofanilli (eds.), *Inflammatory Breast Cancer: An Update*, DOI 10.1007/978-94-007-3907-9_18, © Springer Science+Business Media B.V. 2012

on angiogenesis-related GO-terms was performed on the original data set and on the same data set after removing molecular subtype-specific variation in gene expression. In order to provide an answer to the second question, we identified angiogenesis-related IBC-specific genes that were subjected to Ingenuity Pathway Analysis. In addition, we focused part of our analysis on angiomiRs, microRNA-families that are known to regulate angiogenesis. Comparative analysis of all our data suggests that angiogenesis in IBC is not VEGFA-driven but is merely a consequence of a disturbed balance between proangiogenic and antiangiogenic factors, possibly involving PGF, TSP1 (THBS1) and the miR-221/-222-family. TSP1, a TGFβ-inducible gene that is upregulated in nIBC, is involved in the inhibition of angiogenesis, a process that also involves miR-221/-222. Therefore, we conclude that lack of inhibition of angiogenesis in IBC in conjunction with the increased expression of several angiogenesis-stimulating genes (PGF, mir-221/-222 gene targets) results in increased levels of angiogenesis-related histomorphometrical parameters in IBC.

Keywords Microarray • Affymetrix • Angiogenesis • Lymphangiogenesis • Molecular subtypes • MicroRNAs • Angiomirs • Placental growth factor • Gene ontology • Trombospondin • Gene set enrichment analysis • Ingenuity pathway analysis

18.1   Introduction

Inflammatory breast cancer (IBC) is an aggressive form of locally advanced breast cancer with specific clinicopathological characteristics. One of the pathological hallmarks is the presence of tumour emboli in dermal and parenchymal lymph vessels, although the absence of tumour emboli is not sufficient to rule out the diagnosis. In one study, tumour emboli were found in 34 out of 35 cases (97%) [1].

The tumour emboli are by many regarded as the exponent of the aggressive behaviour observed in IBC. Recent studies have shown that both in patient samples and in the MARY-X model, a stable serial transplantable xenograft, the tumour emboli can be regarded as a stem cell niche [2, 3] and as such the tumour emboli may harbour the molecular traits necessary for therapy resistance. The overexpression of E-Cadherin protein by IBC tumour cells, albeit contra-intuitive as E-Cadherin is widely regarded as a tumour- and metastasis-suppressor, accounts for the formation of this lymphovascular embolus. Recently, the paradoxal overexpression of E-Cadherin by IBC tumour cells has been explained in terms of altered E-Cadherin trafficking, mediated by increased ExoC5 and decreased RAB27 and HRS expression [4]. Once inside the circulation, the tumour emboli might usurp the blood and lymph vessels as highways to spread rapidly throughout the breast gland, explaining the explosive local growth observed in patients with IBC [1]. The characteristic growth pattern of IBC, being tumour cell nests co-localized with tumour emboli and delineated by tumour-free skip zones, as well as and the highly metastatic nature associated with IBC can be explained as such [1].

The exact mechanism of how tumour emboli are formed remains unclear but two theories have been put forward: A. vascular homing of tumour cells or B. vasculogenesis driven by stem cells or tumour cells (i.e. vasculogenic mimicry). Recent data obtained by Mahooti and colleagues on the MARY-X mouse model suggests that the formation of the emboli results from a tumour emboli-induced endothelial differentiation of fibroblasts or myoepithelial cells, lending credit to the theory of vasculogenesis [5]. Either way, the formation of new blood and lymph vessels is a critical factor for both hypotheses.

Evidence from animal models and human samples suggest that IBC is characterized by extensive angiogenesis and lymphangiogenesis. The MARY-X mouse model demonstrates exclusive intravascular tumour growth, both in the primary subcutaneous tumour and in the lung metastases [6]. Vasculogenic mimicry was also observed in two other animal models, a naturally occurring canine inflammatory mammary carcinoma [7, 8] and WIBC9, a second stable serial transplantable xenograft [9, 10]. In case of WIBC9, vasculogenic mimicry was observed in conjunction with peripheral angiogenesis [9, 10]. To our knowledge, lymphangiogenesis has not been studied in these animal models.

Histomorphometrical and molecular analyses of angiogenesis on human tissue samples revealed that IBC, when compared to nIBC, is characterized by elevated microvessel density and elevated endothelial cell proliferation [11]. In addition, approximately 90% of the vessels in both IBC and nIBC are of the immature type [11]. One gene expression study of several angiogenic factors revealed a significantly elevated expression of Flt1, KDR, ANG1, TIE1, TIE2, COX2 and bFGF in IBC, from which COX2 and bFGF were confirmed by immunohistochemistry [12]. Although this study was performed using a limited number of samples, the results were corroborated by high-throughput gene expression profiling studies using both cDNA microarrays and RT-PCR [13, 14]. Histomorphometrical studies focusing on lymphangiogenesis in human tissue samples demonstrated that the fraction of proliferating lymphatic endothelial cells is about 3-fold higher in IBC as compared to nIBC, which strongly suggests ongoing lymphangiogenesis at a higher level in IBC [15]. At the molecular level, the lymphangiogenic factors VEGFC, VEGFD, VEGFR3, PROX1 and LYVE1 were all significantly overexpressed in IBC, corroborating the morphological results [15].

The purpose of this study is to evaluate angiogenesis and lymphangiogenesis in IBC at the molecular level using a gene expression data set of 137 IBC samples and 252 nIBC samples. The latter data set has been constructed by combining different smaller data sets available from research units participating in the IBC consortium. The advantage of using this data set resides in its sample size on the one hand, making statistical analysis more found and allowing for the detection of subtle differences with enhanced statistical power, and in the uniform definition of IBC on the other hand. Using gene ontology analysis, we aim to identify IBC-specific angiogenesis-related processes. In addition, we will evaluate the role of angiogenesis-related microRNAs, called angiomiRs.

18.2   Materials and Methods

18.2.1   Patients and Samples

Tumour samples were obtained from patients with breast adenocarcinoma treated in the Institut Paoli-Calmettes (IPC; Marseille, France), the MD Anderson Cancer Center (MDA; Houston, TX, USA) and the General Hospital Sint-Augustinus (SA; Antwerp, Belgium). Each patient gave written informed consent and this study was approved by the institutional review boards of all three participating centers. The present data set includes 137 samples from patients with IBC ($N_{IPC} = 71$, $N_{MDA} = 25$, $N_{SA} = 41$) and 252 samples from patients with nIBC ($N_{IPC} = 139$, $N_{MDA} = 58$, $N_{SA} = 55$). Patients with IBC were selected by strictly adhering to the consensus diagnostic criteria published by Dawood and colleagues [16]. The nIBC series was non-stage matched (Stage I: 65, Stage II: 97, Stage III: 66 and Stage IV: 24), and not biologically matched. Differences between IBC and nIBC were reported for ER expression ($P < 0.0001$) and age at diagnosis ($P = 0.002$) but not for ErbB2 exprssion ($P = 0.554$). RNA extraction and hybridization onto Affymetrix GeneChips (HGU133-series) were performed as described before [14, 17, 18]. For each of the three data sets separately, probe sets with expression values above log2(100) in at least 1% of the arrays were filtered in. Next, the list of common informative probe sets ($N = 9926$) was identified. This list was used to merge the distinct data sets. Therefore, we performed a regression normalization (limma-package) to remove technical, lab-specific, variation in gene expression between the distinct data sets. All subsequent data analyses were performed using BioConductor in R.

18.2.2   Angiogenesis-Directed Gene Ontology Analysis

Using gene set enrichment analysis (GSEA), all gene ontology terms with at least two genes in common with the informative gene list were analysed. Therefore we calculated an enrichment score (ES) for each term under analysis. Briefly, the list of informative genes was rank-ordered based upon the absolute value of the t-statistic obtained after performing a *t*-test comparing the relative gene expression levels between the groups of patients with and without IBC. Next, for each gene ontology term the positions of the genes belonging to that GO term in the rank-ordered vector were determined. In a second step, a score vector is created by assigning a value that equals the number of informative genes not represented in the gene ontology term to each gene present in gene ontology terms and vice versa. In a third step, a cumulative sum is calculated and the maximum value of this cumulative sum is considered as the enrichment score. As such, gene ontology terms with high numbers of differentially expressed genes associated with them will acquire high enrichment scores and vice versa. The final step was to compare the enrichment scores of the angiogenesis-driven GO terms (GO:0001525, GO:0001946, GO:0002040,

GO:0045765, GO:0045766, GO:0016525, GO:0060055 and GO:0002042) with the enrichment scores of the other GO terms. As the majority of the GO terms are expected not to be enriched for differentially expressed genes, they provide a good reference distribution against which the significance of the angiogenesis-driven GO terms can be assessed.

Next we assessed if the significant angiogenesis-related GO terms are associated with the difference between IBC and nIBC, regardless of the different distribution of the molecular subtypes between both tumour subtypes. Therefore, our data set of 389 samples was classified according to the molecular subtypes using the single sample predictor-method described by Hu and colleagues [19]. In addition, those samples classified as Claudin-low by the nine-cell line Claudin-low predictor [20] were considered as Claudin-low. Next, we corrected the relative gene expression data for molecular subtype-dependent differences using linear regression modeling. After the correction was performed, we recalculated the enrichment scores and reevaluated the significance of the angiogenesis-related GO terms as described above.

Finally, we focused on angiogenesis-related differences between IBC and nIBC at the level of individual genes and pathways. For that purpose, we performed a global test [21] for GO:0001525 on both the original data set and on the data set corrected for molecular subtype-specific differences. We chose to analyze GO:0001525 only as the other GO-terms are siblings from this parental term and as such they represent all genes of interest. The results obtained on the original data set and on the subtype-corrected data set were compared to identify IBC-specific angiogenesis-related genes. Four gene lists were generated: List A. all probe sets with an IBC-specific expression pattern, List B. all probe sets that remained significant after correcting the gene expression data for molecular subtype-specific variation, List C. all probe sets that gained significance after correcting the gene expression data for molecular subtype-specific variation and List D. all probe sets that lost significance after correcting the gene expression data for molecular subtype-specific variation. The identified gene lists were subjected to Ingenuity Pathway Analysis (IPA) to identify associated signal transduction pathways.

18.2.3   AngiomiR-Directed Analysis

Wang [22] and colleagues recently described 13 angiogenesis-related microRNA families (miR-17~92, miR-21, miR-31, miR-126, miR-130a, miR-210, miR-296, miR-378, miR-27b, let-7f, miR-15b/-16, miR-221/-222 and miR-320), collectively called angiomiRs. We evaluated the regulatory effect (RE) of these angiomiRs on the gene expression profiles of IBC and nIBC samples. Therefore, we calculated RE scores for each of these microRNAs and for each sample in our data set by averaging, per sample, the relative gene expression levels of the targets and non-targets [23]. Next, the average relative gene expression level of the targets was subtracted from the average relative gene expression level of the non-targets. A pronounced effect of the investigated microRNAs on the gene expression profile of one sample is exemplified by a lower expression of the mircoRNA-targets and, as such, by an elevated RE score. The RE scores were calculated both on the original data set and on the molecular subtype-corrected data set after which IBC was compared to nIBC.

Next, we aimed to identify relevant mRNA-targets for each of the angiomiR-families. This was done by inspecting three microRNA target databases (PicTar, Miranda and TargetScan) for relationships between the angiomiR-families and the genes annotated by GO:0001525 ("Angiogenesis"). A target was considered for further analysis when an angiomiR/target relationship was present in at least 2/3 databases. Next, we compared the targets with the gene lists containing genes with an IBC-specific expression pattern to identify common targets. For those angiomiRs having significant IBC-specific regulatory effects, a global test was performed on the identified angiogenesis-related targets.

Finally, we evaluated the relevant gene lists of angiomiR-targets using IPA in order to define their role in regulating signal transduction pathways. In addition, the relevant gene lists were compared with the gene lists obtained after the angiogenesis-directed Gene Ontology analysis to identify common themes. More specifically, we sought for signal transduction pathways that were enriched in the relevant angiomiR target gene list and in the lists of angiogenesis-related genes with an IBC-specific expression pattern (i.e. List A through C; *vide supra*), but not in the list of angiogenesis-related genes that lost their significance after correcting the gene expression data for subtype specific variation (i.e. List D; *vide supra*).

18.3 Results

18.3.1 Angiogenesis and Lymphangiogenesis-Directed Gene Ontology Analysis

A total of 11,120 GO terms were analysed. The highest ES was 973,844 and was observed for 104 processes. A total of 8 angiogenesis-associated GO terms were analysed in detail. Four of them ranked amongst the 10% most enriched GO terms (GO:0001525: ES=760,020, Rank=658, P=0.059; GO:0001946: ES=940,030, Rank=257, P=0.023; GO:0002040: ES=913,196, Rank=390, P=0.035; GO:0002042: ES=913,196, Rank=390, P=0.035). Figure 18.1a demonstrates the distribution of the ES of all analysed GO terms. The significant angiogenesis-related GO terms are indicated by coloured vertical lines. GO:0001525 is related to angiogenesis in general, GO:0001946 is related to lymphangiogenesis, GO:0002040 collects genes associated with the extension of new blood vessels from existing capillaries into avascular tissues by proliferation of endothelial cells and GO:0002042 defines genes associated with the orderly movement of endothelial cells into the extracellular matrix in order to form new blood vessels involved in sprouting angiogenesis.

In order to determine to what extent the angiogenesis-related differences between IBC and nIBC are molecular subtype-dependent, we removed molecular

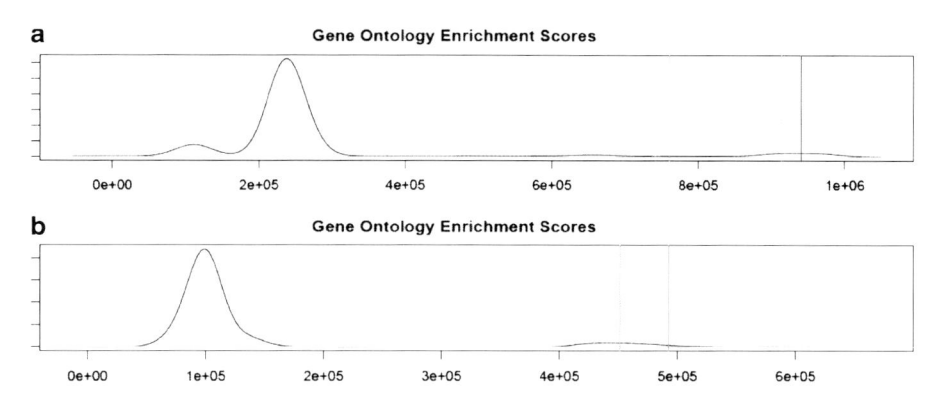

Fig. 18.1 Distribution of the enrichment scores in the original data set (**a**) and the subtype-corrected data set (**b**). The significant angiogenesis-related processes are indicated by *coloured vertical lines*: GO:0001946 in red, GO:0001525 in green and GO:0002040 and GO:0002042 in *yellow*. One can observe that both in the original data set and in the corrected data set, the enrichment scores for the indicated processes lie well outside the range of the enrichment scores for the bulk of the processes

subtype-specific variation in gene expression between IBC and nIBC using linear regression modelling and afterwards reanalysed the data as described before. The highest ES obtained after correction was 630,176, which is about 1.5-fold lower than the highest ES obtained prior to the correction, indicative of the removal of molecular subtype-specific variation in gene expression. The angiogenesis-related GO terms, enriched for differentially expressed genes between IBC and nIBC in our initial screen, remained highly enriched for differentially expressed genes after correction for the differential distribution of the molecular subtypes (GO:0001525: ES = 492,092, Rank = 136, P = 0.012; GO:0001946: ES = 451,500, Rank = 436, P = 0.039; GO:0002040: ES = 451,120, Rank = 444, P = 0.040; GO:0002042: ES = 451,120, Rank = 444, P = 0.040). Figure 18.1b demonstrates the distribution of the ES of all analysed GO terms after correction for the molecular subtype-specific variation.

To analyse angiogenesis-related differences between IBC and nIBC more qualitatively, we performed a global test on the original data set and the subtype-corrected data set for GO:0001525 only. As expected, the global expression pattern of angiogenesis-related genes is significantly associated with the tumour phenotype (IBC *vs.* nIBC) in both data sets (Original data set: Observed Q = 51.52, P < 0.0001; Subtype-corrected data set: Observed Q = 34.80, P = 0.0007). The gene plots for both analyses are provided in Fig. 18.2a and b respectively. In the original data set, 38 angiogenesis-related probe sets were associated with the difference between IBC and nIBC (FDR = 0.12). After correction for subtype-specific variation in gene expression, 29 angiogenesis-related probe sets, corresponding to 23 unique genes, remained significant (List A; FDR = 0.15). The genes are provided in Table 18.1 and were subjected to IPA. In addition, by comparing the global test results before and after molecular-subtype correction we broke down the list of 29 IBC-specific, angiogenesis-related probe sets (List A) in two smaller lists: A. the probe sets that

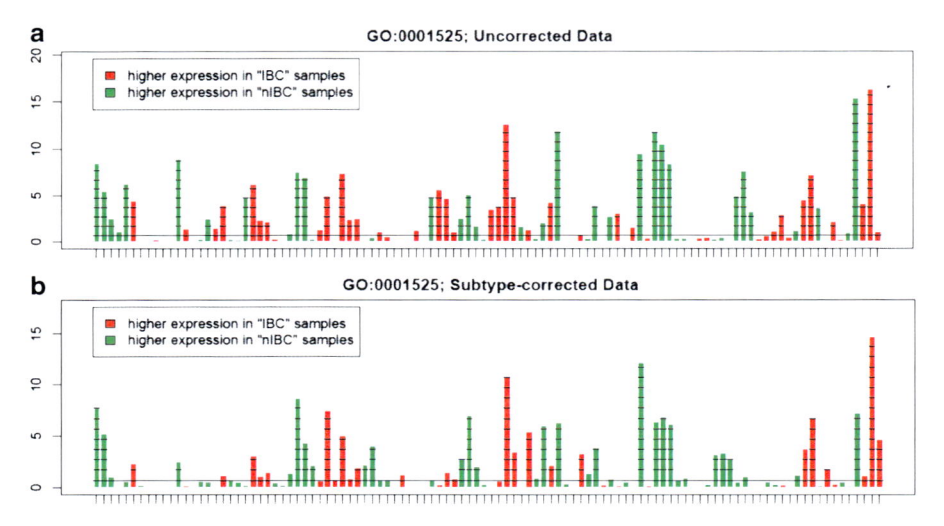

Fig. 18.2 Global tests for the gene set annotated in GO:0001525 ("Angiogenesis") on the original data set (**a**) and on the subtype-corrected data set (**b**). Each vertical bar denotes one gene, a *red bar* indicates a gene with a higher expression in IBC, a *green bar* denotes a gene with a higher expression in nIBC. The Y-axis represents the Z-score. A Z-score of more than 3 indicates a significant gene at an acceptable false discovery rate-level (i.e. ~15%). By comparing both plots we were able to identify angiogenesis-related genes differentially expressed between IBC and nIBC in a subtype independent manner

remained significant after correction (List B; N = 20) and B. the probe sets that gained significance after correction (List C); N = 9. Also the probe sets that lost their significance after correction (List D; N = 18) were identified. Ingenuity pathway analysis performed on List D revealed that IL8-, IL17A- and mTOR-signalling are not involved in IBC-specific angiogenesis. When comparatively analysing all identified gene lists, we sought to identify biological processes or signal transduction pathways enriched in lists A through C but not in list D. Several interesting pathways were identified including: "Inhibition of angiogenesis by TSP1", "TGFβ Signaling", "VEGF Signaling" and "Ephrin Receptor Signaling". Results for these pathways are provided in Table 18.2. Interestingly, most of the molecules associated with each of these pathways are overexpressed in nIBC, except for Placental Growth Factor (PGF), which was highly overexpressed in IBC. TSP1-mediated inhibition of angiogenesis was more pronounced in nIBC, corroborating the increase in angiogenesis observed morphologically in IBC. A diagram of the pathway is provided in Fig. 18.4.

18.3.2   AngiomiR-Directed Analysis

The effect of 13 angiomiR-families on the gene expression profiles of IBC and nIBC samples was evaluated using a RE score-analysis. The results are summarized in Table 18.3. Ten out of 13 (78%) angiomiR-families demonstrated differences in

Table 18.1 IBC-specific angiogenesis-related genes

Id	Symbol	Entrez gene nama	Location	Type	List
201511_at	AAMP	Angio-associated, migratory cell protein	Plasma membrane	Other	B
203935_at	ACVR1	Activin A receptor, type I	Plasma membrane	Kinase	B
218534_s_at	AGGF1	Angiogenic factor with G patch and FHA domains 1	Cytoplasm	Other	B
218671_s_at	**ATPIF1**	ATPase inhibitory factor 1	Cytoplasm	Other	C
211964_at	**COL4A2**	Collagen, type IV, alpha 2	Extracellular space	Other	B
209101_at	CTGF	Connective tissue growth factor	Extracellular space	Growth factor	B
201533_at	CTNNB1	Catenin (cadherin-associated protein), beta 1, 88 kDa	Nucleus	Transcription regulator	B
201289_at	CYR61	Cysteine-rich, angiogenic inducer, 61	Extracellular space	Other	C
210764_s_at	CYR61	Cysteine-rich, angiogenic inducer, 61	Extracellular space	Other	B
201809_s_at	**ENG**	Endoglin	Plasma membrane	Transmembrane receptor	B
216680_s_at	EPHB4	EPH receptor B4	Plasma membrane	Kinase	C
206295_at	**IL18**	Interleukin 18 (interferon-gamma-inducing factor)	Extracellular Space	Cytokine	B
205900_at	**KRT1**	Keratin 1	Cytoplasm	Other	B
206201_s_at	**MEOX2**	Mesenchyme homeobox 2	Nucleus	Transcription regulator	C
211926_s_at	MYH9	Myosin, heavy chain 9, non-muscle	Cytoplasm	Enzyme	C
219158_s_at	**NARG1**	N(alpha)-acetyltransferase 15, NatA auxiliary subunit	Nucleus	Transcription regulator	B
212676_at	NF1	Neurofibromin 1	Cytoplasm	Other	B
215179_x_at	**PGF**	Placental growth factor	Extracellular space	Growth factor	C
211711_s_at	PTEN	Phosphatase and tensin homolog	Cytoplasm	Phosphatase	B
204642_at	**S1PR1**	Sphingosine-1-phosphate receptor 1	Plasma membrane	G-protein coupled receptor	B
204150_at	**STAB1**	Stabilin 1	Plasma membrane	Transporter	B
38487_at	**STAB1**	Stabilin 1	Plasma membrane	Transporter	B
209909_s_at	TGFB2	Transforming growth factor, beta 2	Extracellular space	Growth factor	B
201108_s_at	TSP1	Thrombospondin 1	Extracellular space	Other	B
201109_s_at	TSP1	Thrombospondin 1	Extracellular space	Other	B
201110_s_at	TSP1	Thrombospondin 1	Extracellular space	Other	B

(continued)

Table 18.1 (continued)

Id	Symbol	Entrez gene nama	Location	Type	List
210513_s_at	VEGFA	Vascular endothelial growth factor A	Extracellular space	Growth factor	C
211527_x_at	VEGFA	Vascular endothelial growth factor A	Extracellular space	Growth factor	C
212171_x_at	VEGFA	Vascular endothelial growth factor A	Extracellular space	Growth factor	C

Genes upregulated in IBC are indicated in bold. In addition, for each gene its gene name, function and cellular localisation is provided. Finally, for each gene, the gene sublist (B or C) to which it belongs is indicated

Table 18.2 Ingenuity pathway analysis

Pathway	List A	List B	List C	List D	Genes
Inhibition of angiogenesis by TSP1	P=0.002	P=0.048	P=0.021	P=1.000	TSP1, VEGFA
VEGF signaling	P=0.012	P=1.000	P=0.001	P=0.111	**PGF**, VEGFA
TGFβ signaling	P=0.011	P=0.006	P=1.000	P=1.000	ACVR1, TGFβ2
Ephrin receptor signaling	P=0.004	P=1.000	P<0.001	P=0.201	**PGF**, EPHB4, VEGFA

Signal transduction pathways that are significantly enriched in some of the gene lists with IBC-specific genes (list A through C) but not in the gene list of genes that lost significance after correcting the data for molecular subtype-specific variation in gene expression (list D) are shown. For each pathway, the relevant P-value in the corresponding gene list is reported. The last column indicates the relevant angiogenesis-related genes. Genes upregulated in IBC are indicated in bold

Table 18.3 AngiomiR-directed analysis

Angiomir	Function	Re (uncorrected)	Re (corrected)	Direction	Relevant targets[a]	Reference
miR-17~92	Stimulation	0.0412	NS	No change	23/157 (15%)	[17]
miR-21	Stimulation	0.0235	NS	No change	12/157 (8%)	[17]
miR-31	Stimulation	NS	NS	No change	10/157 (6%)	[17]
miR-126	Stimulation	NS	NS	No change	1/157 (1%)	[17]
miR-130a	Stimulation	0.0571	NS	No change	34/157 (22%)	[17]
miR-210	Stimulation	0.0002	NS	No change	2/157 (1%)	[17]
miR-296	Stimulation	0.0174	0.1039	**Positive**	0/157 (0%)	[17]
miR-378	Stimulation	0.0023	NS	No change	8/157 (6%)	[17]
miR-27b	Stimulation	NS	NS	No change	24/157 (15%)	[17]
let-7f	Stimulation	0.0072	NS	No change	17/157 (11%)	[17]
miR-15b/ miR-16	Inhibition	0.0047	NS	No change	24/157 (15%)	[17]
miR-221/ miR-222	Inhibition	0.0001	0.0041	**Negative**	12/157 (8%)	[17]
miR-320	Inhibition	0.0002	0.0166	**Negative**	0/157 (0%)	[17]

Results from the RE analysis for the angiomiR-families. For each angiomiR-family (column 1), its function in angiogenesis (column 2) is reported together with the P-values resulting from comparing the RE between IBC and nIBC on both the uncorrected (column 3) and the subtype-corrected data set (column 4) and the direction of the RE in IBC relative to nIBC (column 5). The last column reports the number of angiogenesis-related angiomiR targets as a fraction of the total amount of genes present in GO-term GO:0001525 ("Angiogenesis")

RE Regulatory Effect, *NS* Not Significant

[a]Relevant targets were identified by intersecting an angiogenesis-related gene lists (GO:0001525) with the respective microRNA target gene list

their RE scores. After correction for molecular subtype-specific variation in gene expression, 3 angiomiR-families demonstrated an IBC-specific regulatory effect. The IBC-specific RE of these angiomiR-families is consistent with increased angiogenesis in IBC, as the angiogenesis-stimulating miR-296 has a positive regulatory effect on the gene expression profiles of the IBC samples and the angiogenesis-inhibiting miR-221/-222 and miR-320 have a negative regulatory effect on the gene expression profiles of the IBC samples.

For each of the analysed angiomiR-families, we sought to identify relevant mRNA targets by inspecting three databases (PicTar, Miranda and TargetScan) for relationships between the angiomiR-families and the genes represented by GO:0001525 ("Angiogenesis"). For most of the angiomiR-families, angiogenesis-related mRNA-targets could be identified (range: 0–22% of the genes associated with GO:0001525). Unfortunately, from the IBC-specific angiomiRs, only one family (miR-221/-222) was associated with any of the genes annotated by GO:0001525. The results are presented in Table 18.4. For the miR-221/-222 family, we identified two angiogenesis-related targets that have an IBC-specific expression pattern (STAB1: Mean IBC=6.643, Mean nIBC=6.309, P=0.003; NARG1: Mean IBC=8.237, Mean nIBC=7.876, P<0.0001). As expected, both targets are upregulated in IBC, which corroborates the negative regulatory effect of the miR-221/-222 family on the gene expression profile of a highly angiogenic tumor such as IBC. Furthermore, analysis of the miR-221/-222 target gene list with IPA identified the process "Inhibition of angiogenesis by TSP1" as the top ranked biological process (P=0.0003). We performed a global test on the set of miR-221/-222 angiogenesis-related targets to investigate if their combined gene expression profile is related to the difference between IBC and nIBC. Significant results were obtained both on the original data set (P=0.002) and on the subtype-corrected data set (P=0.007). The associated gene plots are provided in Fig. 18.3.

Finally, we evaluated the list of miR-221/-222 angiogenesis-related targets using IPA. Therefore, we compared the list of miR-221/-222 angiogenesis-related targets with the lists of IBC-specific angiogenesis-related genes obtained from the Gene Ontology-driven analysis. "Inhibition of angiogenesis by TSP1" demonstrated an interesting enrichment profile. It was not only enriched with genes belonging to the angiogenesis-related miR-221/-222 target gene list (*vide supra*), but also with angiogenesis-related genes having an IBC-specific expression pattern (Fig. 18.4). In contrast, those angiogenesis-related genes that lost their significance upon correction of gene expression data for molecular subtype-specific variation were not enriched for genes belonging to this process.

18.4 Discussion

In the past, several studies have unambiguously demonstrated that IBC is characterized by increased angiogenesis and lymphangiogenesis [11, 12, 15, 24]. Tissue sections from patients with IBC show a higher degree of vascularisation as compared to nIBC [11, 12]. In addition, the fraction of proliferating (lymphatic) endothelial cells is much more pronounced in IBC as compared to nIBC [11, 15]. Angiogenesis-directed gene expression profiling studies have pressed forward similar conclusions as numerous (lymph-)angiogenic molecules were expressed at a higher level in IBC [12, 15]. Despite these observations, the exact mechanisms by which angiogenesis

Table 18.4 AngiomiR targets

Angiomir	Targets	IBC-Specific targets
miR-17~92	ANGPTL4, AMOT, B4GALT1, CCBE1, COL4A3, **CYR61**, F3, EPAS1, HIF1A, NOX1, PLXDC1, ROBO4, SOX17, SRF, STAB1, TGFB2, APOLD1, TIE1, TYMP, HAND2, ANGPTL3, CSPG4, IL1B	3
miR-21	ARHGAP24, DICER1, IL1A, IL8, JAG1, NPPB, SRF, STAB1, TGFB2, THY1, TNFAIP2, SEMA5A	2
miR-31	APOH, AMOT, COL4A3, KLF5, S1PR1, SHB, THBS1, TNFAIP2, EPAS1, AGGF1,	2
miR-126	TGFB2	1
miR-130a	CDH13, PNPLA6, ANGPT1, ANGPTL3, AMOT, B4GALT1, CCBE1, **CYR61**, F3, DICER1, EPAS1, GHRL, HIF1A, IL8, JAG1, KLF5, LEPR, NOTCH1, NRP1, PLXDC1, PML, S1PR1, SERPINE1, SHB, SHH, SRF, TGFBR2, THBS1, THY1, TNFAIP2, ACVR1, CSPG4, C1GALT1, BTG1	4
miR-210	FGF9, TGFB2	1
miR-296	NA	0
miR-378	AGGF1, ANGPTL3, B4GALT1, BTG1, NRP1, TGFBR2, TYMP, **VEGFA**	2
miR-27b	ANGPT1, ADORA2B, ANGPTL4, APOH, F3, DICER1, ERAP1, GNA13, MAPK14, PF4, DLL4, VEGFC, TGFBR2, THBS1, TIE1, ACVR1, SERPINE1, COL4A2, PLCD3, **PGF**, C1GALT1, ROBO4, AGGF1, PKNOX1	5
let-7f	ANGPT2, COL15A1, AMOT, B4GALT1, FGF9, IL8, TNFRSF12A, NRP1, THBS1, TIE1, IL6, IL1B, STAB1, HAND1, PKNOX1, BTG1, EPAS1	2
miR-15b/ miR-16	COL15A1, ADRA2B, AMOT, ECSCR, FIGF, EPAS1, EREG, GPX1, HTATIP2, KDR, KRT1, KLF5, MAPK14, DLL4, PLG, PLXDC1, PML, TGFB2, THBS1, APOLD1, TNFAIP2, SH2D2A, PNPLA6, ERBB2, CXCL17, JAG1, PTPRM, SEMA5A, THY1	3
miR-221/ miR-222	KDR, NRP1, PML, STAB1, TGFBR2, GNA13, PLXDC1, ELK3, EPAS1, HIF1A, NARG1, SHB	2
miR-320	NA	0

For each angiomiR-family, the relevant angiogenesis-related targets have been reported. In regular type are the angiomiR-targets that are present in list B whereas in bold type are the angiomiR-targets that are present in list C. The last column identifies the number of IBC-specific angiomiR-targets
NA Not Applicable

is induced in IBC remains unknown. In addition, no study has yet addressed the possibility that the increase in angiogenesis observed in IBC might be confounded by the differential distribution of the molecular subtypes in IBC, in particular the low percentage of IBC tumours belonging to the Luminal A subtype (data not shown). Bertucci and colleagues have shown that angiogenesis-related processes are differentially expressed between the luminal- and basal-type of breast tumours [25]. In this study we have used gene expression profiles from 137 IBC samples, all diagnosed

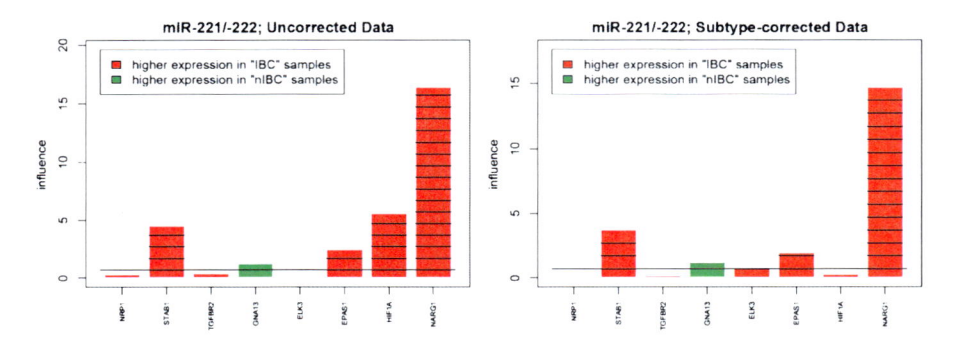

Fig. 18.3 Global tests for the angiogenesis-related targets of the miR-221/-222 family on the original data set (**a**) and on the subtype-corrected data set (**b**). Each vertical bar denotes one gene, a *red bar* indicates a gene with a higher expression in IBC, a *green bar* denotes a gene with a higher expression in nIBC. The Y-axis represents the Z-score. A Z-score of more than 3 indicates a significant gene at an acceptable false discovery rate-level (i.e. ~15%). The miR-221/-222 target gene family is globally overexpressed in IBC, which agrees with the angiogenesis-suppressive effects of the miR-221/-222 family and hence the pro-angiogenic effects of the miR-221/-222 target gene family

by strictly adhering to the consensus diagnostic criteria [16]. These IBC samples were compared with a series of 252 nIBC samples in order to detect molecular angiogenesis-related differences between IBC and nIBC.

In general, we observed that angiogenesis and lymphangiogenesis rank amongst those biological processes most strongly enriched for differential expressed genes, which corroborates the (lymph)angiogenesis-related difference between IBC and nIBC observed in previous studies. In addition, when correcting the gene expression data for molecular subtype-specific variation in gene expression, angiogenesis and lymphangiogenesis remained significantly different between IBC and nIBC. The major drawback about our analysis is that gene set enrichment analysis only takes into account absolute differences between groups and does not incorporate directionality into the result. Therefore, we aimed to investigate the differences between IBC and nIBC with respect to (lymph)angiogenesis more qualitatively. As the Gene Ontology database is structured hierarchically, we decided to focus only on the angiogenesis genes as all the other processes, and hence the associated genes, are represented in their parental term. We identified 29 angiogenesis-related genes that are differentially expressed between IBC and nIBC in a subtype-independent manner. This gene list consisted of 9 gene that gained significance after performing correction for molecular subtype-specific variation in gene expression and 20 genes that retained significance after correction for molecular subtype-specific variation. In addition, 18 genes were identified that lost significance upon correction of the gene expression data for molecular-subtype specific variation. The purpose of the latter gene list was to identify angiogenesis-related pathways that fail to show IBC-specificity. As such, IL8-, IL17A- and mTOR-signaling were ruled out as determinants of IBC-specific angiogenesis. We reasoned that processes that drive angiogenesis in an IBC-specific manner should be enriched in the lists with IBC-specific,

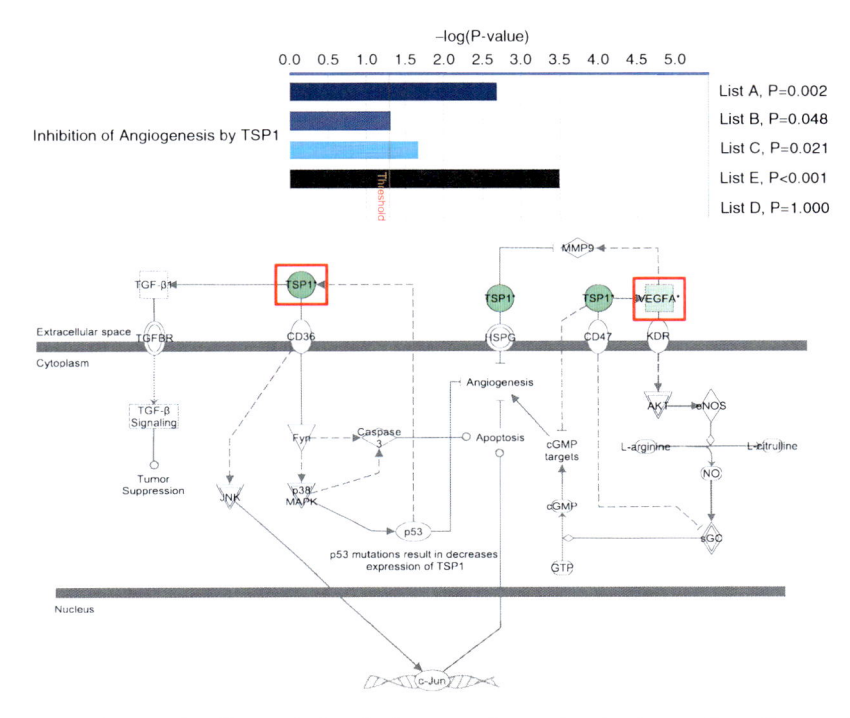

Fig. 18.4 Comparative IPA analysis of relevant angiogenesis-related gene lists. Twenty-nine angiogenesis-related genes with a molecular subtype-independent differential expression profile were identified (*dark blue*, list A). This gene list was broken down into a gene list of 20 genes that remained significant after performing the molecular subtype-correction (*blue*, list B) and a gene list of 9 genes that acquired significance after performing the molecular subtype-correction (*light blue*, list C). In addition, the list of genes that lost significance after performing the molecular subtype-correction (*grey*, list D) and the list of angiogenesis-related miR-221/-222 gene targets (list E, *black*) were also analysed. We focused on pathways that were significantly enriched in the gene lists A through C and E but not in the list D. One pathway, "Inhibition of angiogenesis by TSP1" demonstrated the required pattern. The P-values of enrichment are demonstrated in the bar chart, where the *orange line* denotes the threshold for significance. The nominal P-values are provided on top. A *grey bar* (for list D) is not present as this gene list was not enriched for genes belonging to this pathway. A diagram of the pathway is also provided with the relevant genes (TSP1 and VEGFA) colour-coded green (overexpressed in nIBC)

angiogenesis-related genes but not in the list of genes that lost significance upon correction of the gene expression data for molecular subtype-specific variation. Four interesting pathways, adhering to that pattern, were identified including "Inhibition of angiogenesis by TSP1", "TGFβ signaling", "VEGF signaling" and "Ephrin receptor signaling". Interestingly, most of the associated molecules, including VEGFA, were overexpressed in nIBC, except for PGF. Ephrin receptor signaling is involved in VEGFA-driven angiogenesis [26, 27, 28]. Therefore, these data suggest that angiogenesis in IBC is not VEGFA-driven, but other mechanisms apply. In a study by Van der Auwera and colleagues, VEGFA was not differentially expressed between IBC and nIBC. In fact, the median VEGFA-expression measured in a series of 16 IBC samples and 20 nIBC samples was higher in the nIBC samples [12]. An interesting observation is the increased expression of PGF in IBC. Yoo and colleagues demonstrated that PGF is excreted an IL1-dependent manner by fibroblast-like synoviocytes from patients with the inflammatory condition rheumatoid arthritis, creating a possible link between PGF-mediated angiogenesis and inflammation [29]. Oura and colleagues demonstrated that transgenic mice deficient for PGF have a reduced inflammatory response associated with attenuation of angiogenesis [30]. Interestingly, Carmeliet et al. have shown that a specific synergy exists between VEGFA and PGF in order to induce angiogenesis and that VEGFA actually depends on PGF to induce a specific set of angiogenesis related-target genes via KDR (VEGFR2) [31, 32]. As the matter a fact, pathological angiogenesis critically depended on the role of PGF and VEGFA-induced pathological angiogenesis was attenuated in the absence of PGF [33]. These observations suggest that the overexpression of VEGFA alone in nIBC is not sufficient to induce high levels of angiogenesis whereas in IBC the overexpression of PGF, potentially via inflammatory mediators, is the critical factor for inducing angiogenesis to the levels observed morphologically.

"Inhibition of angiogenesis by TSP1" as process was also enriched in the list of angiogenesis-related target genes of the miR-221/-222 angiomiR-family. The regulatory effect of this microRNA-family was more pronounced on the gene expression profiles of the nIBC samples. The miR-221/-222-family inhibits angiogenesis [22], suggesting that inhibition of angiogenesis is more pronounced in samples from patients without IBC. Our results also demonstrated that STAB1 and NARG1, two miR-221/-222 targets, are upregulated in samples from patients with IBC in a molecular subtype-independent manner. STAB1 or Stabilin-1, is a scavanger receptor that targets advanced glycation end products, such as SPARC, for endocytosis [34, 35]. SPARC is a known inhibitor of angiogenesis [36] and by targeting SPARC for endocytosis, STAB1 acts as a proangiogenic factor. To our knowledge, the role of NARG1 in angiogenesis has not been investigated thoroughly.

Altogether, our data suggest that the increase in the level of angiogenesis-related parameters observed in IBC results from a disturbed balance between proangiogenic factors (PGF, STAB1) and antiangiogenic factors (TSP1, miR-221/-222).

References

1. Vermeulen PB, van Golen KL, Dirix LY (2010) Angiogenesis, lymphangiogenesis, growth pattern, and tumor emboli in inflammatory breast cancer: a review of the current knowledge. Cancer 116(11 Suppl):2748–2754
2. Charafe-Jauffret E, Ginestier C, Iovino F, Tarpin C, Diebel M, Esterni B et al (2010) Aldehyde dehydrogenase 1-positive cancer stem cells mediate metastasis and poor clinical outcome in inflammatory breast cancer. Clin Cancer Res 16(1):45–55
3. Xiao Y, Ye Y, Zou X, Jones S, Yearsley K, Shetuni B et al (2011) The lymphovascular embolus of inflammatory breast cancer exhibits a Notch 3 addiction. Oncogene 30(3):287–300
4. Ye Y, Tellez JD, Durazo M, Belcher M, Yearsley K, Barsky SH (2010) E-cadherin accumulation within the lymphovascular embolus of inflammatory breast cancer is due to altered trafficking. Anticancer Res 30(10):3903–3910

5. Mahooti S, Porter K, Alpaugh ML, Ye Y, Xiao Y, Jones S et al (2010) Breast carcinomatous tumoral emboli can result from encircling lymphovasculogenesis rather than lymphovascular invasion. Oncotarget 1(2):131–147
6. Alpaugh ML, Tomlinson JS, Shao ZM, Barsky SH (1999) A novel human xenograft model of inflammatory breast cancer. Cancer Res 59(20):5079–5084
7. Peña L, Perez-Alenza MD, Rodriguez-Bertos A, Nieto A (2003) Canine inflammatory mammary carcinoma: histopathology, immunohistochemistry and clinical implications of 21 cases. Breast Cancer Res Treat 78(2):141–148
8. Clemente M, Pérez-Alenza MD, Illera JC, Peña L (2010) Histological, immunohistological, and ultrastructural description of vasculogenic mimicry in canine mammary cancer. Vet Pathol 47(2):265–274
9. Shirakawa K, Tsuda H, Heike Y, Kato K, Asada R, Inomata M et al (2001) Absence of endothelial cells, central necrosis, and fibrosis are associated with aggressive inflammatory breast cancer. Cancer Res 61(2):445–451
10. Shirakawa K, Kobayashi H, Sobajima J, Hashimoto D, Shimizu A, Wakasugi H (2003) Inflammatory breast cancer: vasculogenic mimicry and its hemodynamics of an inflammatory breast cancer xenograft model. Breast Cancer Res 5(3):136–139
11. Colpaert CG, Vermeulen PB, Benoy I, Soubry A, Van Roy F, van Beest P et al (2003) Inflammatory breast cancer shows angiogenesis with high endothelial proliferation rate and strong E-cadherin expression. Br J Cancer 88(5):718–725
12. Van der Auwera I, Van Laere SJ, Van den Eynden GG, Benoy I, van Dam P, Colpaert CG et al (2004) Increased angiogenesis and lymphangiogenesis in inflammatory versus noninflammatory breast cancer by real-time reverse transcriptase-PCR gene expression quantification. Clin Cancer Res 10(23):7965–7971
13. Bièche I, Lerebours F, Tozlu S, Espie M, Marty M, Lidereau R (2004) Molecular profiling of inflammatory breast cancer: identification of a poor-prognosis gene expression signature. Clin Cancer Res 10(20):6789–6795
14. Bertucci F, Finetti P, Rougemont J, Charafe-Jauffret E, Nasser V, Loriod B et al (2004) Gene expression profiling for molecular characterization of inflammatory breast cancer and prediction of response to chemotherapy. Cancer Res 64(23):8558–8565
15. Van der Auwera I, Van den Eynden GG, Colpaert CG, Van Laere SJ, van Dam P, Van Marck EA et al (2005) Tumor lymphangiogenesis in inflammatory breast carcinoma: a histomorphometric study. Clin Cancer Res 11(21):7637–7642
16. Dawood S, Merajver SD, Viens P, Vermeulen PB, Swain SM, Buchholz TA et al (2011) International expert panel on inflammatory breast cancer: consensus statement for standardized diagnosis and treatment. Ann Oncol 22(3):515–523
17. Van Laere S, Van der Auwera I, Van den Eynden G, Van Hummelen P, van Dam P, Van Marck E et al (2007) Distinct molecular phenotype of inflammatory breast cancer compared to non-inflammatory breast cancer using Affymetrix-based genome-wide gene-expression analysis. Br J Cancer 97(8):1165–1174
18. Iwamoto T, Bianchini G, Qi Y, Cristofanilli M, Lucci A, Woodward WA et al (2011) Different gene expressions are associated with the different molecular subtypes of inflammatory breast cancer. Breast Cancer Res Treat 125(3):785–795
19. Hu Z, Fan C, Oh DS, Marron JS, He X, Qaqish BF et al (2006) The molecular portraits of breast tumors are conserved across microarray platforms. BMC Genomics 7:96
20. Prat A, Parker JS, Karginova O, Fan C, Livasy C, Herschkowitz JI et al (2010) Phenotypic and molecular characterization of the claudin-low intrinsic subtype of breast cancer. Breast Cancer Res 12(5):R68
21. Goeman JJ, van de Geer SA, de Kort F, van Houwelingen HC (2004) A global test for groups of genes: testing association with a clinical outcome. Bioinformatics 20(1):93–99
22. Wang S, Olson EN (2009) AngiomiRs – key regulators of angiogenesis. Curr Opin Genet Dev 19(3):205–211
23. Van der Auwera I, Limame R, van Dam P, Vermeulen PB, Dirix LY, Van Laere SJ (2010) Integrated miRNA and mRNA expression profiling of the inflammatory breast cancer subtype. Br J Cancer 103(4):532–541

24. McCarthy NJ, Yang X, Linnoila IR, Merino MJ, Hewitt SM, Parr AL et al (2002) Microvessel density, expression of estrogen receptor alpha, MIB-1, p53, and c-erbB-2 in inflammatory breast cancer. Clin Cancer Res 8(12):3857–3862
25. Bertucci F, Finetti P, Cervera N, Charafe-Jauffret E, Buttarelli M, Jacquemier J et al (2009) How different are luminal A and basal breast cancers? Int J Cancer 124(6):1338–1348
26. Wang Y, Nakayama M, Pitulescu ME, Schmidt TS, Bochenek ML, Sakakibara A et al (2010) Ephrin-B2 controls VEGF-induced angiogenesis and lymphangiogenesis. Nature 465(7297): 483–486
27. Das A, Shergill U, Thakur L, Sinha S, Urrutia R, Mukhopadhyay D et al (2010) Ephrin B2/EphB4 pathway in hepatic stellate cells stimulates Erk-dependent VEGF production and sinusoidal endothelial cell recruitment. Am J Physiol Gastrointest Liver Physiol 298(6):G908–G915
28. Krasnoperov V, Kumar SR, Ley E, Li X, Scehnet J, Liu R et al (2010) Novel EphB4 monoclonal antibodies modulate angiogenesis and inhibit tumor growth. Am J Pathol 176(4):2029–2038
29. Yoo S, Yoon H, Kim H, Chae C, De Falco S, Cho C et al (2009) Role of placenta growth factor and its receptor flt-1 in rheumatoid inflammation: a link between angiogenesis and inflammation. Arthritis Rheum 60(2):345–354
30. Oura H, Bertoncini J, Velasco P, Brown LF, Carmeliet P, Detmar M (2003) A critical role of placental growth factor in the induction of inflammation and edema formation. Blood 101(2):560–567
31. Carmeliet P, Moons L, Luttun A, Vincenti V, Compernolle V, De Mol M et al (2001) Synergism between vascular endothelial growth factor and placental growth factor contributes to angiogenesis and plasma extravasation in pathological conditions. Nat Med 7(5):575–583
32. Autiero M, Waltenberger J, Communi D, Kranz A, Moons L, Lambrechts D et al (2003) Role of PlGF in the intra- and intermolecular cross talk between the VEGF receptors Flt1 and Flk1. Nat Med 9(7):936–943
33. Luttun A, Brusselmans K, Fukao H, Tjwa M, Ueshima S, Herbert J et al (2002) Loss of placental growth factor protects mice against vascular permeability in pathological conditions. Biochem Biophys Res Commun 295(2):428–434
34. Adachi H, Tsujimoto M (2002) FEEL-1, a novel scavenger receptor with in vitro bacteria-binding and angiogenesis-modulating activities. J Biol Chem 277(37):34264–34270
35. Tamura Y, Adachi H, Osuga J, Ohashi K, Yahagi N, Sekiya M et al (2003) FEEL-1 and FEEL-2 are endocytic receptors for advanced glycation end products. J Biol Chem 278(15):12613–12617
36. Chlenski A, Liu S, Guerrero LJ, Yang Q, Tian Y, Salwen HR et al (2006) SPARC expression is associated with impaired tumor growth, inhibited angiogenesis and changes in the extracellular matrix. Int J Cancer 118(2):310–316

Chapter 19
Microarray Analysis Identifies an Expression Signature for Inflammatory Breast Cancer

François Bertucci, Pascal Finetti, Max Chaffanet, Patrice Viens, and Daniel Birnbaum

Abstract The molecular bases of inflammatory breast cancer (IBC) are poorly elucidated. Gene expression profiling of small and heterogeneous series of clinical samples revealed the transcriptional heterogeneity of IBC, the existence of molecular subtypes similar to non-IBC (nIBC). Differences in gene expression between IBC and nIBC have been noted but, without gene overlap across the reported signatures. We have recently reported the first integrated analysis of IBC, combining analysis of DNA copy number alterations and RNA expression. We showed the genomic heterogeneity of the disease, and its genomic complexity and instability. We reported 24 potential IBC-specific candidate genes that could explain at least in part the IBC phenotype and/or breast cancer aggressiveness. In the future, larger series of IBC must be profiled calling for urgent international collaborations.

F. Bertucci (✉)
Department of Molecular Oncology, Marseille Cancer Research Center (CRCM), UMR891 Inserm, Institut Paoli-Calmettes (IPC), 232 Bd. Sainte-Marguerite, 13009 Marseille, France

Department of Medical Oncology, IPC, Marseille, France Université de la Méditerranée, Marseille, France
e-mail: bertuccif@marseille.fnclcc.fr

P. Finetti • M. Chaffanet • D. Birnbaum
Department of Molecular Oncology, Marseille Cancer Research Center
(CRCM), UMR891 Inserm, Institut Paoli-Calmettes (IPC), 232 Bd. Sainte-Marguerite, 13009 Marseille, France
e-mail: finettip@marseille.fnclcc.fr; chaffanetm@marseille.fnclcc.fr; daniel.birnbaum@inserm.fr

P. Viens
Department of Medical Oncology, IPC, Marseille, France

Université de la Méditerranée, Marseille, France
e-mail: viensp@marseille.fnclcc.fr

N.T. Ueno and M. Cristofanilli (eds.), *Inflammatory Breast Cancer: An Update*,
DOI 10.1007/978-94-007-3907-9_19, © Springer Science+Business Media B.V. 2012

Keywords Inflammatory breast cancer • Genomics • Microarray • Expression profiling • Array-comparative genomic hybridisation (array-CGH) • Prognosis • Survival

Abbreviations

CGH	comparative genomic hybridization
CNA	copy number alteration
DFS	disease-free survival
ER	estrogen receptor
GSEA	gene set enrichment analysis
IBC	inflammatory breast cancer
nIBC	non-IBC
PR	progesterone receptor
RT-PCR	reverse transcription-polymerase chain reaction
SAGE	serial analysis of gene expression
TNM	tumor node metastasis

19.1 Introduction

Inflammatory breast cancer (IBC) [1] is one of the most lethal forms of breast cancer because of its high metastatic potential [2]. Diagnosis is based on inflammatory clinical signs arising quickly, such as edema, redness, pain, and breast induration [2]. IBC is classified T4d in the TNM classification. The presence of tumor emboli in dermal lymphatics is a pathological hallmark of 50–75% of IBCs. Emboli are non-adherent cell clusters that rapidly spread by continuous passive dissemination [3], and favor both distant and local recurrences. Despite a multi-modality treatment [2, 4], the 3-year survival remains inferior to 50% [5].

Molecular mechanisms underlying IBC are poorly delineated [6, 7]. Analyses of clinical samples and experimental models (human cell lines and xenografts) have revealed that IBCs are more frequently estrogen receptor (ER) and progesterone receptor (PR) negative, ERBB2- and EGFR-positive, and frequently present P53 alterations and WISP3 loss-of-expression [8–14]. IBCs show high angiogenic and angioinvasive capacities and overexpress angiogenic factors [15]. Recently, a role for eIF4G1 has been suggested in the formation of tumor emboli, pointing to the importance of translation control in IBC [16].

High-throughput molecular analyses, developed in the late 1990s, allow the simultaneous analysis of several thousands of molecules in a tumor sample, at different molecular levels, including DNA for genomic profiling with comparative genomic hybridization (CGH) using array-CGH [17], RNA for gene expression profiling with DNA microarrays [18], differential display, SAGE, or multiplex quantitative RT-PCR [19], and proteins [20]. Gene profiling, successfully applied to non-IBC (nIBC) for more than 10 years, was recently applied to IBC, first at the mRNA level, and very recently at the DNA and RNA levels simultaneously. The main goal was to better define the differences between IBC and nIBC. These studies are summarized in the two next sections.

19.2 Expression Profiling of IBC

Gene expression profiling was the first high-throughput approach applied to IBC.

19.2.1 Analysis of Breast Cancer Cell Lines

The pioneering studies from the Ann Arbor's group used differential display to compare the expression profiles of IBC and nIBC cell lines and reported the frequent overexpression of *RHOC* and the underexpression of *WISP3* in IBC [8]. Further functional studies confirmed the role of these proteins in the IBC phenotype [9–12, 21–26].

19.2.2 Analysis of Clinical Samples

Following this initial work, other research groups profiled clinical samples of IBC [27–35] using DNA microarrays essentially. These studies, listed in Table 19.1, have been previously summarized [36]. They showed the feasibility of gene expression profiling from IBC biopsies. Due to their preliminary aspect and the scarcity of the disease, they suffered from some methodological imperfections due to the variety of the technological platforms or to the samples: small (37 IBCs for the largest one) and heterogeneous series with respect to the definition of IBC (clinical and/or pathological), the type of IBC samples (pre- or post-chemotherapy, with or without laser-capture microdissection), the stage of control nIBC samples, and the relative proportions of ER-positive and ER-negative samples in IBCs *vs*. nIBCs. However, they provided informative results. First, they revealed the great transcriptional heterogeneity of IBC, as extensive as that of nIBC, and the existence of the five major molecular subtypes previously described in nIBC. Subtypes displayed the same correlations with histoclinical features as in nIBC. However, basal and ERBB2-overexpressing subtypes were more represented in IBC. The existence of these subtypes in IBC reinforces evidence for the universality of this taxonomy in breast cancer, independently of a specific clinical form, and further suggests that IBCs and nIBCs originate from the same cell subtypes, and that these two characters (subtype and clinical form) are independent at the molecular level, determined by different gene sets.

Table 19.1 Gene expression profiling studies of IBC clinical samples

Ref.	Technological platform	RNAs	IBC definition	Sample	IBC	NIBC	Analyses	Gene expression signature of IBC	Independent validation
[27, 28]	Home-made cDNA microarray	~8.000	Clinical and/or pathological	Whole tissue – before CT	37	44	Whole-genome unsupervised – supervised – molecular subtypes	109 genes	Same study and Boersma's study
[34]	Home-made cDNA microarray	~6.000	Clinical	Whole tissue – before CT	16	18	Whole-genome unsupervised – supervised – molecular subtypes	756 genes	Same study
[33]	Affymetrix oligonucleotide microarray U133+2.0	~40.000	Clinical	Whole tissue – before CT	19	40	Whole-genome unsupervised – supervised – molecular subtypes	1,794 genes	No
[29]	qRT-PCR	538	Clinical	Whole tissue – before CT	36	22	Supervised	48 genes	Same study
[31]	Affymetrix oligonucleotide microarray U133+2.0	~40.000	Clinical and pathological	Whole tissue – before CT	14	23	Supervised	22 genes with little differences in expression	LOOCV
[32]	Affymetrix oligonucleotide microarray U133A	~20.000	Clinical	Whole tissue – before CT	13	12	Supervised – molecular subtypes	No robust signature	

| [30] | Affymetrix oligonucleotide microarray U133A | ~20.000 | Clinical and/or pathological | LCM (epithelium and stroma) – after CT | 15 | 35 | Whole-genome unsupervised – supervised | Little differences but more frequent in the stroma | No |
| [35] | Affymetrix oligonucleotide microarray U133A | ~20.000 | Clinical | Whole tissue – before CT | 25 | 57 | Supervised – IHC subtypes | No robust signature using all samples – signatures per subtype | No |

CT chemotherapy, *LCM* laser-capture microdissection, *LOOCV* leave-one-out cross-validation

Supervised analyses comparing IBCs and nIBCs were reported by four groups. They showed differences in gene expression level variable across studies with sometimes no or very subtle differences, and no gene overlap across the signatures. However, ontology analysis identified some functions commonly represented in at least two of the three tested signatures, such as "Cell Death", and "Molecular Transport" in IBC, and "Connective Tissue Development and Function", and "DNA replication, recombination and Repair" in nIBC.

19.3 Integrated Genome Profiling of Clinical IBC Samples

Overall, the first results of expression profiling remain to date rather inconclusive regarding the molecular differences between IBC and nIBC. Genome profiling may be used to determine DNA copy number alterations (CNAs) that sustain phenotypic and expression differences between the two phenotypes. However, in contrast to nIBCs [37–42], genomic imbalances of IBCs have not yet been analyzed by using high-throughput techniques such as high-resolution array-CGH or SNP-arrays. Similarly, whole-genome integrated studies that combine analysis of DNA CNAs and mRNA expression levels have provided interesting results in nIBCs [37, 42–44] but have not been applied to IBCs. We have recently reported the first study of this type [45]. The main results are summarized below.

19.3.1 Patients and Samples

We studied and compared DNA CNAs and mRNA expression deregulation on a whole-genome scale in a large series of IBCs and nIBCs. We profiled pre-chemotherapy frozen tumor samples collected from 197 patients with invasive adenocarcinomas, who underwent surgical biopsies or initial surgery at the Institut Paoli-Calmettes (IPC, Marseille, France) between 1987 and 2007. The 197 samples comprised 63 IBCs (surgical biopsies) and 134 nIBCs (removed tumors). IBCs were clinically defined as T4d. The control group (nIBCs) was not stage-matched, and included early (121 samples, including 68 with pathological axillary lymph node involvement).and locally-advanced (13 samples) stages. Patients were treated according to standard guidelines. Their main histoclinical characteristics are listed in Table 19.2. As expected, IBCs were associated with unfavorable prognostic features (younger age, higher grade, more frequent ER-negativity and ERBB2- and P53-positivity) and shorter survival than nIBCs. Our objective was the identification of IBC-specific candidate genes, simultaneously altered at the DNA and RNA levels.

Table 19.2 Histoclinical characteristics

Characteristics (N)	IBC N = 63 (%)	nIBC N = 134 (%)	p
Median age, years (range) (197)	48 (24–82)	56 (28–84)	1.26E-03
Pathological tumor size, pT (133)			
pT1	NA	31 (23%)	
pT2	NA	70 (53%)	
pT3	NA	32 (24%)	
Pathological axillary lymph node status, pN (133)			
Negative	NA	57 (43%)	
Positive	NA	76 (57%)	
Grade (190)			1.35E-12
1	0 (0%)	32 (24%)	
2	10 (17%)	62 (47%)	
3	48 (83%)	38 (29%)	
IHC ER status (197)			7.74E-03
Negative	33 (52%)	43 (32%)	
Positive	30 (48%)	91 (68%)	
IHC ERBB2 status (171)			2.16E-04
Negative	30 (61%)	107 (88%)	
Positive	19 (39%)	15 (12%)	
IHC P53 status (163)			5.82E-04
Negative	15 (35%)	79 (66%)	
Positive	28 (65%)	41 (34%)	
Molecular subtype (197)			5.08E-05
Basal	13 (21%)	25 (19%)	
ERBB2	13 (21%)	10 (7%)	
Luminal A	9 (14%)	63 (47%)	
Luminal B	15 (24%)	18 (13%)	
Normal	13 (21%)	18 (13%)	
Genomic pattern (173)			9.30E-04
Complex sawtooth	16 (33%)	23 (19%)	
Complex firestorm	27 (55%)	52 (42%)	
Simplex	6 (12%)	49 (40%)	
5-year MFS (191)	37%	80%	4.40E-10
5-year OS (181)	57%	84%	5.50E-11

NA, not assessable

19.3.2 Genome Profiling

From these 197 samples, DNA was available for 173, including 49 IBCs and 124 nIBCs. Genomic imbalances of the DNA samples were determined by using high-resolution 244K CGH microarrays (Hu-244A, Agilent Technologies, Massy, France). After filtering and normalization, the final dataset contained 225,388 unique probes covering 22,509 genes and intergenic regions according to the hg17/NCBI human genome mapping database (build 35). Our objective was the identification of genes

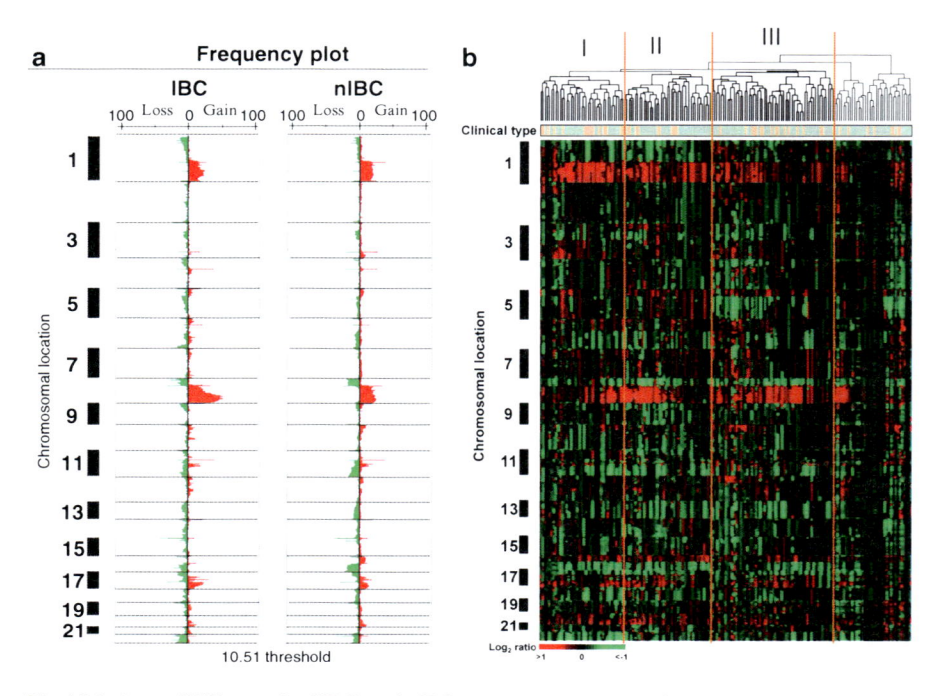

Fig. 19.1 Array-CGH portrait of IBCs and nIBCs. (**a**) Frequency plots of genome CNA. Frequencies (horizontal axis, from 0 to 100%) are plotted as a function of chromosome location (from 1pter to the top, to 22qter to the bottom), for IBCs (N = 49) and nIBCs (N = 124). *Horizontal lines* indicate chromosome boundaries. *Positive* and *negative* values indicate frequencies of tumors showing copy number increase and decrease, respectively, with gains (in *red*) and losses (in *green*). (**b**) Unsupervised hierarchical clustering of genome CNAs measured for 173 breast cancers on 225,388 probes (without X and Y). *Red* indicates increased DNA copy number gain and green indicates decreased copy number. The bars to the *left* indicate chromosome locations ordered like in **a**. The *vertical orange lines* define the three significant tumor clusters (I, II and III). Below the dendrogram, the row indicates the clinical type (*green* for nIBC, and *orange* for IBC)

with more frequent CNA in IBC than in nIBC. Two different threshold values of tumor/normal breast ratio distinguished low level CNAs (log_2 ratio > |0.5|) from high level CNAs (log_2 ratio > |1|).

The frequencies of CNAs, defined by the percent of tumors with a gain or a loss of a given chromosomal region, along each chromosome, were first compared. As shown in Fig. 19.1a, the genomic profiles were globally the same in the two phenotypes, with many similar altered regions and similar frequencies of alterations for most of them, except for some regions more frequently altered in IBC such as the gained 1q, 8q, and 17q regions. This result suggested that CNAs are globally similar, but more frequent for some of them in IBC. This similarity between IBC and nIBC according to their whole-genome profiles is shown in Fig. 19.1b. Clustering of all samples and all probes showed that IBCs were scattered across the three main robust clusters, intermixed with nIBCs, suggesting that, on a whole-genome scale at the DNA level, IBC is as heterogeneous as nIBC, and profiles are globally the same.

Then, we compared the genome stability of both phenotypes. DNA copy number patterns were classified as "simplex" (very few CNAs), "complex sawtooth" (many low-level CNAs), or "complex firestorm" (low-level CNAs and recurrent amplifications) according to a genomic classification [46, 47]. We found that complex patterns were more frequent in IBC (88%: firestorm 55% and sawtooth 33%) than in nIBC (60%: firestorm 42% and sawtooth 18%), whereas simplex patterns were less frequent (12% in IBC *vs.* 40% in nIBC). The median percentage of probe sets displaying a CNA per sample was 3.5% in the whole series, but was higher in IBCs (3.7%, range 0.01–14%) than in nIBCs (1.9%, range 0.01–26%), even if a great variability between samples existed for both phenotypes. Thus, the number and frequency of CNAs were more important in IBCs, clearly suggesting that the genome of IBCs is more unstable, in agreement with their high grade and frequency of *P53* mutations and their aggressiveness. This higher genome instability was further confirmed using gene expression data and Gene Set Enrichment Analysis (GSEA) with an expression signature of genome instability [48].

Then, we sought to identify genes with frequent CNA in IBCs. Frequencies were compared between the two phenotypes using the Fisher's exact test and false discovery rate (FDR) to correct for the multiple testing hypothesis ($p < 0.05$) [49]. A total of 321 genes were amplified in at least 10% of IBCs. They included validated or potential therapeutic targets such as *ANGPT1*, *ERBB2*, *FGFR1*, *GRB7*, *MYC*, *PAK1*, and *STK3*. Other targets such as *ADAM9* (6% of cases), *EGFR*, *FNTA*, and *IKBKB* (4%) were less frequently amplified, but sometimes at a very high level ($\log_2$ ratio > |1|). Conversely, 21 genes were deleted in at least 10% of IBCs. For comparison, many genes, such as the *FGFR1* and *CCND1* genes, were similarly amplified in IBCs and nIBCs in terms of frequency and amplitude. However, amplifications concerned ten times more genes in IBC (n=321) than in nIBC (n=26), with only 19 genes in common; deletions were less frequent in both phenotypes and concerned a similar number of genes (n=21 in IBC; n=16 in nIBC), with 14 genes in common. These results suggested that many more genes are frequently amplified in IBC, and that most of genes altered in nIBC are also altered in IBC.

We then tried to identify, among all altered genes (low or high level CNA), those with CNAs significantly more frequent in one phenotype. We found 628 significant genes, the majority (88%) of which was more frequently altered in IBC, in agreement with the genome instability. Examples include *ERBB2* and *MYC* that were more often amplified in IBCs, or the *RB1* tumor suppressor gene more frequently deleted. Several of the 628 genes code for validated or potential therapeutic targets, which could contribute to enlarge our therapeutic armament in IBC.

19.3.3 Genome and Expression Profiling

The second step was to search for, within these 628 significant genes, those that could be IBC-specific candidate genes, altered at both the DNA and RNA levels. Using whole-genome Affymetrix microarrays (HG-U133 Plus 2.0), we profiled the

63 IBC samples and the 134 nIBC samples. After filtering and normalization, the final dataset contained more than 20,000 probe sets representing more than 17,000 genes. The five molecular subtypes of nIBC were confirmed in our IBC series with 42% of samples being basal or ERBB2-overexpressing. Whole-genome hierarchical clustering confirmed the heterogeneity of IBCs, which were scattered across the different tumor clusters, intermixed with nIBCs.

Our aim was to identify the IBC-specific candidate genes, defined by expression deregulated in relation to CNA and differentially expressed between IBC and nIBC. We thus focused our integrated analysis on the 628 genes with CNA frequencies significantly different between the two phenotypes, and on the 173 tumors profiled on both platforms. Candidate genes had to satisfy three criteria: (i) frequencies of combined alterations (gain associated with overexpression *vs.* other combinations, and conversely, loss associated with underexpression *vs* other combinations) different (Fisher's exact test) between IBCs and nIBCs, (ii) correlation (Student *t*-test) between CNA and expression in the 173 samples, and (iii) expression different (Student *t*-test) between IBCs and nIBCs. In the first above-quoted step, overexpression and underexpression for a given gene were assigned using a threshold of |1| corresponding to twice the expression level found in a normal breast pool. We identified 24 IBC-specific candidate genes (Table 19.3). All were gained and/or amplified and overexpressed in IBC. Most of them were located in 8q22-24 and 17q21 regions, including known cancer-related genes such as *PABPC1*, *RAD21*, *ABCC3*, *SQLE*, or *PTPN2*. Whether these 24 genes are causative or predictive of the IBC phenotype in a biological sense or reflect aggressiveness or another associated phenomenon deserves to be explored by further functional analyses. They are involved in different functions: protein translation (*MRPL27*, *PABPC1*), RNA processing and transcription (*TAF2*, *ATAD2*, *ARID2*, *UTP23*; *INTS2*, *INTS8*), cell cycle (*RBM13/MAK16*, *TAF2*, *ATAD2*, *UTP23*, *MTBP*, *DSCC1*), cell migration (*PTPN2/TC-PTP*, *MTSS1*, *EPN3*, *C17orf37*), DNA repair (*RAD21*, *RAD54B*), in agreement with the hyperproliferative and invasive phenotype of IBC. Of note, some of these functions (protein processing, RNA translation, proliferation and lipid metabolism) have been previously reported as overrepresented among genes or pathways associated with IBC [30, 32]. One of these genes, *PABPC1*, has a link with eIF4G1, recently described as essential in the formation of emboli in IBC. PABPC1 is a poly(A)-binding protein (PABP) required for translation initiation. Its interaction with the translation initiation factor eIF4G is crucial for the translational stimulatory effect conferred by the poly(A) tail. In IBC, eIF4G1 reprograms the protein synthetic machinery for specifically increasing the translation of certain mRNAs, notably that encoding p120 catenin, resulting in an increased stabilization of E-cadherin, and that encoding VEGF [50]. E-cadherin stabilization maintains the structure of tumor emboli, allowing them to survive and to metastasize as entire structures. VEGF expression accounts for high levels of angiogenesis in IBC and resistance to hypoxia. Our result suggests that PABPC1 could also participate and potentiate this process, allowing IBC cells to adapt to the persistent hypoxia they experience as tumor emboli.

We validated this 24-gene signature by analyzing the 24 remaining breast tumors (14 IBCs and 10 nIBCs) only profiled on the Affymetrix platform. First, we derived

Table 19.3 Twenty-four candidate genes with gain or amplification correlated with overexpression showing significant frequency differences between IBCs and nIBCs

Symbol	Name	Cytoband
RBM13	RNA binding motif protein 13	8p12
RAD54B	RAD54 homolog B (S. cerevisiae)	8q22.1
KIAA1429	KIAA1429	8q22.1
INTS8	Integrator complex subunit 8	8q22.1
VPS13B	Vacuolar protein sorting 13 homolog B (yeast)	8q22.2
PABPC1	Poly(A) binding protein, cytoplasmic 1	8q22.3
C8orf53/UTP23	Chromosome 8 open reading frame 53	8q24.11
RAD21	RAD21 homolog (S. pombe)	8q24.11
TAF2	TAF2 RNA polymerase II, TATA box binding protein (TBP)-associated factor, 150 kDa	8q24.12
DCC1	Defective in sister chromatid cohesion homolog 1 (S. cerevisiae)	8q24.12
MTBP	Mdm2, transformed 3T3 cell double minute 2, p53 binding protein (mouse) binding protein, 104 kDa	8q24.12
WDR67	WD repeat domain 67	8q24.13
ATAD2	ATPase family, AAA domain containing 2	8q24.13
MTSS1	CDNA FLJ12372 fis, clone MAMMA1002446	8q24.13
SQLE	Squalene epoxidase	8q24.13
ST3GAL1	ST3 beta-galactoside alpha-2,3-sialyltransferase 1	8q24.22
ARID2	AT rich interactive domain 2 (ARID, RFX-like)	12q12
C17orf37	Chromosome 17 open reading frame 37	17q12
MRPL27	Mitochondrial ribosomal protein L27	17q21.33
LRRC59	Leucine rich repeat containing 59	17q21.33
EPN3	Epsin 3	17q21.33
ABCC3	ATP-binding cassette, sub-family C (CFTR/MRP), member 3	17q21.33
INTS2	Integrator complex subunit 2	17q23.2
PTPN2	Protein tyrosine phosphatase, non-receptor type 2	18p11.21

an IBC/nIBC genomic classifier from the expression data of the 24 genes in the 173 samples (learning set). When applied to the 24-sample validation set (Fig. 19.2a), the classifier correctly classified 75% of samples (10/14 IBCs and 8/10 nIBCs; $p = 0.03$, Fisher's exact test), suggesting its robustness. As additional indirect validation, we hypothesized that, if biologically relevant with respect to the IBC/nIBC distinction, our classifier might be prognostic in nIBC. We thus tested its prognostic value in a series of 1.781 nIBC, collected from five studies [51–55], and the UNC Microarray Database, Based on the classifier, each sample was attributed an "IBC-like" (338 samples) or "nIBC-like" profile (1,323 samples). These two classes displayed different survival (Fig. 19.2b) with a shorter 5-year disease-free survival (DFS) in the "IBC-like" class (61%) than in the "nIBC-like" class (73%; $p = 4.4.E-4$, log-rank test). This prognostic value in nIBC was confronted to that of classical prognostic features. In univariate analysis, the pathological lymph node status, tumor size, and grade, the ER status, and the signature-based classification were significant. Importantly, our IBC signature remained significant on multivariate analysis, suggesting an independent prognostic value in nIBC. This result indirectly validated the association of our classifier with IBC.

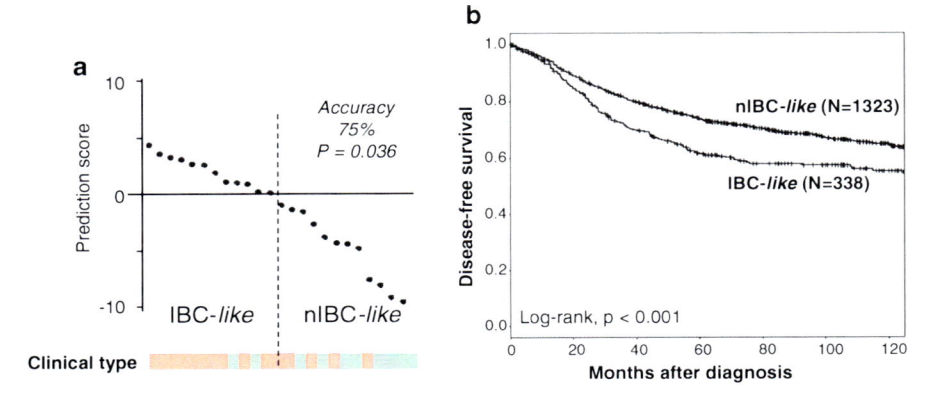

Fig. 19.2 Validation of the 24-gene signature and prognostic value in nIBCs. (**a**) Classification of 24 breast cancers (10 nIBCs and 14 IBCs) of the independent validation set. Samples are ordered from left to right according to the decreasing prediction score defined by the 24-gene model. The *vertical dashed line* indicates the threshold 0 that separates the "IBC-like class" and the "nIBC-like class". The clinical type is indicated under the curve (*green* for nIBC, and *orange* for IBC) (**b**) Kaplan-Meier DFS curves of the two nIBC classes (n = 1,781) defined in by the 24-gene classifier

In conclusion, this study provides the first large-scale and high-resolution repertoire of regions and genes altered at the DNA level in IBC. This repertoire may serve of basis for further studies. Our work also reveals the genomic heterogeneity of IBC, its genomic complexity and instability. It shows that differences between IBC and nIBC are not obvious at the DNA level, even if our analysis was not matched for the molecular subtype. Finally, the study reports 24 potential IBC-specific candidate genes that could explain at least in part the IBC phenotype and/or breast cancer aggressiveness, and which deserve further clinical and functional validation.

19.4   Discussion and Perspectives

We are just at the beginning of deciphering the genomics of IBC. The first work was reported by our group on December 2004, and before our last study, only a few small and heterogeneous studies were available in the literature. As discussed above, the results are rather disappointing regarding the transcriptional differences between IBC and nIBC, but these studies suffer from some methodological imperfections. Our last study reports the largest series of IBCs profiled using high-throughput genomic analytic tools. It is the first high-throughput array-CGH analysis of IBC and the first whole-genome integrated analysis comparing IBC *vs* nIBC. This original approach identifies a 24-gene signature, which does not rule out the likely existence of IBC-specific tumor suppressor genes inactivated by other mechanisms, nor the existence of a gene expression signatures identified by the sole comparison of whole-genome expression data.

Genomic analysis of the tumor, as explored with array-CGH and DNA microarrays, is only one determinant of cancer cell phenotype. Better understanding of IBC may come from the genomic analysis of tumor emboli, tumor microenvironment and host itself (polymorphisms for example), but also from the analysis of epigenetic alterations, gene mutations, microRNAs, or proteins. All these approaches are complementary. Their combination and confrontation in the future will be essential in understanding IBC and unraveling its molecular heterogeneity

Given the genomic complexity and heterogeneity of IBC, given its rarity and the low degree of gene differences observed with nIBCs globally, future studies should ideally compare IBC and nIBC phenotypes within molecular subtypes as recently suggested [35]. This supposes the analysis of large series of samples. To reach these objectives, progresses are ongoing in several directions. The possibility of profiling RNA extracted from formalin-fixed, paraffin-embedded tissues [56] is improving. The availability of data in public repositories will be also essential. But, one of the most important challenges relies in our ability to collect prospectively more IBC samples through international collaborations and using homogeneous selection criteria. This is a major objective of the IBC International Consortium that was set up during the first International Inflammatory Breast Cancer Conference in Houston on December 2008. We are currently analyzing an international series of 150 IBCs collected in Marseille, Houston and Antwerp. Larger series will allow also to address two major translational issues of IBC, which have been addressed by only two groups to date, but in small series and without any independent validation set : the prediction of response to primary chemotherapy [28] and the prognosis [29].

In conclusion, today, none of the genomic results has yet modified the clinical management of IBC, and the approach remains in the research field. Progresses are expected from the set up of international collaborations. The stakes are important, at the scientific, medical, and pharmaceutical levels, and could transform IBC management into a structured and logical science and a more successful medicine.

References

1. Hance KW, Anderson WF, Devesa SS, Young HA, Levine PH (2005) Trends in inflammatory breast carcinoma incidence and survival: the surveillance, epidemiology, and end results program at the National Cancer Institute. J Natl Cancer Inst 97:966–975
2. Singletary SE, Cristofanilli M (2008) Defining the clinical diagnosis of inflammatory breast cancer. Semin Oncol 35:7–10
3. Alpaugh ML, Tomlinson JS, Kasraeian S, Barsky SH (2002) Cooperative role of E-cadherin and sialyl-Lewis X/A-deficient MUC1 in the passive dissemination of tumor emboli in inflammatory breast carcinoma. Oncogene 21:3631–3643
4. Dawood S, Ueno NT, Cristofanilli M (2008) The medical treatment of inflammatory breast cancer. Semin Oncol 35:64–71
5. Woodward WA, Cristofanilli M (2009) Inflammatory breast cancer. Semin Radiat Oncol 19:256–265
6. Charafe-Jauffret E, Tarpin C, Viens P, Bertucci F (2008) Defining the molecular biology of inflammatory breast cancer. Semin Oncol 35:41–50

7. Houchens NW, Merajver SD (2008) Molecular determinants of the inflammatory breast cancer phenotype. Oncology 22:1556–1561
8. van Golen KL, Davies S, Wu ZF, Wang Y, Bucana CD et al (1999) A novel putative low-affinity insulin-like growth factor-binding protein, LIBC (lost in inflammatory breast cancer), and RhoC GTPase correlate with the inflammatory breast cancer phenotype. Clin Cancer Res 5:2511–2519
9. van Golen KL, Wu ZF, Qiao XT, Bao L, Merajver SD (2000) RhoC GTPase overexpression modulates induction of angiogenic factors in breast cells. Neoplasia 2:418–425
10. van Golen KL, Wu ZF, Qiao XT, Bao LW, Merajver SD (2000) RhoC GTPase, a novel transforming oncogene for human mammary epithelial cells that partially recapitulates the inflammatory breast cancer phenotype. Cancer Res 60:5832–5838
11. Kleer CG, Zhang Y, Pan Q, van Golen KL, Wu ZF et al (2002) WISP3 is a novel tumor suppressor gene of inflammatory breast cancer. Oncogene 21:3172–3180
12. Kleer CG, Zhang Y, Pan Q, Merajver SD (2004) WISP3 (CCN6) is a secreted tumor-suppressor protein that modulates IGF signaling in inflammatory breast cancer. Neoplasia 6:179–185
13. Huang W, Zhang Y, Varambally S, Chinnaiyan AM, Banerjee S et al (2008) Inhibition of CCN6 (Wnt-1-induced signaling protein 3) down-regulates E-cadherin in the breast epithelium through induction of snail and ZEB1. Am J Pathol 172:893–904
14. Zhang Y, Pan Q, Zhong H, Merajver SD, Kleer CG (2005) Inhibition of CCN6 (WISP3) expression promotes neoplastic progression and enhances the effects of insulin-like growth factor-1 on breast epithelial cells. Breast Cancer Res 7:R1080–R1089
15. Vermeulen PB, van Golen KL, Dirix LY (2010) Angiogenesis, lymphangiogenesis, growth pattern, and tumor emboli in inflammatory breast cancer: a review of the current knowledge. Cancer 116:2748–2754
16. Silvera D, Arju R, Darvishian F, Levine PH, Zolfaghari L et al (2009) Essential role for eIF4GI overexpression in the pathogenesis of inflammatory breast cancer. Nat Cell Biol 11:903–908
17. Pinkel D, Segraves R, Sudar D, Clark S, Poole I et al (1998) High resolution analysis of DNA copy number variation using comparative genomic hybridization to microarrays. Nat Genet 20:207–211
18. Phimister B (1999) The chipping forecast. Nat Genet 21(Supplement):1–60
19. Wittwer CT, Herrmann MG, Gundry CN, Elenitoba-Johnson KS (2001) Real-time multiplex PCR assays. Methods 25:430–442
20. Bertucci F, Birnbaum D, Goncalves A (2006) Proteomics of breast cancer: principles and potential clinical applications. Mol Cell Proteomics 5(10):1772–1786
21. Wu M, Wu ZF, Kumar-Sinha C, Chinnaiyan A, Merajver SD (2004) RhoC induces differential expression of genes involved in invasion and metastasis in MCF10A breast cells. Breast Cancer Res Treat 84:3–12
22. van Golen KL, Bao LW, Pan Q, Miller FR, Wu ZF et al (2002) Mitogen activated protein kinase pathway is involved in RhoC GTPase induced motility, invasion and angiogenesis in inflammatory breast cancer. Clin Exp Metastasis 19:301–311
23. Kleer CG, Griffith KA, Sabel MS, Gallagher G, van Golen KL et al (2005) RhoC-GTPase is a novel tissue biomarker associated with biologically aggressive carcinomas of the breast. Breast Cancer Res Treat 93:101–110
24. Kleer CG, van Golen KL, Zhang Y, Wu ZF, Rubin MA et al (2002) Characterization of RhoC expression in benign and malignant breast disease: a potential new marker for small breast carcinomas with metastatic ability. Am J Pathol 160:579–584
25. van Golen KL, Bao L, DiVito MM, Wu Z, Prendergast GC et al (2002) Reversion of RhoC GTPase-induced inflammatory breast cancer phenotype by treatment with a farnesyl transferase inhibitor. Mol Cancer Ther 1:575–583
26. Kleer CG, Zhang Y, Pan Q, Gallagher G, Wu M et al (2004) WISP3 and RhoC guanosine triphosphatase cooperate in the development of inflammatory breast cancer. Breast Cancer Res 6:R110–R115
27. Bertucci F, Finetti P, Rougemont J, Charafe-Jauffret E, Cervera N et al (2005) Gene expression profiling identifies molecular subtypes of inflammatory breast cancer. Cancer Res 65:2170–2178

28. Bertucci F, Finetti P, Rougemont J, Charafe-Jauffret E, Nasser V et al (2004) Gene expression profiling for molecular characterization of inflammatory breast cancer and prediction of response to chemotherapy. Cancer Res 64:8558–8565
29. Bieche I, Lerebours F, Tozlu S, Espie M, Marty M et al (2004) Molecular profiling of inflammatory breast cancer: identification of a poor-prognosis gene expression signature. Clin Cancer Res 10:6789–6795
30. Boersma BJ, Reimers M, Yi M, Ludwig JA, Luke BT et al (2008) A stromal gene signature associated with inflammatory breast cancer. Int J Cancer 122:1324–1332
31. Dressman HK, Hans C, Bild A, Olson JA, Rosen E et al (2006) Gene expression profiles of multiple breast cancer phenotypes and response to neoadjuvant chemotherapy. Clin Cancer Res 12:819–826
32. Nguyen DM, Sam K, Tsimelzon A, Li X, Wong H et al (2006) Molecular heterogeneity of inflammatory breast cancer: a hyperproliferative phenotype. Clin Cancer Res 12:5047–5054
33. Van Laere S, Van der Auwera I, Van den Eynden G, Van Hummelen P, van Dam P et al (2007) Distinct molecular phenotype of inflammatory breast cancer compared to non-inflammatory breast cancer using Affymetrix-based genome-wide gene-expression analysis. Br J Cancer 97:1165–1174
34. Van Laere S, Van der Auwera I, Van den Eynden GG, Fox SB, Bianchi F et al (2005) Distinct molecular signature of inflammatory breast cancer by cDNA microarray analysis. Breast Cancer Res Treat 93:237–246
35. Iwamoto T, Bianchini G, Qi Y, Cristofanilli M, Lucci A et al (2011) Different gene expressions are associated with the different molecular subtypes of inflammatory breast cancer. Breast Cancer Res Treat 125(3):785–795
36. Bertucci F, Finetti P, Birnbaum D, Viens P (2010) Gene expression profiling of inflammatory breast cancer. Cancer 116:2783–2793
37. Pollack JR, Sorlie T, Perou CM, Rees CA, Jeffrey SS et al (2002) Microarray analysis reveals a major direct role of DNA copy number alteration in the transcriptional program of human breast tumors. Proc Natl Acad Sci USA 99:12963–12968
38. Fridlyand J, Snijders AM, Ylstra B, Li H, Olshen A et al (2006) Breast tumor copy number aberration phenotypes and genomic instability. BMC Cancer 6:96
39. Loo LW, Grove DI, Williams EM, Neal CL, Cousens LA et al (2004) Array comparative genomic hybridization analysis of genomic alterations in breast cancer subtypes. Cancer Res 64:8541–8549
40. van Beers EH, Nederlof PM (2006) Array-CGH and breast cancer. Breast Cancer Res 8:210
41. Bergamaschi A, Kim YH, Wang P, Sorlie T, Hernandez-Boussard T et al (2006) Distinct patterns of DNA copy number alteration are associated with different clinicopathological features and gene-expression subtypes of breast cancer. Genes Chromosomes Cancer 45:1033–1040
42. Chin K, DeVries S, Fridlyand J, Spellman PT, Roydasgupta R et al (2006) Genomic and transcriptional aberrations linked to breast cancer pathophysiologies. Cancer Cell 10:529–541
43. Adelaide J, Finetti P, Bekhouche I, Repellini L, Geneix J et al (2007) Integrated profiling of basal and luminal breast cancers. Cancer Res 67:11565–11575
44. Andre F, Job B, Dessen P, Tordai A, Michiels S et al (2009) Molecular characterization of breast cancer with high-resolution oligonucleotide comparative genomic hybridization array. Clin Cancer Res 15:441–451
45. Bekhouche I, Finetti P, Adelaide J, Ferrari A, Tarpin C et al (2011) High-resolution comparative genomic hybridization of inflammatory breast cancer and identification of candidate genes. PLoS One 6:e16950
46. Geyer FC, Marchio C, Reis-Filho JS (2009) The role of molecular analysis in breast cancer. Pathology 41:77–88
47. Hicks J, Krasnitz A, Lakshmi B, Navin NE, Riggs M et al (2006) Novel patterns of genome rearrangement and their association with survival in breast cancer. Genome Res 16:1465–1479
48. Carter SL, Eklund AC, Kohane IS, Harris LN, Szallasi Z (2006) A signature of chromosomal instability inferred from gene expression profiles predicts clinical outcome in multiple human cancers. Nat Genet 38:1043–1048

49. Hochberg Y, Benjamini Y (1990) More powerful procedures for multiple significance testing. Stat Med 9:811–818
50. Silvera D, Schneider RJ (2009) Inflammatory breast cancer cells are constitutively adapted to hypoxia. Cell Cycle 8:3091–3096
51. Loi S, Haibe-Kains B, Desmedt C, Lallemand F, Tutt AM et al (2007) Definition of clinically distinct molecular subtypes in estrogen receptor-positive breast carcinomas through genomic grade. J Clin Oncol 25:1239–1246
52. Miller LD, Smeds J, George J, Vega VB, Vergara L et al (2005) An expression signature for p53 status in human breast cancer predicts mutation status, transcriptional effects, and patient survival. Proc Natl Acad Sci USA 102:13550–13555
53. van de Vijver MJ, He YD, van't Veer LJ, Dai H, Hart AA et al (2002) A gene-expression signature as a predictor of survival in breast cancer. N Engl J Med 347:1999–2009
54. van 't Veer LJ, Dai H, van de Vijver MJ, He YD, Hart AA et al (2002) Gene expression profiling predicts clinical outcome of breast cancer. Nature 415:530–536
55. Wang Y, Klijn JG, Zhang Y, Sieuwerts AM, Look MP et al (2005) Gene-expression profiles to predict distant metastasis of lymph-node-negative primary breast cancer. Lancet 365:671–679
56. Hoshida Y, Villanueva A, Kobayashi M, Peix J, Chiang DY et al (2008) Gene expression in fixed tissues and outcome in hepatocellular carcinoma. N Engl J Med 359:1995–2004

Chapter 20
Cell Gene Expression Signatures in Inflammatory Breast Cancer

Wendy A. Woodward

Keywords Gene expression • Microarray • Stem cells • IBC • Intrinsic subtypes • Aldefluor • CD44 • Claudin-low

Abbreviations

ALDH1	aldehyde dehydrogenase
AJCC	American Joint Committee on Cancer
DLI	dermal lymphatic invasion
ER	estrogen receptor
IBC	inflammatory breast cancer
IGS	invasive gene signature
NF-κB	nuclear factor–kappaB
RT-PCR	reverse-transcription polymerase chain reaction

20.1 Introduction

Since publication of the landmark report by Al-hajj et al. provocatively suggesting that breast cancers may be organized in a cellular hierarchy similar to that described for hematogenous malignancies [1], numerous studies have sought to characterize the small, undifferentiated fraction of cells at the top of the hierarchy purported to give rise to all of the others. It is speculated that if these cells are in fact responsible

W.A. Woodward, M.D., Ph.D. (✉)
Department of Radiation Oncology, The University of Texas
MD Anderson Cancer Center, Houston, TX, USA
e-mail: wwoodward@mdanderson.org

N.T. Ueno and M. Cristofanilli (eds.), *Inflammatory Breast Cancer: An Update*,
DOI 10.1007/978-94-007-3907-9_20, © Springer Science+Business Media B.V. 2012

for repopulating the tumor, the represent a critical target in cancer eradication. Many of the studies describing the phenotype of putative cancer stem cells suggest that they possess aggressive characteristics associated with treatment resistance, invasion, and metastases [2–5]. More recently, these cells have been described as most prevalent in tumors with poor prognostic features, including estrogen receptor (ER)–negative breast cancer, metaplastic breast cancer, and inflammatory breast cancer (IBC) [6–8]. Gene expression array analysis has become a valuable tool for grouping tumor types with similar features and prognosis and for elucidating the biology of specific subtypes. This chapter focuses on the progression of studies examining the gene expression profiles of IBC and the intersection of these efforts with similar work exploring the biology of cancer stem cells.

20.2 Inflammatory Breast Cancer

As well described elsewhere in this book, IBC is a clinically defined variant of breast cancer characterized by its presentation and associated with poor overall survival. The nomenclature "inflammatory breast cancer" was initially ascribed because of the swollen, erythematous, and edematous presentation of the breast, which shares some cardinal features of inflammation secondary to infection. While gene array and other studies may ultimately demonstrate a role for classic inflammatory pathways in IBC, it is important to recognize this moniker as somewhat of a misnomer, as no pathologic evidence of inflammation or infection is characteristic of IBC. While many unknowns remain in the etiology of the skin erythema and edema associated with IBC, most believe that the presence of tumor emboli in the dermal lymphatics as well as the diffuse distribution of the tumor cells within the breast parenchyma functionally obstruct the lymphatics, leading to the clinical sequelae of erythema and edema of the skin and breast. If, indeed, the propensity for migration through dermal lymphatics mediates the clinical presentation and outcome for this cohort, understanding the biology that mediates emboli migration and of the emboli themselves will likely be critical in understanding this disease. It might be said that a limitation of the published gene array studies in IBC to date is the inclusion of tissue samples likely to contain both tumor and breast stroma, but not explicitly focused on dermal emboli. Efforts to examine these cells by laser capture microdissection are ongoing, and the findings will be very interesting.

20.3 What Can We Learn from Cell Lines?

Although the value of cell line studies has been hotly debated by stem cell biologists, numerous studies have now demonstrated concordance between cell lines and patient samples, and while appropriate limitations are of course noted, it seems that many initial advances have been demonstrated in cell lines. To this end, Neve et al. recently reported a comprehensive comparison of the molecular and biological features of a collection of 51 breast cancer cell lines to those of primary breast tumors [9]. Importantly, this analysis showed that the cell lines display the same heterogeneity in copy number and expression abnormalities as the primary tumors, and they carry almost all of the recurrent genomic abnormalities associated with clinical outcome in primary tumors. The authors reported that breast cancer cell lines cluster into basal-like and luminal expression subsets, as do primary tumors, and the cell lines exhibit heterogeneous responses to targeted therapeutics, paralleling clinical observations.

Similar comprehensive examinations of putative cancer stem cell markers in cell lines have been undertaken by several authors [10–12]. Stuelten et al. examined multiple single markers and combinations in the NCI60 cell line panel and reported a complex pattern of expression largely clustered by tumor type rather than clonogenicity [12]. Charafe-Jauffret et al. characterized a panel of breast cancer cell lines by gene expression analysis and demonstrated clustering by aldefluor positivity vs negativity, although aldefluor positivity was also correlated with ER-negative status and specifically with basal/mesenschymal subtypes. Interestingly, the IBC cell lines in this analysis, SUM190 and SUM149, did not cluster together [10]. Fillmore et al. similarly demonstrated that a widely used putative stem cell marker, $CD44^+CD24^-$, distinguishes only basal subtype, not tumorigenicity, but they also showed that $CD44^+CD24^-ESA^+$ cells can prospectively isolate tumorigenic cells from cell lines, including SUM149 [11]. Overall, while the variability of markers in varying conditions and across cell lines makes interpretation of cell line results somewhat difficult, the use of cell lines has had a substantial impact on cancer research for years and seems a prudent place to begin to explore the expression profiles of IBC.

Human breast cancer has been classified into six subtypes based on gene expression profiling, and this system is believed to cluster patients based on similarities in the cells from which their tumors were derived [8, 13–15]. These six types are Luminal A, Luminal B, *Her2-neu* enriched, basal, normal-like, and claudin low. The claudin low subtype was identified most recently and is characterized by low expression of the genes encoding for tight junction proteins claudin 3, 4, and 7, E-cadherin, and a calcium-dependent cell-cell adhesion glycoprotein [14]. These subtypes have been reproduced across cell lines and animal models [8, 9, 16]; the two most widely used IBC cell lines, SUM-149 and SUM-190, fall into the basal subgroup [9, 14]. Interestingly, in an unsupervised analyses for intrinsic subtype by Prat et al., SUM149 and SUM190 segregated together [14]. No IBC cell lines fell into the claudin low subgroup, perhaps not surprisingly given the low E-cadherin status of this subgroup. Indeed, clinical sample analysis has revealed that the claudin low subtype is associated predominantly with metaplastic breast cancers [7, 14].

Two separate reports have suggested that the claudin low phenotype is most strongly associated with cancer stem cell–based array signatures. SUM159, a metaplastic cell line derived from a primary tumor, demonstrates a striking correlation with a gene signature associated with the claudin low phenotype, and expresses the cell surface markers shown to represent human mammary stem cells $CD49f^+/EpCAM^-$ [17]. This is perhaps a bit surprising given the strong data for stem cell phenotypes in IBC cell lines and samples [10, 17–19]. Interestingly, the SUM149

IBC cell line, which is classified in the basal subtype, is composed of two populations of cells, CD49f+/EpCAM- (a phenotype associated with stem cells in the normal mammary gland) and CD49f+/EpCAM+ (associated with progenitor cells of the normal human mammary gland). Gene array analysis of both populations revealed that the CD49f+/EpCAM- population shares a significantly greater correlation with the claudin low signature [14], potentially suggesting that IBC is maintained by the stem cell population but is not blocked from differentiation during progression. A separate study of the IBC cell line SUM149 also demonstrated two distinct populations—putative cancer stem cells vs. not—based on the flow cytometry ALDEFLUOR Kit assay for aldehyde dehydrogenase 1 (ALDH1) activity (STEMCELL Technologies, Vancouver, BC, Canada). Aldefluor expression correlated with tumor-initiation capacity in SUM149 cells, with successful outgrowths from 500 positive cells but not from 50,000 negative cells [20].

These authors described the same findings from the only reported IBC animal model to recapitulate the dermal lymphatic emboli characteristic of IBC, the Mary-X model. They also reported that ALDH1 expression in tumor cells from patient biopsies is correlated with poorer overall survival in IBC patients. Xiao et al. further evaluated the stem cell phenotype in IBC and reported that the lymphovascular embolus from the Mary-X model of IBC expresses a stem-like phenotype. They reported the expression of several previously reported stem cell surface marker profiles and demonstrated tumor recapitulation from as few as 100 cells derived from a Mary-X spheroid cell [21]. Together, these data suggest a stem cell phenotype in IBC, and highlight a role for therapies targeting cancer stem cells.

20.4 Gene Expression from IBC Patient Samples

While the rarity of IBC limits the prospects for large analyses of patent samples, several studies have examined gene expression signatures in tumors from IBC patients in an effort to identify a molecular determinant of this clinically variable disease [22–28]. Several issues independent of the technical considerations inherent in array-based studies challenge the development of such an IBC discriminator. The diffuse nature of IBC, which often presents without a dominant mass, makes it likely that the ratio of tumor to nontumor cells will differ between IBC and non-IBC biopsy specimens unless laser capture microdissection is performed. It remains unclear, furthermore, whether unselected non-IBC patients or stage-matched T4a-c non-IBC patients represent the ideal comparison group. Finally, the dominance of the basal subtype in the IBC cohort makes it difficult to distinguish IBC-specific signatures from those merely selecting for differences in subtype. Ultimately a rigorous signature would be expected to classify IBC vs. non-IBC basal cancers to clearly demonstrate independence from subtype.

Prior to the description of the claudin low subtype, two authors examined the prevalence of the four initially described intrinsic subtypes in patients with IBC [23, 28] and determined that while most IBC cancers are of the basal subtype, all subtypes are represented. Using DNA microarrays containing ~8,000 genes, Bertucci et al. profiled breast cancer samples from 81 patients, including 37 with IBC and 44 with non-IBC [23]. IBC cases were classified as such based on T4d staging by the American Joint Committee on Cancer (AJCC) criteria and/or the presence of dermal lymphatic invasion (DLI) on pathologic examination. The investigators did not mention the number of patients whose disease was not staged T4d but who were included on the basis of DLI, and it could be argued that this cohort should not be included. Global unsupervised hierarchical clustering was able to some extent to distinguish IBC and non-IBC cases (60% IBC cases in one main cluster and 31% in the other) and revealed subclasses of IBC; most of the IBC samples were of the basal subtype. Ultimately, basal and luminal gene clusters were the two most discriminating clusters in this portion of the analysis [23]. These authors then performed a supervised analysis that identified a 109-gene set whose expression discriminated IBC from non-IBC samples. This molecular signature was validated in an independent series of 26 samples, with an overall performance accuracy of 85%. Discriminator genes were associated with various cellular processes possibly related to the aggressiveness of IBC, including signal transduction, cell motility, adhesion, and angiogenesis.

Van Laere et al. performed a similar analysis using cDNA microarrays and ultimately identified ~8,500 informative genes in pretreatment tumor samples of 16 patients with IBC and 18 patients with non–stage-matched non-IBC [28]. IBC samples were staged as T4d according to the AJCC TNM classification. Unsupervised hierarchical clustering accurately distinguished IBC and non-IBC samples. A set of 50 discriminator genes was identified in a learning group of tumor samples and was successful in diagnosing IBC in a validation group of samples (accuracy 88%) (Table 20.1). Interestingly, although these authors noted a correlation between IBC samples and *ER*-negative/basal gene expression using the genes from the set of *Perou* et al. [13] that were available in their gene set, the authors reported that exclusion of *ER*-related or *HER2*-related genes did not alter this discriminatory accuracy, suggesting that expression of other genes in addition to *ER* and *HER2* characterizes the IBC phenotype. The molecular signature of IBC revealed overexpression of a large number of nuclear factor-kappaB (NF-κB) target genes, highlighting a potential target for IBC treatment [27].

Van Laere et al. further developed this analysis using an independent Affymetrix-based platform and reported on gene expression of 19 IBC and 40 non-IBC specimens subjected to clustering and principal component analysis [26]. This analysis included four samples from the previous study and after filtering left more than 18,000 informative genes. IBC vs. non-IBC principal component analyses revealed two clearly distinct groups, although the IBC global gene expression pattern was surprisingly more like that of non-IBC T1/T2 tumors than that of locally advanced non-IBC. The authors speculated that comparison to stage-matched non-IBC samples may be less valuable than to unselected cases. Cell-of-origin subtypes were formally examined using the full signatures for the first time, and this confirmed that all subtypes are represented in IBC, although 13 of 19 were of the basal or ErbB2 subtype. The 756 genes capable of discriminating IBC in the first study [28] were compared to this list, and the 739 genes common to both lists were examined

Table 20.1 Genes most often differentially expressed in three published data sets comparing IBC to non-IBC: blue [24], orange [29], green [28]. There is remarkably little overlap.

Symbol	Name
CALML4	Calmodulin-like 4
AKR1B10	Aldo-keto reductase family1, member B10
RAB3D	RAB3D, member RAS oncogene family
CLGN	Calmegin
AQP3	Aquaporin 3
PITPNC1	Phosphatidylinositol transfer protein, cytoplasmic 1
CKB	Creatine kinase, brain
CHST5	Carbohydrate (N-acetylglucosamine 6-O)sulfotransferase 5
	Similar to KIAA0563 gene product
TFCP2L1	Transcription factor CP2-like 1
G1P2	IFN-α–inducible protein (clone IFI-15 K)
PEX14	Peroxisomal biogenesis factor 14
GCHFR	GTP cyclohydrolase I feedback regulator
TAF6	TAF6 RNA polymerase II
	TATA box binding protein–associated factor
	Ribosomal protein S4-like (RPS4L)
RNF24	Ring finger protein 24
NCOR1	Nuclear receptor co-repressor 1
SULT1E1	Sulfotransferase family 1E, estrogen-preferring, member 1
SIAT7E	Sialyltransferase 7
ZNF496	Zinc finger protein 496
	EST
CHST12	Carbohydrate (chondroitin 4) sulfotransferase 12
Symbol	Name
JUN	Jun oncogene
EGR1	Early growth response 1 (Krox-24)
DUSP1	Dual specificity phosphatase 1 (CL100, MKP-1)
JUNB	Jun B oncogene
FOS	Fos oncogene
FOSB	Fos B oncogene
VEGF	Vascular endothelial growth factor
DTR/HB-EGF	Diphtheria toxin receptor/heparinbinding EGF-like growth factor
TBXA2R	Thromboxane A2 receptor
PTGS2/COX2	Prostaglandin-endoperoxide synthase 2/COX-2
IGFBP7	Insulin-like growth factor binding protein 7
IL6	Interleukin 6
NOS3	Nitric oxide synthase 3, endothelial (ENOS)
MAP3K8/COT	Mitogen-activated protein kinase kinase kinase 8
RASGRF1	Ras protein-specific guanine nucleotide-releasing factor 1
KAI1	Kangai 1 (CD82 antigen)
THBD	Thrombomodulin
PPARGC1	Peroxisome proliferative activated receptor, gamma, coactivator 1
ANGPT2	Angiopoietin 2
EREG	Epiregulin

(continued)

Table 20.1 (continued)

Symbol	Name
TNFRSF10A	Tumor necrosis factor receptor superfamily, member 10a
ROBO2	Roundabout homolog 2
CCL3/MIP1A	Chemokine (C-C motif) ligand 3
MYCN	N-myc oncogene
CCL5/RANTES	Chemokine (C-C motif) ligand 5
SNAIL1	Snail homolog 1
H19	H19, imprinted maternally expressed untranslated mRNA
MKI67	Proliferation-related Ki-67 antigen
ESR1/Erα	Estrogen receptor 1

Symbol	Name[a]
mt2	Metallothionein 2A
mtp	Microsomal triglyceride transfer protein
dj515n1	
p2y5	ILsophosphatidic acid receptor 6
ngk2d	
capl	S100 calcium binding protein A4
c1qb	Complement component 1, q subcomponent, B chain
apoer2	Apolipoprotein E receptor 2
flj10339	TBC1 domain family, member 12
ppp1a	Protein phosphatase 1, catalytic subunit, alpha isozyme
fgl2	Fibrinogen-like 2
rie2	Ring finger protein 10
kiaa0270	Paralemmin
pa28b	Proteasome (prosome, macropain) activator subunit 2
atp1b	ATPase, Na+/K+ transporting, beta 1
ugtrel1	Solute carrier family 35, member B1
cosmid r34382	
clone 24,700	
gs3686	Interferon-induced protein 44-like
lox1	Lysyl oxidase
ndp	Norrie disease (pseudoglioma)
ppic	Peptidylprolyl isomerase C (cyclophilin C)
chc11	
cdc25b	Cell division cycle 25 homolog B (S. pombe)
kiaa0218	
aclp	Adipocyte enhancer binding protein 1
pdgfa	Platelet-derived growth factor alpha
sgcg	Sarcoglycan, γ
hfe	Hemochromatosis
ctps	Cytidine 5'-triphosphate synthetase
col3a1	Collagen, type III, alpha 1
pim	Pim1 oncogene
dora	Immunoglobulin superfamily member 6
clone23785	

(continued)

Table 20.1 (continued)

Symbol	Name[a]
acvrl1	Activin A receptor type II-like 1
nubp1	Nucleotide binding protein 1
clone tua8	
ws2a	Waardenburg syndrome, type 2A
selplg	Selectin P ligand
1r20	Regulator of G-protein signaling 1
clone tua8	
grx	Glutaredoxin (thioltransferase)
ny-co-33	Teashirt zinc finger homeobox 1
pbf2	Complement factor B
kiaa0119	
fut1	Fucosyltransferase 1
ikap	IkappaB kinase complex-associated protein
mpp10	M-phase phosphoprotein 10
polr2g	Polymerase (RNA) II polypeptide G

[a]Gene names for this data set were identified using GeneCard

for independent platform validation. Unsupervised clustering revealed a group enriched for IBC patients: 12 of the 18 patients in the cluster had IBC. Part of the gene-expression differences between IBC and non-IBC were attributable to the differential presence of the cell-of-origin subtypes, since IBC primarily segregated into the basal-like or ErbB2-overexpressing group. Gene ontology analysis of the commonly overexpressed genes suggests that the insulin-like growth factor signaling pathway contributes to the biology of IBC. Validation of the previous findings regarding NF-κB signaling was less clear, since an NF-κB gene signature largely segregated the IBC samples into one group, but no clear overexpression of NF-κB genes was reported in the IBC signature derived from this study. The NF-κB signature ultimately seemed to separate ER-negative cases rather than cases of IBC.

Bieche et al. examined the largest group of IBC patients ($n = 37$) and compared their tumor gene expression to that of 22 stage II or III non-IBC tumor samples [29]. All tumors were clinically staged. These authors used real-time quantitative reverse-transcription polymerase chain reaction (RT-PCR) to quantify the mRNA expression of 538 selected genes in IBC relative to non-IBC. They reported that 27 (5.0%) of the 538 genes were significantly upregulated in IBC compared with non-IBC (Table 20.1). None were downregulated. The 27 upregulated genes mainly encoded for transcription factors (*JUN, EGR1, JUNB, FOS, FOSB, MYCN*, and *SNAIL1*), growth factors (*VEGF, DTR/HB-EGF, IGFBP7, IL6, ANGPT2, EREG, CCL3/ MIP1A*, and *CCL5/ RANTES*), and growth factor receptors (*TBXA2R, TNFRSF10A/TRAILR1*, and *ROBO2*). Factors previously reported to be differentially expressed in IBC, including *RhoC, E-cadherin*, and *Wisp3*, were not different in this dataset. Certainly, RT-PCR has a different sensitivity and dynamic range of mRNA detection than gene expression arrays and may give disparate results.

Using a different approach to match patients, Iwamoto et al. compared gene expression analyses of 25 T4d IBC patients and 57 stage-matched T4a-c non-IBC patients [30]. Fine-needle aspirations were performed prior to any therapy, and gene expression profiling was performed using the Affymetrix U133A gene chip. After filtering, ~19,000 genes were informative. Genes that were differentially expressed between IBC and non-IBC specimens were identified using the t-test, and differential expression of gene sets was assessed using gene set analysis. Three distinct clinical subtypes of IBC and non-IBC were compared: *ER* positive/*HER2* normal, *HER2* amplified, and *ER* negative/*HER2* normal. Unlike the prior reports, comparing expression data from all IBC and all non-IBC revealed no significant differences after adjusting for multiple testing. Further, none of the previously described IBC gene signatures effectively segregated these samples into IBC and non-IBC, possibly highlighting the inherent limitations of signatures based on small numbers as well as the heterogeneity in samples of IBC as defined clinically. Interestingly, when IBC and non-IBC tumors were compared by clinical subtype, significant differences emerged. The IBC metagene identified by Bieche et al. [29] was expressed at a significantly higher level in *ER*-positive/*HER2*-normal IBC than in non-IBC of the same phenotype, while the gene set identified by Bertucci et al. [22] was expressed at significantly higher levels in *HER2*-amplified IBC. Complement and immune system–related pathways were overexpressed in *ER*-positive/*HER2*-normal IBC. Protein translation and mTOR signaling were overexpressed in *HER2*-amplified IBC. Apoptosis-, neural-, and lipid metabolism-related pathways were overexpressed in *ER*- negative/*HER2*-normal IBC compared with non-IBC of the same receptor phenotype.

This was not the only study that did not find a clear signature in unsupervised analysis. Nguyen et al. compared 14 IBC samples (IBC was clinically defined as rapid-onset cancer associated with erythema and skin changes) to samples of 20 non-IBC stage III breast cancers, using the Affymetrix HG-U133A microarrays. Like the study by Iwamoto et al., this study found no significant differences at the individual gene level but observed some differences at the gene set level [31]. Gene expression analyses indicated that IBC had higher expression of genes associated with increased metabolic rate, lipid signaling, and cell turnover than non-IBC tumors.

A final study using the Affymetrix U133 platform examined the gene expression of 14 IBC and 26 stage II or III non-IBC [24]. IBC was defined as erythema covering more than 30% of the breast, breast edema, and DLI. The authors do not comment as to how many non-IBC patients met the clinical criteria without DLI (also appropriately classified T4d based on AJCC staging). Using a Bayesian statistical analysis to avoid false discovery, a binary regression model was generated to analyze the difference in IBC (yes vs. no) in this data set. Cross-validation using the leave-one-out prediction method revealed a set of 22 genes that characterized the phenotype of IBC (Table 20.1). Gene ontology analysis of the genes enriched in IBC revealed largely genes that encode for stromal proteins, including a variety of proteoglycans.

Overall, several studies have reported identification of an IBC-specific signature, but this appears to be highly variable and potentially related to selection of patients for the comparison, inclusion criteria for IBC, platform or approach used, and statistical rigor. The genes most frequently observed to be differentially expressed between IBC and non-IBC from publications that present this data are listed in Table 20.1. The enrichment of basal and ErbB2 subtypes in IBC tumors further complicates the statistical power in small studies. A larger study, ideally facilitated by the ongoing global collaborations in IBC, would potentially refine our understanding of this problem.

20.5 Stem Cell Signatures in IBC Gene Array Studies

While the reportedly stem-like claudin low subtype has not been clearly associated with IBC in the limited data examining this, several of the studies already discussed have also examined stem cell–based signatures in IBC vs. non-IBC comparisons and reported compelling enrichment in IBC samples consistent with the *in vitro* data described by numerous authors [10, 14, 20]. An *in vitro* study comparing the expression profile of Mary-X spheroids to signatures isolated from cultures enriched for putative stem cell markers (CD44+ immunosorted cells [32] and CD44+ mammospheres/neurospheres [33]) revealed three genes present in all three signatures: Complement component 1 (r subcomponent), Chitinase 3-like 1, and Notch homologue 3 [21]. Additional overexpressed genes were common in the Mary-X cells and one (as opposed to both) of the two stem cell–sorted signatures. These included genes involved in extracellular matrix, immunity, metabolism, and transcription, among others.

Iwamoto et al. examined the CD44+ signature [32] as well as a novel Wnt-based lung metastasis signature derived from the SUM1315 breast cancer skin metastasis–derived cell line [34] in the intrinsic subtypes in the analysis described in the previous section. They reported that the CD44+ stem cell signature had borderline significance, while the Wnt gene set was significantly overexpressed in *ER*-negative/*HER2*-normal IBC. Van Leare et al. provided an even more comprehensive comparison with stem cell signatures, examining seven published signatures derived from cells isolated on the basis [10, 32, 35–37]. Significant overexpression of six of these seven stem cell signatures was noted in the IBC samples relative to the non-IBC samples. Interestingly, these signatures were also largely associated with the basal or ErbB2 subtypes. Specifically examining the invasiveness gene signature (IGS) that distinguishes CD44+CD24− tumorigenic breast cancer cells vs. normal breast epithelium, the authors demonstrated that unsupervised clustering by IGS generated two clusters, one enriched for IBC samples (66%) and one enriched for non-IBC samples (92%). Furthermore, the gene expression profiles of the IBC samples were more significantly associated with the IGS signature. Similar centroid-mediated classification comparisons with the other stem cell signatures showed that 74% of IBC samples were expected to have a stem cell compartment [18]. Finally, comparing the list of genes differentially expressed between IBC and non-IBC in this study revealed significant overlap between the IBC gene set and most of the stem cell signatures, except for those not associated with breast cancer [18].

20.6 Conclusion

The clinical course of IBC, an aggressive disease associated with treatment resistance and poor outcome, strongly mirrors the expected hallmarks of a cancer stem cell–driven cancer. Both preclinical and clinical gene array studies support this association. While metaplastic, claudin low subtypes may represent disease related to the most primitive stem cells, IBC appears to share the biology associated with normal and cancer stem cells, strongly supporting the ongoing efforts to target IBC using anti–cancer stem cell therapies. While a definitive IBC signature remains elusive, overlaps in genes related to metabolism, extracellular matrix, and stem cell signaling are prevalent, and future larger studies taking intrinsic subtypes into account will certainly add significantly to the existing literature.

References

1. Al-Hajj M, Wicha MS et al (2003) Prospective identification of tumorigenic breast cancer cells. Proc Natl Acad Sci USA 100(7):3983–3988
2. Lacerda L, Pusztai L et al (2010) The role of tumor initiating cells in drug resistance of breast cancer: implications for future therapeutic approaches. Drug Resist Updat 13(4–5):99–108
3. Woodward WA, Chen MS et al (2005) On mammary stem cells. J Cell Sci 118(Pt 16):3585–3594
4. Woodward WA, Sulman EP (2008) Cancer stem cells: markers or biomarkers? Cancer Metastasis Rev 27(3):459–470
5. Xu W, Debeb BG et al (2010) Potential targets for improving radiosensitivity of breast tumor-initiating cells. Anticancer Agents Med Chem 10(2):152–156
6. Creighton CJ, Li X et al (2009) Residual breast cancers after conventional therapy display mesenchymal as well as tumor-initiating features. Proc Natl Acad Sci USA 106(33):13820–13825
7. Hennessy BT, Gonzalez-Angulo AM et al (2009) Characterization of a naturally occurring breast cancer subset enriched in epithelial-to-mesenchymal transition and stem cell characteristics. Cancer Res 69(10):4116–4124
8. Herschkowitz JI, Zhao W et al (2011) Breast cancer special feature: comparative oncogenomics identifies breast tumors enriched in functional tumor-initiating cells. Proc Natl Acad Sci USA June 1, PMID: 21633010
9. Neve RM, Chin K et al (2006) A collection of breast cancer cell lines for the study of functionally distinct cancer subtypes. Cancer Cell 10(6):515–527
10. Charafe-Jauffret E, Ginestier C et al (2009) Breast cancer cell lines contain functional cancer stem cells with metastatic capacity and a distinct molecular signature. Cancer Res 69(4):1302–1313
11. Fillmore CM, Kuperwasser C (2008) Human breast cancer cell lines contain stem-like cells that self-renew, give rise to phenotypically diverse progeny and survive chemotherapy. Breast Cancer Res 10(2):R25
12. Stuelten CH, Mertins SD et al (2010) Complex display of putative tumor stem cell markers in the NCI60 tumor cell line panel. Stem Cells 28(4):649–660
13. Perou CM, Sorlie T et al (2000) Molecular portraits of human breast tumours. Nature 406(6797):747–752
14. Prat A, Parker JS et al (2010) Phenotypic and molecular characterization of the claudin-low intrinsic subtype of breast cancer. Breast Cancer Res 12(5):R68
15. Sorlie T, Perou CM et al (2001) Gene expression patterns of breast carcinomas distinguish tumor subclasses with clinical implications. Proc Natl Acad Sci USA 98(19):10869–10874

16. Prat A, Perou CM (2010) Deconstructing the molecular portraits of breast cancer. Mol Oncol 5(1):5–23
17. Lim E, Vaillant F et al (2009) Aberrant luminal progenitors as the candidate target population for basal tumor development in BRCA1 mutation carriers. Nat Med 15(8):907–913
18. Van Laere S, Limame R et al (2010) Is there a role for mammary stem cells in inflammatory breast carcinoma?: a review of evidence from cell line, animal model, and human tissue sample experiments. Cancer 116(11 Suppl):2794–2805
19. Woodward WA, Debeb BG et al (2010) Overcoming radiation resistance in inflammatory breast cancer. Cancer 116(11 Suppl):2840–2845
20. Charafe-Jauffret E, Ginestier C et al (2010) Aldehyde dehydrogenase 1-positive cancer stem cells mediate metastasis and poor clinical outcome in inflammatory breast cancer. Clin Cancer Res 16(1):45–55
21. Xiao Y, Ye Y et al (2008) The lymphovascular embolus of inflammatory breast cancer expresses a stem cell-like phenotype. Am J Pathol 173(2):561–574
22. Bertucci F, Finetti P et al (2005) Gene expression profiling identifies molecular subtypes of inflammatory breast cancer. Cancer Res 65(6):2170–2178
23. Bertucci F, Finetti P et al (2004) Gene expression profiling for molecular characterization of inflammatory breast cancer and prediction of response to chemotherapy. Cancer Res 64(23):8558–8565
24. Dressman HK, Hans C et al (2006) Gene expression profiles of multiple breast cancer phenotypes and response to neoadjuvant chemotherapy. Clin Cancer Res 12(3 Pt 1):819–826
25. Van Laere SJ, Van den Eynden GG et al (2006) Identification of cell-of-origin breast tumor subtypes in inflammatory breast cancer by gene expression profiling. Breast Cancer Res Treat 95(3):243–255
26. Van Laere S, Van der Auwera I et al (2007) Distinct molecular phenotype of inflammatory breast cancer compared to non-inflammatory breast cancer using Affymetrix-based genome-wide gene-expression analysis. Br J Cancer 97(8):1165–1174
27. Van Laere SJ, Van der Auwera I et al (2006) Nuclear factor-kappaB signature of inflammatory breast cancer by cDNA microarray validated by quantitative real-time reverse transcription-PCR, immunohistochemistry, and nuclear factor-kappaB DNA-binding. Clin Cancer Res 12(11 Pt 1):3249–3256
28. Van Laere S, Van der Auwera I et al (2005) Distinct molecular signature of inflammatory breast cancer by cDNA microarray analysis. Breast Cancer Res Treat 93(3):237–246
29. Bieche I, Lerebours F et al (2004) Molecular profiling of inflammatory breast cancer: identification of a poor-prognosis gene expression signature. Clin Cancer Res 10(20):6789–6795
30. Iwamoto T, Bianchini G et al (2011) Different gene expressions are associated with the different molecular subtypes of inflammatory breast cancer. Breast Cancer Res Treat 125(3):785–795
31. Nguyen DM, Sam K et al (2006) Molecular heterogeneity of inflammatory breast cancer: a hyperproliferative phenotype. Clin Cancer Res 12(17):5047–5054
32. Shipitsin M, Campbell LL et al (2007) Molecular definition of breast tumor heterogeneity. Cancer Cell 11(3):259–273
33. Dontu G, Abdallah WM et al (2003) In vitro propagation and transcriptional profiling of human mammary stem/progenitor cells. Genes Dev 17(10):1253–1270
34. DiMeo TA, Anderson K et al (2009) A novel lung metastasis signature links Wnt signaling with cancer cell self-renewal and epithelial-mesenchymal transition in basal-like breast cancer. Cancer Res 69(13):5364–5373
35. Dontu G, Wicha MS (2005) Survival of mammary stem cells in suspension culture: implications for stem cell biology and neoplasia. J Mammary Gland Biol Neoplasia 10(1):75–86
36. Honeth G, Bendahl PO et al (2008) The CD44+/CD24- phenotype is enriched in basal-like breast tumors. Breast Cancer Res 10(3):R53
37. Liu R, Wang X et al (2007) The prognostic role of a gene signature from tumorigenic breast-cancer cells. N Engl J Med 356(3):217–226

Chapter 21
The Effect of Systemic Chemotherapy on Minimal Residual Disease in the Blood and Bone Marrow of Patients with Inflammatory Breast Cancer

Luc Y. Dirix, Dieter Peeters, Steven Van Laere, and Peter B. Vermeulen

Abstract Inflammatory breast cancer (IBC) is a particularly aggressive subtype of breast cancer that affects approximately 2.5% of patients with breast cancer in the industrialized countries, with a higher incidence reported in some other regions of the world [1–3]. Circulating tumour cells (CTCs) and disseminated tumor cells (DTCs) have become increasingly accepted as independent prognostic factors both in patients with primary and with metastatic breast cancer [8–12]. Several research groups have reported on the enumeration of CTCs and DTCs in patients with IBC [22-23, 27-29]. Although particularly data in metastatic IBC are limited, the probability of detecting CTCs and DTCs in untreated IBC seems higher than what has been reported in any other subgroup of patients with breast cancer. These observations are in line with the purported prognostic significance of CTCs and DTCs in breast cancer and the well-known aggressive clinical course of IBC. Furthermore, they provide a reasonable explanation for the necessity of chemotherapy in the management of these patients and lend support to the hypothesis that improvement in IBC can only arise from superior systemic agents.

Keywords Disseminated tumor cells • Circulating tumor cells • Inflammatory breast cancer • Bone marrow •

21.1 Introduction

Inflammatory breast cancer (IBC) is a particularly aggressive subtype of breast cancer that affects approximately 2.5% of patients with breast cancer in the industrialized countries, with a higher incidence reported in some other regions of the world [1–3].

L.Y. Dirix (✉) • D. Peeters • S. Van Laere • P.B. Vermeulen
Translational Cancer Research Unit, Oncology Center, General Hospital Sint-Augustinus, Antwerp, Belgium
e-mail: luc.dirix@telenet.be

N.T. Ueno and M. Cristofanilli (eds.), *Inflammatory Breast Cancer: An Update*,
DOI 10.1007/978-94-007-3907-9_21, © Springer Science+Business Media B.V. 2012

It is characterized by a rapid onset and diffuse local progression, a tendency to affect younger women, with a significant proportion of patients presenting with local and/or distant metastases and often with the pathological hallmark of lymphovascular, E-cadherin positive tumoremboli [4, 5]. Despite the fact that various methods have been proposed to more accurately describe IBC, the final diagnosis remains primarily a clinical one. Although associated with a poorer prognosis than other subtypes of breast cancer, the advent of combined multimodality therapy has altered the natural course of this disease from being historically uniformly fatal to approximately one third of women diagnosed with IBC eventually becoming long term survivors [6, 7].

Both circulating tumor cells (CTCs) aswell as disseminated tumor cells (DTCs) have become increasingly accepted as independent prognostic factors both in patients with primary and with metastatic breast cancer [8–12]. For CTCs this also holds true for patients with metastatic colorectal and castrate-refractory prostate cancer [13–15]. In patients with breast cancer the prognostic significance of CTC number after systemic chemotherapy, both in the adjuvant setting and after primary systemic treatment, has been reported [16–18]. This seems similar to the prognostic significance of the residual tumor burden after primary systemic chemotherapy.

The more widespread introduction of the standardized CellSearch technique has been instrumental in the majority of these studies [19].

The clinical phenotype of IBC is one of rapid evolution both locally and at distant organ sites. This suggests that one would predict a higher yield for both CTCs and DTCs compared to the numbers obtained in patients affected with non-IBC breast cancer.

21.2   Circulating Tumour Cells in Inflammatory Breast Cancer

Two research groups have reported data on the enumeration of CTCs in patients with IBC (Table 21.1). The data are mainly based on the large French cooperative group experience as part of an extensive clinical trials program in IBC. The single institution Antwerp experience is included in this analysis. Both labs have contributed to an external quality control system, justifying their combined analysis [20]. The CellSearch system is described in numerous publications [11, 12, 18, 21]. Briefly, CTCs are isolated and enumerated in 7.5 ml venous blood (PVB). Blood samples are drawn in CellSave Preservative Tubes (Immunicon, Huntingdom Valley, USA), stored at room temperature and are processed within 72 h. The samples are analysed using the CellSearch Circulating Tumour Cell kit (Veridex). CTCs are positively selected using an immunomagnetic bead system with antibodies directed at EPCAM. Criteria for an EpCAM positive object to be defined as a CTC include a round-to-oval morphology, a visible nucleus (DAPI+), a positive staining for cytokeratin and a negative staining for CD45. A threshold of 5 CTCs per 7.5 mL blood was used to evaluate results, with poor prognosis indicated by 5 or more CTCs and good prognosis defined by <5 CTCs.

The two French multicenter trials Beverly1 and Beverly2 of neoadjuvant chemotherapy both combined with bevacizumab in patients with IBC, included the enumeration of CTCs prior to the start of treatment [22, 23]. In the Beverly1 study,

Table 21.1 CTCs in patients with non-metastatic IBC

		Beverly1	Beverly2	Antwerp	Antwerp	All
N		92 HER2-	52 HER2+	15 HER2-	8 HER2+	167
CTC	> or = 1	37 (40%)	18 (35%)	5 (30%)	3 (37%)	63 (37.7%)
CTC	> or = 5	17 (18.5%)	7 (13%)	2 (13.3%)	2 (25%)	28 (16.7%)
	Range	1–559	0–92	0–103	0–43	–
	Median	12	0	0	0	–

patients with HER2 negative IBC were included. They all received 4 cycles of 5-fluorouracil, cyclophosphamide and epirubicine (FEC100) followed by 4 cycles of docetaxel, both in combination with bevacizumab (15 mg/kg q3w). Of the 101 patients included in this study, 92 were evaluable for CTC. At baseline 37/92 or 40% had > or at least 1 CTC and 17/92 had more than or equal to 5 CTCs/7.5 mL (18.5%). In the Beverly2 study of similar design, but in HER2 overexpressing IBC, treatment included the use of trastuzumab. Seven (13%) patients with non-metastatic IBC had at baseline more or equal to 5 CTCs, and in total 18 patients (35%) had at least one CTC at baseline.

The Antwerp group reported on 23 patients with non-metastatic IBC. In this cohort of patients with locoregional disease, 8 (34%) had one or more CTCs, and 4 (17%) had >5 CTCs.

In analyzing these data together, it seems fair to conclude that CTCs can be detected in over one third of patients with non-metastatic IBC. This number is clearly more elevated than in other patient cohorts sampled prior to treatment [24]. This observation combined with the fact that inflammatory breast cancers are enriched in HER2 amplified and basal-like subtypes, is also reassuring for the sensivity of this Epcam-based assay. The observed differences in CTC number between the HER2 positive and HER2 negative disease are similarly reassuring in this respect. If anything, both the frequency of positivity and the actual count seem more elevated in the HER2 negative group.

21.3   Influence of Treatment on Circulating Tumour Cells in Inflammatory Breast Cancer

Primary systemic chemotherapy (PST) in the management of IBC is accepted as the standard of care. This is mainly based on the observed change in prognosis in comparison with historical pre-chemotherapy data. Currently all patients with IBC should be treated with consecutive regimens consisting of anthracyclines and taxanes. The need for a reliable surrogate of response is probably most pressing in IBC as prognosis remains poor with 5 year survival figures around 40%. Any major progress will unavoibdably be the result of more effective systemic therapies.

The Antwerp group has reported on the evolution of CTC count during chemotherapy in 15 patients with HER2 negative IBC. These patients received 4 cycles of FEC100 followed by four cycles of docetaxel. These data need to be

Table 21.2 Influence of FEC chemotherapy on CTCs in HER2 negative IBC

		Beverly1	Beverly 1	Antwerp	Antwerp
		Baseline	Post 4x FEC + Bev	Baseline	Post 4x FEC
N		92 HER2-	82 HER2-	15 HER2-	15 HER2-
CTC	> or = 1	37/92 (40%)	5/82 (6%)	5/15 (30%)	3/15 (20%)
CTC	> or = 5	17 (18.5%)	1/82 (1%)	2 (13.3%)	1/15 (6.6%)
	Range	1–559	1–6	1–58	1–9

Table 21.3 Influence of chemotherapy and Trastuzumab on CTCs in HER2 positive IBC

		Beverly2	Beverly2	Beverly2	Antwerp	Antwerp
N HER2+		52 baseline	48 4xFEC + Bev	43 4xFEC + Bev + 4xDoc + Bev + Tras	8 baseline	8 4xDoc + Tras
CTC	> or = 1	18 (35%)	6 (13%)	3 (7%)	3 (37%)	1 (12%)
CTC	> or = 5	7 (13%)	0	0	2 (25%)	0
	Range	0–92	0–4	0–2	0–43	0–3
	Median	0	0	0	0	0

distinguished from the more extensive Beverly1 data. All the Beverly1 patients received another targeted agent; bevacizumab and this from the start of the chemotherapy (Table 21.2).

The Beverly1 data show a very rapid change in the number of patients with an increased CTC count from 37/92 to 5/82. Similarly, the actual number of CTCs dropped most impressively. Taken into account all the potential caveats of across datasets comparisons, the patients not treated with the bevacizumab combination, had a more limited CTC clearance, with an identical chemotherapy regimen. This is at least in agreement with the well established influence of bevacizumab on the response rate in patients treated with first line chemotherapy for metastatic breast cancer [25].

Table 21.3 summarizes the results of the Beverly2 study and the Antwerp cases. Both data sets are very similar; over one third of patients had detectable CTCs. And after 4 cycles of chemotherapy; FEC100 + Bevacizumab and Docetaxel and Trastuzumab, respectively, CTCs decrease very rapidly. The Beverly2 data suggest that this is mainly a chemotherapy effect, or at least the contibution of trastuzumab might not be critical to explain this rapid and steep fall in CTC number. Again these data are in concordance with other observations in non-IBC breast cancer [26].

21.4   CTCs in Patients with Metastatic IBC

The MD Anderson Cancer Center retrospectively compared the CTC number in 42 patients with metastatic IBC with the results obtained in 107 patients with metastatic non-IBC breast cancer [27]. This report included only patients with metastatic disease and 15 out of 42 patients were scheduled to receive second line chemotherapy. Moreover, nine IBC (69%) patients with HER2-amplified disease were pretreated by anti-HER2 therapy before CTC measurement. Ten (23.8%) IBC patients had 5 or more CTCs per 7.5 mL blood compared to 48 (44.9%) non-IBC patients. Importantly, none of the 13 IBC patients with HER2 amplified disease had more than 5 CTCs per 7.5 mL blood. Survival was not different according to this threshold of 5 CTCs in the IBC population, but it was in the non-IBC population.

Our own group has made similar observations in 14 patients with IBC with only 6 patients with one or more CTCs and 3 with 5 or more CTCs.

These data suggest that these numbers are lower than in non-IBC metastatic breast cancer, however these data seem premature to draw firm conclusion and seem contradictory to the data obtained in untreated patients with non-metastatic IBC.

21.5 Disseminated Tumor Cells in IBC

At least a number of the circulating tumor cells are considered the initiating cells or group of cells, responsible for the emergence of metastasis at distant sites. These cells capable of completing this entire process, i.e. leaving the primary tumor, invading the surrounding stroma, intravasation, surviving in the circulation, extravasating at an organ site and initiating secondary growth at that site, are considered rare members of the collection of tumor cells in the primary site. Their actual number or better the proportion of cells capable of accomplishing this process remains unclear. The cells that have finished this sequence but prior to becoming a clinically detectable metastasis, can be identified as disseminated tumor cells or DTCs. These cells are most often detected in bone marrow, mainly because of the relative ease of bone marrow sampling. Their presence is unequivocal proof of spread of the tumor outside the boundaries of its site of origin. It has been shown in numerous studies that their presence is a relevant prognostic factor. It is yet unclear whether they can be used as a means of monitoring the efficacy of a particular treatment, nor whether they represent a specific target for agents aimed at these putative tumor initiating cells.

In our unit we performed a study on DTCs in bone marrow in 33 patients presenting with untreated, non-metastatic IBC between June 2002 and January 2009 [28, 29]. In addition to routine examinations all patients underwent a more extensive work-up including computed tomographic imaging of the chest and the abdomen. All these patients underwent a posterior iliac crest bone marrow aspiration prior to the initiation of systemic chemotherapy. In 18 patients a second bone marrow sample was obtained after the completion of the systemic treatment and prior to surgery and/or radiotherapy. In brief, a total 10 ml of bone marrow was aspirated from the posterior iliac crest under local anaesthesia. Mononuclear cells (MNC) were isolated by density-gradient centrifugation through Ficoll-Paque (Amersham Pharmacia Biotech). Cell suspension was counted and cytocentrifuged onto glass slides at a concentration of 5×10^5 per spot. Immunostaining to detect cytokeratin-positive cells was done with the Epimet®-kit (Baxter). This kit uses the monoclonal antibody A45-B/

Table 21.4 RT-PCR results for CK19 and MAM in 33 patients with M0 IBC

RT-PCR marker	CK19+	MAM+	CK19+/MAM+	CK19+ or MAM+
N	33	33	33	33
Positive	21	16	13	24
% Positive	63.5	48	39.3	72.7

B3, which is a pancytokeratin marker. For the immunocytochemical (ICC) analysis a total of two million cells per patient were screened microscopically by two pathologists. Cells were identified as disseminated epithelial cells according to the European ISHAGE Working group for Standardisation of Tumor Cell Detection [30]. Results are expressed as the number of positive cells per million MNC. From the other half of the bone marrow aspirate total RNA was extracted from the MNC using a RNeasy kit (Qiagen). The amount of RNA was measured spectrophotometrically. All samples had an OD 260/280 nm ratio >1.8, indicating high purity. For generation of first strand cDNA, 2 μg of total RNA was reverse transcribed with the high-Capacity cDNA Archive Kit (Applied Biosystems) in a total volume of 100 μl. Details of the RT-PCR reaction for cytokeratin-19 (CK19) and mammoglobin (MAM) have been described in detail [28, 29].

All patients were treated with primary systemic chemotherapy consisting of four cycles of FEC100 followed by four cycles of docetaxel 100 mg. Treatment with trastuzumab was administered in 5 patients after the end of chemotherapy, and after mastectomy was performed. As such this does not affect results of DTCs in bone marrow samples.

In the BM aspirate prior to chemotherapy, in 20/33 (61%) patients ICC CK+ cells were detected. Their number ranged from 1 to 29 cells/2×10^6 MNC. The median number of DTCs was 3 cells/2×10^6 MNC. Using an identical technique to enumerate the number of DTCs in 117 patients with non-IBC localized breast cancer, the median number of DTCs was 0 with a range between 0 and 7 cells/2×10^6 BM. Only 27 out of 117 patients had detectable DTCs. This makes up some 23% compared to 61% in patients with M0 IBC. In this same cohort of 117 patients the BM was CK19+ and/or MAM+ in 36 patients which amounts to 30%.

The RT-PCR data are summarized in Table 21.4.

Of the 18 patients who underwent a second bone marrow aspirate after the completion of the PST, 12 patients had an initial positive BM. ICC detected DTC numbers decreased in all 12. In 1 patient out of 6 initially negative patients, BM became positive with one ICC detected cell (1 DTC/2×10^6 MNC). All patients underwent mastectomy with a pCR rate of 10/33 (30%). Of the 4 out of the 18 patients who underwent a second BM aspirate that had a pCR, 3 had a positive initial BM (4, 8, 9 DTCs /10^6), with the second becoming negative in all three.

This study remains small and it is not justified to draw firm conclusions, other than the observation that both the frequency of bone marrow positivity for DTCs and the actual number of DTCs in patients with apparently localized IBC, is substantially higher than the proportion and number observed in patients with non-IBC localized breast cancer. These observations are in keeping with those from a pooled analysis combining DTC data from nine European studies including 4,703 stage I-III breast cancer patients [9]. DTC were detected in 22/46 (48%) IBC patients as opposed to 30% of non-IBC patients. This is agreement with higher number and higher frequency of detecting CTCs in these patients. It is also a reasonable explanation of the necessity for the need for chemotherapy in the management of these patients and lends support to the hypothesis that improvement in IBC can only arise from superior systemic agents.

21.6   Conclusions

The probability of detecting CTCs and DTCs in untreated IBC is higher than what has been reported in any other subgroup of patients with breast cancer. This is true for the proportion of patients with detectable CTCs and DTCs and for the actual number of CTCs and DTCs. This observation is in line with the purported prognostic significance of CTCs and DTCs in breast cancer and the well-known aggressive clinical course of inflammatory breast cancer. The comparison between the Beverly studies and the Antwerp data, confirm previous observations of the contribution of both bevacizumab and trastuzumab in increasing the clearance rate and kinetics of CTCs above those obtained with chemotherapy alone.

The increased proportion of the genomically defined basal-like subtype of breast cancer in HER2 negative IBC, does not seem to affect the probability of the Epcam based CellSearch assay to detect CTCs in this group.

The patients with IBC are in urgent need for improved systemic treatment options. The current data on CTCs and DTCs in IBC are suggestive of a continuous role for CTC and DTC detection and phenotyping in order to define treatment targets and speed up drug development.

Acknowledgments This work was supported by a grant from the "Stichting tegen Kanker-Foundation contre le Cancer" entitled "Evaluation of the importance of stem/progenitor cells for the biology of inflammatory breast cancer and breast cancer metastasis". We sincerely thank all patients who gave blood and bone marrow samples for research intentions. We acknowledge all staff members of the Clinical Trials Organisation and Translational Cancer Research Unit from GZA Hospitals Sint-Augustinus, Antwerp, Belgium for their assistance. Dieter Peeters is research assistant of the Fund for Scientific Research Flanders and the University of Antwerp.

References

1. Robertson FM, Bondy M, Yang W, Yamauchi H, Wiggins S, Kamrudin S, Krishnamurthy S, Le-Petross H, Bidaut L, Player AN, Barsky SH, Woodward WA, Buchholz T, Lucci A, Ueno NT, Cristofanilli M (2010) Inflammatory breast cancer: the disease, the biology, the treatment. CA Cancer J Clin 60(6):351–375
2. Dawood S, Merajver SD, Viens P, Vermeulen PB, Swain SM, Buchholz TA, Dirix LY, Levine PH, Lucci A, Krishnamurthy S, Robertson FM, Woodward WA, Yang WT, Ueno NT, Cristofanilli M (2011) International expert panel on inflammatory breast cancer: consensus statement for standardized diagnosis and treatment. Ann Oncol 22(3):515–523

3. Dirix LY, Van Dam P, Prové A, Vermeulen PB (2006) Inflammatory breast cancer: current understanding. Curr Opin Oncol 6:563–571
4. Vermeulen PB, van Golen KL, Dirix LY (2010) Angiogenesis, lymphangiogenesis, growth pattern, and tumor emboli in inflammatory breast cancer: a review of the current knowledge. Cancer 116(11 Suppl):2748–2754
5. Van Laere S, Van der Auwera I, Van den Eynden G, Van Hummelen P, van Dam P, Van Marck E, Vermeulen PB, Dirix L (2007) Distinct molecular phenotype of inflammatory breast cancer compared to non-inflammatory breast cancer using Affymetrix-based genome-wide gene-expression analysis. Br J Cancer 97(8):1165–1174
6. Ueno NT, Buzdar AU, Singeltary SE et al (1997) Combined modality treatment of inflammatory breast carcinoma: twenty years of experience at M.D Anderson Center. Cancer Chemother Pharmacol 40:321–329
7. Cristofanilli M, Gonzalez-Angulo AM, Buzdar AU et al (2004) Paclitaxel improves the prognosis in estrogen receptor negative inflammatory breast cancer: the M.D Anderson Cancer Center experience. Clin Breast Cancer 4:415–419
8. Bidard FC, Vincent-Salomon A, Gomme S, Nos C, de Rycke Y, Thiery JP, Sigal-Zafrani B, Mignot L, Sastre-Garau X, Pierga JY, Institut Curie Breast Cancer Study Group (2008) Disseminated tumor cells of breast cancer patients: a strong prognostic factor for distant and local relapse. Clin Cancer Res 14(11):3306–3311
9. Braun S, Vogl FD, Naume B, Janni W, Osborne MP, Coombes RC, Schlimok G, Diel IJ, Gerber B, Gebauer G, Pierga JY, Marth C, Oruzio D, Wiedswang G, Solomayer EF, Kundt G, Strobl B, Fehm T, Wong GY, Bliss J, Vincent-Salomon A, Pantel K (2005) A pooled analysis of bone marrow micrometastasis in breast cancer. N Engl J Med 353(8):793–802
10. Janni W, Vogl FD, Wiedswang G, Synnestvedt M, Fehm T, Jückstock J, Borgen E, Rack B, Braun S, Sommer H, Solomayer E, Pantel K, Nesland J, Friese K, Naume B (2011) Persistence of disseminated tumor cells in the bone marrow of breast cancer patients predicts increased risk for relapse – a European pooled analysis. Clin Cancer Res 17(9):2967–2976
11. Cristofanilli M, Hayes DF, Budd GT, Ellis MJ, Stopeck A, Reuben JM, Doyle GV, Matera J, Allard WJ, Miller MC, Fritsche HA, Hortobagyi GN, Terstappen LW (2005) Circulating tumor cells: a novel prognostic factor for newly diagnosed metastatic breast cancer. J Clin Oncol 23:1420–1430
12. Cristofanilli M, Budd GT, Ellis MJ, Stopeck A, Matera J, Miller MC, Reuben JM, Doyle GV, Allard WJ, Terstappen LW, Hayes DF (2004) Circulating tumor cells, disease progression, and survival in metastatic breast cancer. N Engl J Med 351:781–791
13. Olmos D, Arkenau HT, Ang JE, Ledaki I, Attard G, Carden CP, Reid AH, A'Hern R, Fong PC, Oomen NB, Molife R, Dearnaley D, Parker C, Terstappen LW, de Bono JS (2009) Circulating tumour cell (CTC) counts as intermediate end points in castration-resistant prostate cancer (CRPC): a single-centre experience. Ann Oncol 20(1):27–33
14. Morgan TM, Lange PH, Porter MP, Lin DW, Ellis WJ, Gallaher IS, Vessella RL (2009) Disseminated tumor cells in prostate cancer patients after radical prostatectomy and without evidence of disease predicts biochemical recurrence. Clin Cancer Res 15(2):677–683
15. Tol J, Koopman M, Miller MC, Tibbe A, Cats A, Creemers GJ, Vos AH, Nagtegaal ID, Terstappen LW, Punt CJ (2010) Circulating tumour cells early predict progression-free and overall survival in advanced colorectal cancer patients treated with chemotherapy and targeted agents. Ann Oncol 21(5):1006–1012
16. Pierga JY, Bidard FC, Mathiot C, Brain E, Delaloge S, Giachetti S, de Cremoux P, Salmon R, Vincent-Salomon A, Marty M (2008) Circulating tumor cell detection predicts early metastatic relapse after neoadjuvant chemotherapy in large operable and locally advanced breast cancer in a phase II randomized trial. Clin Cancer Res 14(21):7004–7010
17. Bidard FC, Mathiot C, Delaloge S, Brain E, Giachetti S, de Cremoux P, Marty M, Pierga JY (2010) Single circulating tumor cell detection and overall survival in nonmetastatic breast cancer. Ann Oncol 21(4):729–733
18. Rack BK, Schindlbeck C, Andergassen U, Schneeweiss A, Zwingers T, Lichtenegger W, Beckmann M, Sommer HL, Pantel K, Janni W, Study Group SUCCESS (2010) Use of circulating

tumor cells (CTC) in peripheral blood of breast cancer patients before and after adjuvant chemotherapy to predict risk for relapse: the SUCCESS trial. J Clin Oncol 28:1003

19. Allard WJ, Matera J, Miller MC, Repollet M, Connelly MC, Rao C, Tibbe AG, Uhr JW, Terstappen LW (2004) Tumor cells circulate in the peripheral blood of all major carcinomas but not in healthy subjects or patients with nonmalignant diseases. Clin Cancer Res 10:6897–9047

20. Kraan J, Sleijfer S, Strijbos MH, Ignatiadis M, Peeters D, Pierga JY, Farace F, Riethdorf S, Fehm T, Zorzino L, Tibbe AG, Maestro M, Gisbert-Criado R, Denton G, de Bono JS, Dive C, Foekens JA, Gratama JW (2011) External quality assurance of circulating tumor cell enumeration using the Cell Search(®) system: a feasibility study. Cytometry B Clin Cytom 80(2):112–118

21. Riethdorf S, Fritsche H, Muller V, Rau T, Schindlbeck C, Rack B, Janni W, Coith C, Beck K, Janicke F, Jackson S, Gornet T, Cristofanilli M, Pantel K (2007) Detection of circulating tumor cells in peripheral blood of patients with metastatic breast cancer: a validation study of the Cell Search system. Clin Cancer Res 13:920–928

22. Pierga J-Y, Bidard F-C, Andre F, Petit T, Dalenc F, Delozier T, Romieu G, Bonneterre J, Ferrero J, Kerbrat P, Martin A, Viens P (2011) Early drop of circulating tumor cells (CTC) and increase of circulating endothelial cells (CEC) during neoadjuvant chemotherapy (CT) combined with bevacizumab in HER2 negative inflammatory breast cancer (IBC) in multicentre phase II trial BEVERLY 1. J Clin Onc 29 (suppl):abstract 10510

23. Pierga J-Y, Bidard F-C, Petit T, Delozier T, Ferrero J-M, Campone M, Gligorov J, Lerebours F, Roche H, Kraemer S, Mathiot C, Viens P (2011) Monitoring Circulating Tumor Cells (CTC) and Circulating Endothelial Cells (CEC) during neoadjuvant combination of trastuzumab and bevacizumab with chemotherapy in HER2 overexpressing Inflammatory Breast Cancer (IBC): an ancillary study of BEVERLY 2 multicenter phase II trial. Cancer Res 70:PD04–PD07

24. Riethdorf S, Müller V, Zhang L, Rau T, Loibl S, Komor M, Roller M, Huober J, Fehm T, Schrader I, Hilfrich J, Holms F, Tesch H, Eidtmann H, Untch M, von Minckwitz G, Pantel K (2010) Detection and HER2 expression of circulating tumor cells: prospective monitoring in breast cancer patients treated in the neoadjuvant GeparQuattro trial. Clin Cancer Res 16(9):2634–2645

25. Miles DW, Chan A, Dirix LY, Cortés J, Pivot X, Tomczak P, Delozier T, Sohn JH, Provencher L, Puglisi F, Harbeck N, Steger GG, Schneeweiss A, Wardley AM, Chlistalla A, Romieu G (2010) Phase III study of bevacizumab plus docetaxel compared with placebo plus docetaxel for the first-line treatment of human epidermal growth factor receptor 2-negative metastatic breast cancer. J Clin Oncol 28(20):3239–3247

26. Slamon DJ, Leyland-Jones B, Shak S, Fuchs H, Paton V, Bajamonde A, Fleming T, Eiermann W, Wolter J, Pegram M, Baselga J, Norton L (2001) Use of chemotherapy plus a monoclonal antibody against HER2 for metastatic breast cancer that overexpresses HER2. N Engl J Med 344(11):783–792

27. Mego M, De Giorgi U, Hsu L, Ueno NT, Valero V, Jackson S, Andreopoulou E, Kau SW, Reuben JM, Cristofanilli M (2009) Circulating tumor cells in metastatic inflammatory breast cancer. Ann Oncol 11:1824–1828

28. Benoy IH, Elst H, Van der Auwera I, Van Laere S, van Dam P, Van Marck E, Scharpe S, Vermeulen PB, Dirix LY (2004) Real-time RT-PCR correlates with immunocytochemistry for the detection of disseminated epithelial cells in bone marrow aspirates of patients with breast cancer. Br J Cancer 91:1813–1820

29. Benoy IH, Elst H, Philips M, Wuyts H, van Dam P, Scharpe S, Van Marck E, Vermeulen PB, Dirix LY (2006) Real-time RT-PCR detection of disseminated tumour cells in bone marrow has superior prognostic significance in comparison with circulating tumour cells in patients with breast cancer. Br J Cancer 94:672–680

30. Borgen E, Naume B, Nesland JM, Kvalheim G, Beiske K, Fodstad O, Diel I, Solomayer EF, Theocharous P, Coombes RC, Smith BM, Wunder E, Marolleau JP, Garcia J, Pantel K (1999) Standardization of the immunocytochemical detection of cancer cells in BM and blood: I. establishment of objective criteria for the evaluation of immunostained cells. Cytotherapy 1(5):377–388

Chapter 22
Perspective of Patient Advocacy

Michelle Esteban and Patti Bradfield

Keywords Family • Daughter • Patient • Parent • Advocacy

Inflammatory Breast Cancer (IBC) for decades has been a small paragraph narrative in medical journals. "Doctors learn about it in medical school, but most never see a patient", stated one breast oncologist when urged to explain why IBC is misdiagnosed and misunderstood so often. Through the looking glass of time we know those same doctors probably did see patients who presented with clinical symptoms, but believing that IBC was so rare, they, the physicians, disregarded the possibility. Only with the advent of the internet with information at the fingertips of anyone with a computer, has this deadly disease been brought out of the dusty tombs of literature and now is being looked at under a microscope. Between a defiant retired reporter whose daughter tried to fight the odds, and an active reporter that pushed the camera lights into those unilluminated recesses of medical knowledge did the world sit up and take a closer look at what was once thought to be too rare to even contemplate.

22.1 Perspective of Michelle Esteban KOMO TV, Seattle WA Reporter

For too long, IBC has been what I call the 'Rodney Dangerfield' of breast cancer, it got no respect.

M. Esteban (✉)
KOMO TV
e-mail: MEsteban@komotv.com

P. Bradfield
Chief Education Officer/Founder, The Inflammatory Breast Cancer Foundation
e-mail: p.thewriter@frontier.com

N.T. Ueno and M. Cristofanilli (eds.), *Inflammatory Breast Cancer: An Update*,
DOI 10.1007/978-94-007-3907-9_22, © Springer Science+Business Media B.V. 2012

To me it appeared to be an inconvenient truth, just too uncommon of a cancer to care about.

In my opinion, it didn't fit the short and simple breast cancer message that we all know so well; look for a lump, get a mammogram.

It wasn't until a group of Washington State women got so fed up, that we finally learned of this Silent Killer. At KOMO-TV I started interviewing those women and quickly dubbed IBC the Silent Killer. Silent because the patients never heard of IBC until they got it. It's also a Silent Killer because it rarely attacks with a tell tale lump and is almost never detected on a mammogram and even more frightening most patients were misdiagnosed. Their doctors didn't recognize the Silent Killer either.

The majority of women I interviewed were initially mis-diagnosed; told they had a breast infection or a bug bite, when in fact, they were all fighting the most aggressive and lethal form of breast cancer, but didn't know it.

Each of them considered their diagnosis cruel and shocking. How could they have a breast cancer they never heard of?

I hope what the medical community and breast cancer awareness advocates have done for traditional breast cancer survival, we can also do for inflammatory breast cancer.

While there have been enormous strides in the treatment of traditional breast cancer, there's still so much more IBC awareness work to do.

When I did a special report on IBC in May of 2006 – what happened next stunned me. Never in the 22 years that I've been working as a reporter has one story made such an impact. The response was overwhelming. Hundreds of emails not just from my state in Washington, but from all over the U.S. and around the world.

My report shocked viewers, especially women because I told them something most of them had never heard. There's more than one kind of breast cancer.

The news was so shocking that men and women clamored for more information. The demand was so overwhelming that our website komotv.com http://komotv.com/ crashed, repeatedly. We set up phone banks, they crashed too. The calls kept coming long after our phone banks closed.

We know my report was downloaded more than 20 million times and that it was embedded in countless email threads. It created an email frenzy of mostly women passing the information on and demanding the recipients share the information with every woman they know.

Because of the brave IBC patients of Washington who told me their stories, I heard from women from around the world who insisted this new information saved their lives. Many insisted those personal stories touched them and at the same time taught them about this Silent Killer. They now knew not to just ask a doctor if they had IBC, but to demand that the doctor rule out IBC.

To this day, five years later people are still circulating the video clip in mass emails- the subject usually says something like: 'Forward this to every woman you know, they must watch this video'.

I've probably made 100 DVD copies for advocacy groups, cancer centers, education centers, and women who want to share it with their friends.

In addition to that initial report, I also produced a 30 minute prime time Special Report on IBC and the online version still gets regular viewings and generates viewer emails and phone calls. Many of them say the same thing:

"I never heard of IBC until I saw the KOMO-TV News report" or even sadder they compared themselves to our Washington IBC patients, explaining they too, "never heard of IBC" until they were fighting it.

All but two patients that I interviewed told me they were initially misdiagnosed because their doctors insisted they were suffering from a bug bite or a breast infection.

There was a time when some doctors and national cancer organizations criticized me for making what they called a big deal out of 'such a rare type of breast cancer.' They accused me of needlessly scaring women.

Like me, our viewers were stunned that they were learning about inflammatory breast cancer from a TV reporter, a shell shocked mother and a string of IBC patients, mostly in their thirties.

If their doctor didn't know – how many others didn't know?

Too many.

IBC desperately needs exactly what teams of oncologists and medical researchers around the world are giving it: respect.

The lives of countless women are counting on it.

I'm so proud of Dr. Massimo Cristofanilli and his leadership. I remember how touched I was to learn that Dr. C was inspired by an IBC patient too. He carries a photo daily of Morgan Welch in his pocket as a reminder of the work yet to be done on IBC diagnosis and treatment. Welch, a new bride, was just 24 when she lost her IBC battle. On her death bed she begged Dr. C to promise to save other women and search until he found a faster and better way to diagnosis and treat patients. He's keeping that promise.

But for me, our IBC story began with one determined and angry Redmond mother, Patti Bradfield.

If it hadn't been for her determination the IBC story I got to tell may never have been told. When Patti, a former newspaper reporter learned her daughter Tina Turk had been diagnosed with a cancer she never heard of, she was crushed, incensed, and hell-bent on learning everything she could about it and finding a way to spread the word.

Before I met Patti and her daughter, Patti stood on street corners handing out fliers willing to talk to strangers in hopes of telling them something they may never hear from their doctor. There's more than one kind of breast cancer and this type is so aggressive, you have to act fast.

We're both journalist and we both were shocked to learn of a breast cancer we never heard of, especially one so scary and lethal.

As journalists we knew we had to tell this story – but as a mother, Patti knew it was a matter of life and death, not just for her daughter but for every woman yet to be diagnosed.

That mother's love touched me. I'll never forget Tina's funeral, how I was in a daze. As I drove across back and forth from Seattle to Yakima for her memorial, I just kept hearing Tina over and over in my head saying what she told me the day I met her, "If I had heard of it prior, I probably would have been more suspect that something was wrong rather than just being young and dumb."

It wasn't her fault. Like so many women, she didn't know. She never heard of IBC, until she was diagnosed with it.

A husband's love motivated me too.

Phil Willingham broke my heart when he told me the story of his wife Marilyn being misdiagnosed. He beams when he describes how he fell in love with her in the 4th grade and by chance years later he saw her standing on the sidewalk and asked her out on a date. They dated and were soon married.

In the spring of 2003 Marilyn thought she had a spider bite. Her doctor said it was a breast infection. A second doctor knew just by looking at Marilyn's breast that it was Inflammatory Breast Cancer. Her breast was swollen, red, hot to the touch and itchy. Marilyn had a brief remission, but the cancer came back. Marilyn died in December of 2005, just 2 weeks before Christmas and a few days after her 65th birthday.

Phil and Patti both reached out to me and to Washington Governor Chris Gregoire. In 2006 the Governor, a survivor of a rare breast cancer agreed to proclaim October, IBC Awareness Month in our state. She has every year since and credited the diligence of Patti, Phil and all the IBC advocates in our state with making the proclamation a reality.

Lori Davider learned about IBC through one of my TV reports. A relative encouraged her to check out our website to see if her symptoms matched up.

"That's me, that's me, that's me," said the late Davider as she watched my report and matched up with every IBC symptom listed.

Lori was a 40 something, mother of two and had just remarried. She told me she was having 'the time of her life.'

IBC changed everything.

Because she worked in a doctor's office – she was miffed that she of all people never heard of IBC until she watched my report.

Lori's cancer quickly spread to her brain. She had multiple operations, surgery limited her speech, at one point she could not talk.

A few months later, IBC took another friend, Lori Davider, left behind a new husband and two heartbroken children.

Two other Washington women; Deena McIlroy (mcilroy) and Alison Score both left behind husbands, children and their stories.

Deena's unbreakable hope is what I'll remember about her, and, I'll always remember her great sense of style and how good she looked with just a touch of peach fuzz on her head. She let me spend five hours with her as she happily endured each painful hour of chemotherapy. Her fingernails were on fire, submerged deep in a plastic bowl of ice, yet she happily prattled on as if we were sitting at a cafe in the sunshine. She had only two concerns; family and warning other women about IBC. She took an entire summer off from work to spend with her kids. That day in the Cancer Center she told me, "I don't know how much time I have. What's my number one priority? It's my children."

She confessed she thought she was too young to get breast cancer.

"I never in a million years thought it was cancer, I had no idea," said told me, "I wasn't even 40 yet, I was fit, active, thought I did a good job of taking care of myself."

And unlike many IBC patients, changes to Deena's breast were subtle, not obvious like these women with IBC.

"It didn't look bad, in fact, it looked pretty good! It was firm, it was perky and it had a nice rosy glow." Deena and Patti's daughter Tina were the only two women who told me by the time they thought to go to the doctor, they got an immediate and correct diagnosis. In the spring of 2007 I learned I won an Emmy for some of my IBC reports, I dedicated it to Deena.

Alison Score, a mother of two young daughters was just 35 when diagnosed with IBC. I remember her telling me about the time she sat around with 7 other girlfriends talking about a scary statistic; one in 8 women will be diagnosed with breast cancer in Washington. She said at that moment she said that's one of us. How shocked she was just a few years later to find out she was that one. Five years ago she told me, "I thought breast cancer was you have to have a lump, you get it removed, that's it. When they say the words to you, 'you have breast cancer' you think, but I'm only 35."

In 2003 Alison was told she had a breast infection and antibiotics should clear it up. She was breast feeding her 9 month old daughter, Morgan at the time. Her daughter Courtney was just three years old. 10 days after antibiotics – her breast was still swollen, red, hard and the stabbing pain got worse.

By the time the IBC was diagnosed, the cancer in her breast was so involved that it actually showed up on a mammogram.

Alison had to rely on family to take care of her children, while she battled IBC for months. Unlike traditional breast cancer – IBC patients like Alison get chemo first followed by a mastectomy.

Then her chest wall was blasted with radiation. Alison had 33 separate radiation treatments before the doctors were able to say she's NED, no evidence of disease. Because the cancer could come back at any time, she knew she was never in remission. Her hope was to see IBC taught in high school health care curriculums nationwide. Even while she was battling IBC, like so many of the IBC Warriors I've had the honor of knowing, Alison took time to tell her story. She had such a sweet disposition, always unassuming and just a kind, kind person. I was moved and surprised when she agreed to be interviewed and then repeatedly agreed to work our KOMO-TV phone banks to answer questions about IBC. Thank you Alison. We are all richer and better for knowing her. Alison was snatched from us last year.

In February of 2010 another IBC patient, this time a wonderful woman with an infectious laugh from California, Christina Hicks reached out to me. She told me in an email there were no more chemotherapies left to try and that she would be coming to Seattle to take part in a clinic trial at the University of Washington. "I will do every study they will have me for, cause I want to be the guinea pig. I want to be the last person in my family who has this illness, I don't want to meet another person who has to go through this", she insisted as we sat on a park bench in downtown Seattle.

Christine like so many other women was blind-sided by IBC. She said she learned more about IBC thru my reporting than her primary care physician. "This should have never happened, if they told women, ya they tell us about lumps, but tells us about a rash, inverted nipples tell us about the stuff that IBC does," said Christina Hicks in August of 2009. The first sign of trouble revealed itself when Christine's areola turned white, then a rash appeared on her breast. Her doctors thought it was a bug bite.

Before her battle with IBC Christine was living the California dream; loving family, great home, wonderful friends. She got her dose of sunshine playing beach volleyball with the 30-something's. She was healthy, happy and always laughing. Even in her Seattle hospital bed as she rolled up her sleeves to be a 'guinea pig' for two long weeks every month, she laughed. She brought a small collection of wind-up toys to keep her, the other participants and the staff amused. She insisted on laughter.

"It may not be lifesaving for me, though disappointing, it's okay, at least I'm giving a framework for who it will help."

IBC didn't get all her tears. She told me only months before she died, that research and laughter would be her legacy.

I'm going to repeat something IBC survivor Nancy Key told me, "Not one more woman should say 'I didn't know.'"

She wasn't the only one. That sentiment was the dying wish of Morgan Welch, Angie Elliot, Tina Turk, Deena McIlroy, Marilyn Willingham, Lori Davider, Christine Hicks and Allison Score. Eight women who I profiled who are now no longer with us.

I've watched too many woman die and all of them have asked me not to let them die in vain, begged me to do everything we can to warn others, to understand this most lethal form of breast cancer.

IBC deserves and it desperately needs our respect.

"It's not something most women know about. It's not something most primary care physicians think about."

When Seattle Breast Specialist Dr. Julie Gralow said those words to me during an interview in 2006; I was stunned.

How can a breast cancer be so deadly, yet most of us have never heard of it. Shouldn't we know? Shouldn't somebody tell us, warn us, I thought.

And even more frightening; how can a breast cancer as lethal as IBC not be on every Primary Care Physician's medical radar? Gralow told me although doctors learn about IBC in Medical School, she suspected that most had never knowingly encountered a case.

Back in 2006, the National Cancer Institute deemed IBC 'rare' insisting it accounted for just 1% of all breast cancer. Now 5 years later the NCI puts it closer to 5%. Even before Dr. Gralow and I met, I was beginning to see an alarming pattern just in Western Washington; misdiagnosed patients.

It got to the point in my interviews where I could actually finish a patient's sentence. They'd tell me how their breast swelled over night so they went to the doctor who told them it's nothing to worry about. Let me guess, I'd say. 'Your doctor told you, it's a breast infection and prescribed antibiotics'.

In some cases, patients were put on antibiotics for six long weeks. As I've learned from IBC patients the right diagnosis and immediate treatment is their best defense. A number of IBC patients are like Nancy Key. She and her doctor thought the mark on her breast was just a nasty 'bug bite', but when her breast wouldn't heal, Nancy finally got the right diagnosis.

'I was, what do you mean, I have the worst breast cancer there is, I don't have a lump, how can that be?' asked Nancy.

She learned by the time IBC gets to the breast, it's already traveled through the body. That's what makes it so deadly.

And like so many IBC patients Nancy never heard of IBC, until she got it.

'I was furious and at the same time, terrified, that I was going to die, because I didn't know.'

Every patient I've interviewed has the same wish; that they would have known about IBC prior to their diagnosis. While they were getting regular mammograms and looking for a lump, they had no idea that IBC is rarely found on a mammogram or self breast exam. Nancy had no idea that an MRI and biopsy are the best catch.

She was diagnosed in July, 1998. Ever since she's been warning women and working with doctors.

"I have such a passion, for not one more woman to be surprised, I don't want another one to say how come I didn't know, how come I didn't know," says Nancy.

Kathryn Gordon didn't know.

'That it's unusual isn't a good reason not to know about it,' insists Kathryn, 'My physician who I consider a well-prepared woman didn't have a clue either.'

Kathryn never heard of IBC until her diagnosis.

'I wish someone had scared me early, I'm still angry my life is threatened by something I never heard of.'

Kathryn shared her story with me because she's determined to help create IBC awareness. Although she believes more women know about IBC than back when she was diagnosed 8 years ago; she still worries that not enough doctors will recognize the symptoms. Her family doctor said her symptoms: a red blotchy, swollen breast, hot to the touch was a reaction to hormone replacement therapy.

Kathryn went back to work and forgot about it.

3 months later, a radiologist thought Kathryn's breast looked suspicious – a biopsy confirmed the IBC.

'I told her don't tell me to go home and get my life in order, cause I'm not ready.'

Kathryn is N.E.D, but with a distinction, she's changed it from No-Evidence-of-Disease to No-Expiration-Date.

'I have no plan to expire,' laughed Kathryn.

IBC got their attention and their respect, as advocates our hope is that IBC gets the attention of every primary care physician, ever oncologist, gynecologist and radiologist, so that no woman ever has to ask, 'How come I didn't know?'

22.2 Perspective of Patti Bradfield, Mother and Retired Newspaper Reporter, President of the Inflammatory Breast Cancer Foundation

On August 29, 2007 at exactly 3:05 a.m. my beautiful daughter Tina died from metastasized liver complications from Inflammatory Breast Cancer, fifteen days short of four years since her diagnosis. My life, as you can imagine, turned upside down. The reality of her passing hit my heart first, but my brain could not conceive the reality until later.

My daughter said to me from the very beginning, "Science is great Mom, but who is helping the women who need help after their diagnosis"? That question is still elusive as too many physicians even though they may diagnose IBC correctly, still do not know the proper treatment, and even though they have the same capabilities of the internet as their patient, will not try to find a specialist to call and consult. It is maddening.

Like my daughter, there were hundreds of women whom I come in contact with who are fighting their own doctors to get diagnosed with whatever is going on within their bodies which they know is not normal. They have to fight until they either are diagnosed with IBC, or have IBC ruled out. Many, too many to count, are not with us anymore. Many of those did not have to die. If they had been diagnosed when they first went to their primary care doctors or OBGYN physicians, they could possibly still be with us. So I have to ask, "How far have we come since September of 2003?" How far have we come since I first started my own personal crusade to alert women about this breast cancer that was misdiagnosed or mistreated from its very earliest stages.

Daily I talk with women who have the symptoms of IBC, who have traversed the medical system with no luck, being told either "let's try another antibiotic", or "your pregnant and this is normal", or "let's watch this and see in a couple of months if it resolves itself". Those reading this journal might be shaking their combined heads at this point, but these are actual statements frustrated women relate.

There have been many times I have personally stepped over the invisible barrier to a proper diagnosis, only to find an angry physician who refuses to accept that "such a rare condition could just pop up overnight". It is those times that I relate how my own daughter woke one morning to a swollen breast. And yes, it had "popped up overnight" as so many women with IBC can attest.

For readers of this journal, test this theory: Ask a woman who has fought and won over 'regular' breast cancer, if she knows what 'Inflammatory Breast Cancer' is. The usual answer is: "I know everything about breast cancer".

Seventy-five percent of the time, she has never heard of IBC and is shocked her physician(s) have not alerted her to the possibility that she could recur with IBC. True, not an every day occurrence, but physicians should make their patients aware of the symptoms of this lethal disease.

I have continued my (what I would call) rampage of awareness campaigns about Inflammatory Breast Cancer, because it was the only thing that kept my mind working. Just three months prior to Tina's passing, Dr. Massimo Cristofanilli, Jenee Bobbora and I, started a foundation, with the hope we could make a difference in the way this disease was perceived by the public and the medical community. We started on a course of education on May 25th, 2007, and have not veered from that to this day.

We can say with certainty that there are IBC specific clinics which have opened; there are IBC specific doctors who have dedicated their careers to finding the science and possibly the treatments to stop or (dare I say possibly) cure IBC. There is now a world conglomerate of physicians and scientists who have come together to study and treat this disease; There are Continuing Educational courses on IBC; There are new treatment protocols and vaccines for women who are in the thick of the battle against this deadly form of breast cancer; there are scientists who work daily on finding the root cause of IBC, though at this writing this 'root' is still elusive and controversial.

Our foundation has pushed ahead, sometimes too slow for this writer, trying to get a foothold into the bigger institutions to scream the message that mammograms are not the answer. And we will continue through our educational material which we give away; through our radio show once a month where we interview the doctors and researchers who are the most knowledgeable about IBC, and our talks to large groups where we have to loudly vocalize over the top of the bigger breast cancer groups that mammograms are not the end all, when it comes to this disease.

But, we cannot do this alone. We badly need more people to join our team of non-paid volunteers to spread much needed education before any science can be achieved. Without education and public awareness, science can only do so much. For if we cannot get doctors to realize that this disease, Inflammatory Breast Cancer, is in a class all by itself and needs immediate diagnosis and quicker turnaround from diagnosis to treatment, our passionate speeches are going to be useless. The more people that can join our cause and help with the education, the more lives we can save. It is that simple.

*Note: The 'Silent Killer' piece is still actively shared on the internet in blogs and news reports, hopefully saving women from lingering in limbo without a correct diagnosis. I know Michelle's piece has changed lives, as one woman told me, "that story saved my life…a friend emailed me the 'Silent Killer' and I took the story to my doctor, on my laptop, and made him watch and learn".

There is not enough room to list ALL the women who have called, written and stated loudly that if it hadn't been for the piece Michelle Esteban did, and all her follow-up stories on all the women in our area, they would never have known about IBC.

One thing Michelle didn't say is the reaction from her piece in 2006, nationally. ABC's Good Morning America called KOMO TV in Seattle shortly after the piece ran and said "because so many news stations around the country are doing stories on IBC (where before they wouldn't touch anything 'so rare'), they wanted to interview Michelle. And they did. CNN followed up, as did MSNBC with their own stories. IBC was finally out of the closet.

Thank you Michelle. And my Tina would thank you too if she were still alive, as do all the women and families your words and courage have touched.

What have we learned since we started this journey of educating the masses, which includes the medical community?

"Ignorance is causing death", is what I (Patti) said into the KOMO television cameras in May of 2006. At that time I thought it was women who didn't know or hadn't been educated, but now seven years later I could say the same, only now it would be aimed at physicians. I know that sounds harsh, but sadly it is a reality that the most glaring point that stands out today is the remaining lack of education of the symptoms of IBC in the medical community. Second only to the correct treatment after a correct diagnosis. We need a national mandate, similar to what happened with HIV, that doctors MUST take a CME on IBC for their yearly medical license. That would be, in this writers mind, the only way to be assured that ALL physicians have the same current data that the IBC specialists do, today. If the layperson can go onto the internet and find recent data, does it not follow that a physician with all his or her training can find the same data?

Patients across the country, are still relating the lack of knowledge by their own physicians thus in many cases a stage IIIB case of IBC on first clinical observation, becomes a stage IV by the time the patient is finally treated. This also holds true for nurses and medical educators who have to have this information to stay current on physical symptoms that they could be presented with, and the current treatment protocols that prolong if not save their patients life. This is an urgent need, and needs immediate attention in all aspects of the medical community.

Index